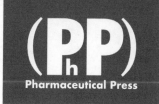

Pharmacy Management of Long-term Medical Conditions

Editors
Ross Ferguson
Jonathan Burton

Published by the Pharmaceutical Press
66-68 East Smithfield, London E1W 1AW, UK

© Pharmaceutical Press 2021

(P,P) is a trade mark of Pharmaceutical Press
Pharmaceutical Press is the publishing division of the Royal Pharmaceutical Society

First edition published 2021

Printed in Great Britain by TJ Books Limited, Padstow, Cornwall

ISBN 978 0 85711 405 1

A catalogue record for this book is available from the British Library.

I'd like to dedicate this book to my two amazing children, Juliet and Hugo, and my wife, Janie.

Ross Ferguson, 2021

Table of Contents

Preface

The day-to-day challenges faced by the NHS (increasing demand as a result of the growing elderly population and the relentless pressure on the currently dwindling numbers of GPs) are well documented.

It makes sense that other healthcare professionals, including pharmacists and pharmacy technicians, suitably qualified, competent and confident, contribute more to patient care when they have the appropriate skills and experience.

This means not only diagnosing and treating common acute clinical conditions, but also helping people to manage their long-term medical conditions, enabling them to live longer and have better quality lives.

People with long-term medical conditions aren't only facing the consequences and complications of the disease itself, but they are also dealing with the possible harms associated with the treatments.

Multimorbidity, defined as having two or more long-term medical conditions, is almost universal in adults and prevalence increases with age, so with a growing elderly population, it is clear that the challenge of meeting demand will continue.

The prevalence of multimorbidity in England is around 27 per cent, with 33 per cent of these people having both a physical and mental morbidity. This is starker in younger people with multimorbidity, where more than half have a physical-mental comorbidity.[1]

Meanwhile, in Scotland, a study of nearly 2 million people found that more than half of people with multimorbidity and nearly two-thirds with physical-mental health comorbidity were younger than 65 years, and the onset of multimorbidity occurred 10-15 years earlier in people in areas of socioeconomic deprivation. By age 50 years, half of the population had at least one morbidity, and by age 65 years most were multimorbid.[2]

These statistics paint a grim picture for the individuals affected and their families, not to mention the demands on the NHS. However, with the right treatment managed well, prognosis and quality of life can be improved. There is a lot of work to do.

Yet, we know that 50 per cent of people taking medicines for long-term medical conditions do not take prescribed medicine as intended,[3] and in a meta-analysis[4] which assessed the percentage of people with preventable adverse drug reactions among outpatients and people admitted to hospital, approximately half were preventable.

Conducting a regular patient-centred pharmacy review is essential to ensure that treatment is optimised. This includes asking about adherence, monitoring disease progression, ensuring there is therapeutic benefit and managing drug interactions and adverse effects.

Moreover, providing patient education about their condition, and the treatments, and signposting to resources that can help and support them and their family are equally important elements of care.

It is obvious that regardless of the setting in which they work, there is enough scope for pharmacists to help people manage their long-term medical conditions. The setting shouldn't be a barrier to the development of professional skills and knowledge, but instead help to provide easy access to healthcare professionals with expertise in medicines. However, some settings by their nature can make this more challenging where there is professional isolation, lack of time and perhaps lack of confidence and experience too.

The aim of this book is to support pharmacists and pharmacy technicians to provide pharmaceutical care to people with long-term medical conditions to help improve patient outcomes.

It focuses on the most prevalent long-term medical conditions where pharmacists can have a positive impact on care and takes a stepwise approach to reflect possible contributions to patient care depending on the level of knowledge, from input that all pharmacists should be able to provide to more advanced interventions. It is then down to the individual to consider which level of care they are competent to provide. This will vary depending on the condition being treated, the resources available and experience. What is certain though is that all pharmacists can make a positive contribution and that's the important part.

The final chapter on multimorbidity and polypharmacy is a reminder that we need to focus on the individual as a whole, not view them as a series of separate diseases to be managed one by one – it provides some invaluable advice and information on how to manage people with multimorbidity and consider deprescribing in a patient-centred way.

There is a wealth of talent within the pharmacy profession with specialists in a whole range of medical conditions and consultant levels posts throughout the UK. Pharmacists have many thousands of interactions with patients every day – we must make these count, so we need to learn from our colleagues so we as a profession can have more of a positive impact, and that means sharing knowledge and expertise. Hopefully, this book is a useful step in that direction.

Ross Ferguson
BSc (Hons), MFRPSI MRPharmS

References

1. Cassell A *et al.* The epidemiology of multimorbidity in primary care: a retrospective cohort study. *Br J Gen Pract* 2018; 68(669): e245-e251.

2. Barnett K *et al.* Epidemiology of multimorbidity and implications for health care, research, and medical education: a cross-sectional study. *Lancet* 2012; 380(9836): 37-43.

3. Sabaté E, ed. Adherence to Long-Term Therapies: Evidence for Action. Geneva, Switzerland: World Health Organization; 2003.

4. Hakkarainen KM *et al.* Percentage of patients with preventable adverse drug reactions and preventability of adverse drug reactions – a meta-analysis. *PloS ONE* 2012; 7(3): e33236.

● ● ●

It has often been said that good care starts with a conversation. My experience as a pharmacist has taught me that this is very much the truth. As pharmacists, we are privileged to be the custodians of a great deal of medical and pharmaceutical knowledge, but this knowledge and associated expertise needs to be shared with patients and the public for us to make a positive impact on their lives.

I hope this book, with chapters authored by expert pharmacists in their respective fields, will serve as a tool to inspire and support many conversations between pharmacists and people with long-term conditions in our care. The information and advice within the text can then be augmented by expert advice and mentorship from colleagues in practice. As the clinical role of pharmacists and pharmacy technicians increases in a variety of care settings, I cannot emphasise enough the value of learning from and collaborating with colleagues, both from within the pharmacy profession and from the many other healthcare disciplines with which we interact.

It is very important never to assume that another member of the multidisciplinary healthcare team, perhaps in another setting, has already done a particular job or performed a particular check when it comes to the safe use of medicines or the general management of their condition. This mantra can be applied to all long-term conditions.

Take asthma as an example. Who has responsibility for checking the patient's inhaler technique and understanding? Or perhaps demonstrating how to use a spacer device or peak flow meter properly? Who asks the patient the simple questions to help ascertain whether their asthma is adequately controlled and if therapies need to be adjusted, added or removed? The answer is that this is predominantly a shared responsibility, and we as pharmacists and pharmacy technicians have a key role to play.

We will always be presented with an endless stream of opportunities to start the conversation to help and safeguard people with long-term conditions who need to use medication. We need to take these opportunities whenever they present themselves.

In the community pharmacy setting the opportunity could be an acute symptom presentation (e.g. a sore mouth, ankle swelling or gastric pain) where a long-term condition or associated medication may be a potential underlying causative factor. People may present to the pharmacy with suspected adverse drug reactions, or issues relating to long-term conditions may surface during a more structured medication review process or when speaking to a patient when they present a new prescription.

In GP practice and hospital settings there will be myriad scenarios where pharmaceutical care can be provided, as part of both unscheduled and planned interventions, and pharmacists will often be intimately involved with the initiation, monitoring and review of medication regimens in these settings.

Once these conversations begin and the therapeutic relationship between pharmacist and patient develops, by listening to people with long-term conditions and showing empathy with the impact disease has on people's lives, we can then start to learn aspects of pharmaceutical care that are not found in textbooks, the aspects only a patient can teach.

Jonathan Burton
MBE, BPharm (Hons), MFRPSII FRPharmS

Acknowledgement

I'd like to thank the many authors involved in the production of this book for taking the time in their busy schedules to contribute their expertise, and the team at the Pharmaceutical Press for their help in publishing it.

I'd also like to thank Jonathan Burton MBE for his invaluable input and unique insight into every chapter which has helped shape the content, and for his help and support throughout the process.

About the contributors

Editors

Ross Ferguson BSc (Hons) MFRPSI MRPharmS has been a pharmacist for over 25 years. He has practised in community pharmacies in England, Scotland and Wales, and has owned a pharmacy. He has been involved in pharmacy publishing for over 20 years and is currently Assistant Editor at Clarity Informatics where he authors clinical knowledge summaries for the NICE CKS website, as well as e-learning material for primary healthcare professionals.

Jonathan Burton MBE MFRPSII FRPharmS is a community pharmacist based in Stirling, Scotland. He is the co-founder and co-owner of the Right Medicine Pharmacy group and served as their Superintendent Pharmacist for 15 years. He now practices as a patient-facing community pharmacist and independent prescriber, with particular interests in common conditions, dermatology, mental health, sexual health and vaccination services. He is an experienced pre-registration tutor and also enjoys mentoring and teaching undergraduate students and pharmacists wishing to develop their clinical assessment and prescribing skills. He was awarded an MBE for services to healthcare in 2018.

Contributors

Jayne Agnew BSc MSc IPresc, MPSNI MRPharmS
Consultant Pharmacist for Older People, Southern Health and Social Care Trust, Craigavon Area Hospital

Professor Nina L Barnett JP, PhD IPresc, FFRPS FRPharmS
Consultant Pharmacist, Care of Older People, Pharmacy, Northwick Park Hospital
London North West University Healthcare NHS Trust & NHS Specialist Pharmacy Service
Visiting Professor, Kingston University, London

Delia Bishara BPharm (Hons) MSc
Consultant Pharmacist for Mental Health of Older Adults and Dementia, South London & Maudsley NHS Foundation Trust and Institute of Psychiatry, Psychology & Neuroscience, King's College London

Nabil Boulos BSc PGDip clinical pharmacy practice MSc IPresc
Senior Clinical Pharmacist
University Hospital Southampton NHS Foundation Trust

Dr Toby G D Capstick BSc DipClinPharm DPharm, MRPharmS
Consultant Pharmacist - Respiratory Medicine, Medicines Management and Pharmacy Services, Leeds Teaching Hospitals NHS Trust

Paula Crawford BSc MSc, MPSNI
Consultant Pharmacist Older People, Belfast HSC Trust

Carmel Darcy BSc MSc IPresc, MPSNI MRPharmS
Consultant Pharmacist Older People
Western Health and Social Care Trust

Fiona Dorrington BSc MSc Clinical Pharmacy IPresc, MRPharmS
Macmillan Principal Pharmacist Palliative Care - Frimley Health NHS Trust and Thames Hospice

Ann Dougan BSc MPharm PGDip IPresc, MRPharmS
Highly Specialist Pharmacist, Surgery/Neurosciences, Bart's Health NHS Trust

Georgina Ell PgDip Clinical Pharmacy PgCert Psychiatric Pharmacology IPresc, MRPharmS
Advanced Specialist Pharmacist – Park Royal (Brent) Lead Pharmacist Learning Disabilities
Central and North West London NHS Foundation Trust (CNWL)
Member of the College of Mental Health Pharmacy (CMHP)

Lynn Elsey MPharm MSc
Lead Respiratory/ Severe Asthma Pharmacist Pharmacy Department, Wythenshawe Hospital, Manchester
NHS Foundation Trust.
Member of the BTS Special Advisory Group

Paul Forsyth MPharm MSc (Primary Care)
Lead Pharmacist - Clinical Cardiology (Primary Care)/Heart Failure Specialist, NHS Greater Glasgow &
Clyde

Nicola Greenhalgh PgCert Psychiatric Therapeutics PgDip Pharmacy Practice IPresc
Lead Pharmacist – Mental Health Services, North East London NHS Foundation Trust

Rachel Howatson BPharm, DipClinPharm, IPresc
Senior CVD Pharmacist for South London
Member of the UKCPA, GPhC and support to Pharmacy Management CVD advisory group

Emyr Jones MPharm (Hons) IPresc, MRPharmS
Consultant Pharmacist, National lead for Wales: Community Healthcare
Honorary Lecturer - School of Pharmacy and Pharmaceutical Sciences, Cardiff University
Honorary Clinical Senior Lecturer - College of Human and Health Sciences, Swansea University

Hilary McKee MSc IPresc, MPSNI
Consultant Pharmacist, Northern Health and Social Care Trust
Clinical Lead, Rheumatology Pharmacists UK

Helen Meynell BPharm DipClinPharm PhD IPresc, MRPharmS FFPS
Consultant Pharmacist with an interest in Respiratory Medicine and Palliative Care
Doncaster and Bassetlaw Teaching Hospitals NHS Foundation Trust
UKCPA Respiratory Group Committee Member

Karen Miller BSc PhD, MPSNI
Consultant Pharmacist (Older People)
Southern Eastern Health and Social Care Trust

Philip Newland-Jones MPharm MSC IPresc, MRPharmS MFRPSADVII
Consultant Pharmacist – Diabetes and Endocrinology, Clinical Director Diabetes & Endocrinology UHS
University Hospital Southampton NHS Foundation Trust

Lelly Oboh BPharm PGCert Pharmacy Practice PGDip Clinical Pharmacy IPresc, FRPharmS
Consultant Pharmacist Guys & St Thomas NHS Foundation Trust AND Medicines Use and Safety, NHS
Specialist Pharmacy Services
Chair, Specialist Clinical Pharmacists Group, Primary Care Pharmacist Association (PCPA) Member,
London Frailty Clinical Leadership Group

David Rogalski MPharm PG Dip GPP Psychiatric Therapeutics PgCert MSc (APP) IPresc, MRPharmS
Lead Pharmacist - Practice Based Mental Health Team
Camden and Islington NHS Foundation Trust

Suzanne Saunders MPharm PG Dip (Clin Pharm) IPresc, MRPharmS
Specialist Pain Pharmacist, Fife Pain Management Service

Heather Smith BPharm (Hons) MSc Clinical Pharmacy, FFRPS MRPharmS
Consultant Pharmacist: Older People / Interfaces of Care
Medicines Management & Pharmacy Services
Leeds Teaching Hospitals NHS Trust

Karen Somerville BSc (Hons) PG Dip Advanced Pharmacy Practice IPresc, MRPharmS
Specialist Pain Pharmacist, Fife Pain Management Service

Deborah Steven BSc (Hons) PG Dip Clin Pharm MSc Pain Management IPresc, MRPharmS
Lead Pharmacist, Fife Pain Management Service, Lynebank Hospital
Postgraduate Tutor Robert Gordon University

Helen Williams FFRPS FRPharmS
Consultant Pharmacist for CVD, NHS Southwark CCG
Clinical Network Lead for CVD, NHS Lambeth CCG
National Clinical Adviser for AF, AHSNs Network
Clinical Director for AF, Health Innovation Network
Clinical Lead for AF (NCL), UCL Partners

CHAPTER 1

Anxiety and depression in adults

David Rogalski

Overview

Depression and anxiety are common mental health problems, and 'Depression and anxiety' will often be the diagnosis recorded in the GP patient records instead of distinguishing between both.

The overlap is greatest when the symptoms are mild and may be classified as mixed anxiety and depressive disorder. However, depression and anxiety are distinct diagnoses in the International Classification of Diseases (ICD-10) or Diagnostic and Statistical Manual of Mental Disorders (DSM-V);[1] although in the world of real people, many suffer from symptoms of both – surveys show up to 60-70% of those with depression also have anxiety.[2]

Depression has an annual incidence in industrialised countries of approximately 5%.[3] Prevalence is similar across the age range 18-64 years, with women having 1.5-2.5 times higher prevalence than men.[4] Men may be particularly affected by a lack of diagnosis or by not seeking help. Depression is mainly treated in primary care with about 5% of patients referred for specialist treatment and 2% of those admitted for in-patient care.

Depression is more than simply feeling unhappy or fed up for a few days – it is a condition that can affect people differently and cause a wide variety of distressing symptoms, ranging from lasting feelings of unhappiness and hopelessness, to losing interest in the things they enjoy and feeling very tearful. There can also be physical symptoms too, such as feeling constantly tired, sleeping badly, having no appetite or sex drive, and various aches and pains. Depression can lead to relationship and family breakdown, increase the likelihood of drug or alcohol addiction, reduce the ability to overcome serious illness and increase mortality rates – not just from the risk of suicide.

Depression significantly increases the risk and rate of suicide, which itself remains the leading cause of death for males aged 35 to 49 years in England and Wales.[5]

With appropriate treatment, 70-80% of individuals with major depressive disorder can achieve a significant reduction in symptoms, although as many as 50% of patients may not respond to the initial treatment trial.

There are many factors which need to be considered in relation to the aetiology of depression including psychological, genetic and biological. These factors do not interact in a simple additive manor but modify each other directly and indirectly. Certain adverse circumstances can increase the probability that a person will experience an episode of depression.[6] These include:

- life events such as bereavement, or even positive events such as having a baby
- the presence of continuing psychological stressors, for example problems at work
- adverse developmental experiences, such as abuse.

Individual genes have not yet been identified for the cause of depression, but there is strong evidence of a genetic basis for a vulnerability to depression. Two biological aspects have received most attention:

1. Hormonal influences – the role of cortisol (hydrocortisone), the body's major stress hormone
2. The behaviour of the monoamine neurotransmitters – the monoamine hypothesis

Diagnosis

Although there are several ways to diagnose depression, all cases are based on a biopsychosocial assessment. This is a qualitative assessment of someone presenting with suspected depression that considers the various domains of symptoms, which can be physical, psychological or social. Although the International Classification of Disease 10th Edition (ICD-10) can be used, the National Institute for Health and Care Excellence (NICE) guidelines on depression currently use the Diagnostic and Statistical Manual of Mental Disorders (DSM-4) criteria to standardise the diagnosis and treatment of depression (see *Table 1.1*). Note: while DSM-5 has been published, at the time of publication of this book, NICE guidance has not yet been updated, but the criteria remain the same.

Table 1.1: *Diagnostic and Statistical Manual of Mental Disorders, 4th Edition, (DSM-IV) Classification system*[1]

Key symptoms	Associated symptoms
Persistent sadness or low mood Marked loss of interests or pleasure At least one of these, most days, most of the time for at least 2 weeks	• Disturbed sleep (decreased or increased compared to usual) • Decreased or increased appetite and/or weight • Fatigue or loss of energy • Agitation or slowing of movements • Poor concentration or indecisiveness • Feelings of worthlessness or excessive or inappropriate guilt • Suicidal thoughts or acts
Subthreshold depressive symptoms	• Fewer than 5 symptoms of depression
Mild depression	• Few, if any, symptoms in excess of the 5 required to make the diagnosis, and symptoms result in only minor functional impairment
Moderate depression	• Symptoms or functional impairment are between 'mild' and 'severe'
Severe depression	• Most symptoms, and the symptoms markedly interfere with functioning • Can occur with or without psychotic symptoms

Depression is not always easy to define, describe or identify; this in part is due to the heterogeneity of the condition. The DSM diagnosis of major depression is made when a patient has any 5 out of 9 symptoms, several of which are opposites.

There can be both psychological and physical symptoms accompanied by changes in behaviour. Central to making a diagnosis of depression is depressed mood and/or loss of pleasure in most activities. Severity of the disorder is determined by the number and severity of symptoms, as well as the degree of functional impairment. Duration of symptoms is also important.

Management

NICE advises a stepwise approach to treating depression based on the severity of symptoms (see *Table 1.2*).

The routine use of antidepressants for mild and subthreshold depressive symptoms among adults is not generally recommended. They do not typically provide benefit for patients with subthreshold depressive symptoms or mild depression. However, prescription may be considered when clinically indicated (i.e. patients with a history of moderate or severe depression; initial presentation of subthreshold depressive symptoms that have been present for a long period, typically at least 2 years; subthreshold depressive symptoms or mild depression that persist(s) after other interventions).[7]

SSRI antidepressants are considered first-line options when pharmacological treatments are required because of their relatively tolerable side effect profile and safety in overdose compared to other antidepressant classes (see *Table 1.3* for preferred treatment options). Treatment should be taken at minimum effective doses, at least, to treat and maintain recovery.

Table 1.2: *Stepped care model for depression[7]*

Step	Clinical features	Interventions
1	• All known and suspected presentations of depression	• Assessment • Support • Psychoeducation • Active monitoring • Referral for further assessment and interventions
2	• Persistent subthreshold depressive symptoms • Mild to moderate depression	• Low-intensity psychosocial interventions • Psychological interventions • Medication • Referral for further assessment and interventions
3	• Persistent subthreshold depressive symptoms • Mild to moderate depression with inadequate response to initial interventions • Moderate and severe depression	• Medication • High-intensity psychological interventions • Combined treatments • Collaborative care • Referral for further assessment and interventions
4	• Severe and complex depression • Risk to life • Severe self-neglect	• Medication • High-intensity psychological interventions • Electroconvulsive therapy • Crisis service • Combined treatments • Multi-professional and inpatient care

Table 1.3: *NICE: Medicine choice in the management of depression[7]*

Options	Medicine choice
First line	• Serotonin reuptake inhibitors
Second line	• Alternative serotonin reuptake inhibitor, or • A better tolerated newer generation antidepressant (e.g. mirtazapine)
Third line (with specialist advice)	• Venlafaxine, or • A tricyclic antidepressant, or • Moclobemide, phenelzine, or vortioxetine
Fourth line (with specialist advice)	Combination treatments: • SSRI plus mirtazapine, or • Venlafaxine plus mirtazapine
	Augmentation treatments: • Antidepressant plus lithium • Antidepressant plus an antipsychotic (aripiprazole, olanzapine, quetiapine or risperidone)

It should also be noted that adolescents and young adults (up to the age of 25 years) may be more at risk of increased suicidality, especially during the initial two weeks of treatment, and therefore they require more frequent monitoring of their symptoms at this stage.[7]

Antidepressants should be taken for at least four weeks before considering their full efficacy; however, improvements are usually seen within two weeks of initiation if a person is responsive to that particular treatment.[8,9] See *Box 1.1* for information on the minimum effective doses of commonly used antidepressants and *Box 1.2* for general minimum treatment duration recommendations.

Box 1.1: The minimum effective doses of antidepressants for adults[8]*

Medicines should be started at lower doses and be increased to at least these doses:
- Tricyclics 75-100 mg/day
- Citalopram 20 mg/day
- Sertraline 50 mg/day
- Fluoxetine 20 mg/day
- Paroxetine 20 mg/day
- Mirtazapine 30 mg/day

Variations in doses should take into account age, pharmacokinetic changes, drug interactions and comorbidities.

*Adapted from the Maudsley Prescribing Guidelines in Psychiatry, 13th edition[8]

Box 1.2: General minimum antidepressant treatment durations[9]*

1st episode: 6 months post-recovery
2nd episode: 1-3 years
3rd episode: 5 years or longer
4th episode: the person should have a very good reason to stop

*Adapted from the Psychotropic Drug Directory 2018, Chapter 1.14[9]

Anxiety disorders

Anxiety is an unpleasant emotional state characterised by fearfulness and unwanted and distressing physical symptoms. Short-term anxiety is a natural emotional response that can help drive performance and improve alertness; however, when anxiety becomes prolonged or severe it can be distressing and disabling. It is then considered to be pathological, requiring treatment to enable the sufferer to resume and maintain a normal lifestyle. Individuals vary in the amount of anxiety they generate or can handle, in the same way that people vary in their response to stressful events.

Pooled analysis of European populations suggests that approximately one in five people will fit the diagnostic criteria for an anxiety disorder at some point in their adult lives.[10] Specific phobias have a lifetime prevalence of 13.2% and are the most common anxiety disorder. This is followed by social anxiety disorder (5.8%) and generalised anxiety disorder (GAD; 5.1%).[11] In general, twice as many women than men are affected by anxiety; however, this ratio varies between disorders. Although anxiety disorders can occur at any age, many patients develop symptoms during childhood that tend to persist if left untreated.

Emerging data suggest that having an anxiety disorder can reduce quality of life and worsen outcomes for patients with chronic physical illnesses. Notably, strong associations have been identified between anxiety disorders and irritable bowel syndrome, asthma and chronic pain.[12]

As with depression, the aetiology of anxiety is complex and multifaceted including psychological, genetic and biological components.

Diagnosis

The main components of anxiety are:

- Psychological - the essential feeling of dread and apprehension and accompanied by restlessness, narrowing of attention to focus on the source of danger, worrying thoughts, increased alertness (with insomnia) and irritability. Symptoms include disturbed sleep, fear, irritability, restlessness and poor concentration.
- Somatic - muscle tension and respiratory increase. Symptoms include nausea, poor appetite, breathlessness, tinnitus and headache.
- Autonomic - heart rate and sweating increase, the mouth becomes dry and there may be an urge to urinate or defecate. Symptoms include palpitations, sweating and tightness over the chest.
- Avoidance of danger - a phobia is a persistent, irrational fear of a specific object or situation.

Although all the symptoms can occur in any of the anxiety disorders, there is a characteristic pattern in each disorder, see *Table 1.4*. The disorders share many features of their clinical picture and aetiology but there are also differences.

Table 1.4: *Anxiety disorders*

Disorder	Description	Time course of symptoms
Generalised anxiety disorder	Excessive worry about a number of different events associated with heightened tension (although may fluctuate in intensity). Patients have physical anxiety symptoms and key psychological symptoms. Symptoms should be present for at least 6 months and should cause clinically significant distress or impairment in social, occupational or other important areas of functioning.	Continuous over several months or several years
Panic disorder (with or without agoraphobia)	Presence of recurring, unforeseen panic attacks followed by at least 1 month of persistent worry about having another panic attack and concern about the consequences of a panic attack, or a significant change in behaviour related to the attacks. At least two unexpected panic attacks are necessary.	Intermittent
Social phobia (social anxiety disorder)	Marked, persistent and unreasonable fear of being observed or evaluated negatively by other people, in social or performance situations, which is associated with physical and psychological anxiety symptoms. Feared situations (such as speaking to unfamiliar people or eating in public) are either avoided or are endured with significant distress.	Intermittent or infrequent
Post-traumatic stress disorder	History of exposure to trauma (actual or threatened death, serious injury, or threats to the physical integrity of the self or others) with a response of intense fear, helplessness or horror; with the later development of intrusive symptoms (such as recollections, flashbacks or dreams), avoidance symptoms (e.g. efforts to avoid activities or thoughts associated with the trauma), negative alterations in cognitions and mood, and hyper-arousal symptoms (including disturbed sleep, hypervigilance and an exaggerated startle response).	Usually arises within 6 months of a serious traumatic event
Obsessive-compulsive disorder	Recurrent obsessive ruminations, images or impulses, and/or recurrent physical or mental rituals which are distressing, time-consuming and cause interference with social and occupational function. Common obsessions relate to contamination, accidents, and religious or sexual matters; common rituals include washing, checking, cleaning, counting and touching.	Continuous over several months or even years
Body dysmorphic disorder	A preoccupation with an imagined defect in one's appearance, or in the case of a slight physical anomaly, the person's concern is markedly excessive. BDD is characterised by time-consuming behaviours such as mirror gazing, comparing particular features to those of others, excessive camouflaging tactics to hide the defect, skin picking and reassurance seeking.	Continuous over several months or even years

Treatment

Antidepressants are recommended treatment options for GAD, panic disorder, OCD and social anxiety disorder. Choice of antidepressant depends on the type of disorder, supporting evidence and the UK marketing authorisation of the medicine. Antidepressants with serotonin-enhancing properties are preferred and selective serotonin reuptake inhibitors (SSRIs) should be tried first (see *Table 1.5*).

Table 1.5: *First-line medicine choice in the treatment of anxiety disorders*

First-line antidepressants	Type of anxiety disorder
Sertraline	Generalised anxiety disorder
SSRI	Panic disorder, obsessive compulsive disorder
SSRI or venlafaxine	Social phobia
Fluoxetine	Body dysmorphic disorder
Paroxetine or mirtazapine	Post-traumatic stress disorder

Other treatment options may include:
- Benzodiazepines – these provide rapid symptomatic relief from acute anxiety states. They should only be used to treat anxiety that is severe, disabling or subjecting the individual to extreme distress. A very small number of patients with severely disabling anxiety may benefit from long-term treatment with a benzodiazepine with a plan in place by a specialist and these patients should not be denied treatment.[8]
- Buspirone – licensed for short-term use in anxiety. There is some evidence supporting its use for when the anxiety symptoms of GAD first appear.[11] It may be an option for patients with GAD who refuse SSRIs due to their sexual adverse effects. Despite being licensed, buspirone is not considered an option for the treatment of anxiety by NICE.
- Antipsychotics – should not be offered for the treatment of anxiety in primary care. Specialist input is required.
- Beta blockers – not recommended but used occasionally to manage the physical symptoms of anxiety, such as tremor, palpitations, sweating and shortness of breath.[9] When stopping a beta blocker, it should be reduced gradually as abrupt withdrawal may precipitate or result in severe exacerbation of angina pectoris, acute myocardial infarction, sudden death, malignant tachycardia, sweating, palpitation and tremor.[11]
- Antihistamines – hydroxyzine is licensed for the treatment of short-term anxiety and has been found to be more effective at treating GAD than placebo.[13] It may be particularly useful in people with a history of misusing benzodiazepines and who may have become tolerant to their effects as a result of such action.
- Pregabalin – licensed in the UK for the treatment of GAD. However, it is not licensed or recommended by NICE for social anxiety disorder. NICE has recommended pregabalin as a treatment option for GAD when SSRIs and SNRIs have not been tolerated.

Talking therapy

Talking therapies, such as counselling, psychotherapy and coaching, offer a safe, confidential place to talk to a trained professional about feelings and concerns. Talking therapies alone seem most effective in milder forms of depression and anxiety disorders, but combinations of talking therapies with an antidepressant seems to have a synergistic effect at the more severe end of the spectrum.

There is robust research on the benefits of treating anxiety disorders and depression with talking therapies, such as cognitive behavioural therapy (CBT).[14] CBT is only one of many therapy options but probably the most common and used in the Improving Access to Psychological Therapies (IAPT) services. IAPT services provide evidence-based talking therapies to people with anxiety disorders and depression.

Pharmacy input

In 90% of cases, depression and anxiety are treated in primary care and non-specialist settings. Furthermore, out of 130 cases of depression (including those considered mild) per 1,000, only 80 consult their GP.[15] Community-based primary care staff – and especially the pharmacy team – have many contact opportunities to identify people who may be suffering and offer effective interventions or signposts to other sources of help if appropriate.[16]

Roles that can be undertaken by the pharmacy team include:

- Encourage self-management approaches (See *Box 1.3*)
- Signpost to local or online support groups
- Assist patients in self-referral to the local IAPT service and forge links with these organisations
- Offer advice and about mindfulness-based practices such as meditation
- Offer specific advice about medication
- Support the adherence by using their skills and knowledge to manage a patient's expectation of medicines, and offering motivation and support when starting and continuing treatment[16]
- Manage adverse effects

Box 1.3: Practice point: self-management approaches

- Establish regular sleep and wake times and avoid daytime naps.
- Avoid excessive eating, smoking or drinking of alcohol.
- Abstain from recreational drug use.
- Avoid caffeine-containing products 3-6 hours before bed.
- Create a suitable environment for sleep: sleep in a darkened room, avoid extremes of temperature and background noise.
- Take regular physical exercise during the day (which may promote sleep).
- Avoid 'screen-time' from back-lit screens, such as mobile devices or the television (the blue-based light emitted inhibits melatonin release).

Your approach, interventions and management of people with depression and anxiety will depend on your knowledge and skills; some suggested roles depending on your skill level are outlined in *Table 1.6*. You must always act within your level of competency and know when to refer to a healthcare professional with more experience.

Table 1.6: *Skill level and appropriate management of patients with depression and anxiety*

Skill level	Management
Foundation (all pharmacists can do this)	• Consider pragmatic solutions to the difficulties • Provide general information about medication, mental health, and direct to resources • Signpost the patient back to GP or mental health team • If urgent, get in touch with appropriate team directly • Address unwanted effects
Advanced (pharmacists with enhanced clinical skills/knowledge)	In addition to above: • If a change in medication is indicated and feel confident, can discuss other first- and second-line treatments
Specialist (pharmacist with expertise in specific condition) Consultant (national or international expert)	In addition to above: • Further in-depth reviews • Consideration of third- and fourth-line treatments • Advanced multidisciplinary team working • If independent prescriber in area of practice can make changes to medication treatment

Pharmacy review

It is thought that between a third and a half of all medicines prescribed for long-term conditions are not taken as recommended.[17] For people with anxiety or depression this may be for a vast number of reasons such as the prominent sexual dysfunction side effects. Exploring these reasons is an important task during the consultation.

NICE[7] recommends that for people started on antidepressants who are not considered to be at increased risk of suicide, normally see them after 2 weeks. See them regularly thereafter, for example at intervals of 2 to 4 weeks in the first 3 months, and then at longer intervals if response is good. A person with depression started on antidepressants who is considered to present an increased suicide risk or is younger than 30 years should normally be seen after 1 week and frequently thereafter as appropriate until the risk is no longer considered clinically important.

In the consultation with people who have a mental health diagnosis there is emphasis on the quality of the consultation. Try to allow yourself to be in the position of the patient in front of you and use your own feelings to interpret what is being conveyed is essential to the work.

A good consultation can be therapeutic in itself and can affect the therapeutic outcome.[17] Building a good therapeutic relationship is important,[18] but may not always feel like it is possible. Part of your role is ensuring boundaries, and while setting boundaries can be challenging, if they are not set the therapeutic alliance is doomed to fail. During the consultation you will be using consultation skills such as:

- active listening
- using a non-judgemental attitude
- demonstrating empathy
- offering people an opportunity to voice their concerns and expectations.

Time is always a challenge when reviewing people with anxiety and depression. It is helpful to have some understanding of the context of the diagnosis and who made the diagnosis (e.g. was the diagnosis made by a specialist?). When conducting a review be alert to cues in appearance and behaviour – this can provide important information to signs of how they are currently managing. Screening questions can be used to identify areas that may require more detailed assessment.

There are many questionnaires/scales available to detect depression. In primary care, screening is relatively easy to conduct. The most common ones are:

- The Patient Health Questionnaire (PHQ-9) – often used in primary care to monitor the severity of depression and response to treatment. It is not a screening tool but it can be used to make a tentative diagnosis of depression. It scores each of the nine DSM-IV criteria on a range from zero (not at all) to 3 (nearly every day).
- Generalised Anxiety Disorder Assessment (GAD-7) – a seven item instrument that is used to measure or assess the severity of generalised anxiety disorder (GAD). Each item asks the individual to rate the severity of his or her symptoms over the past two weeks.
- The General Health Questionnaire (GHQ-12) – can be given to patients when they register at a new GP surgery. This rating scale is commonly used in primary care settings to help identify potentially depressed patients.
- Edinburgh Postnatal Depression Scale (EPDS) – health visitors often use this for postnatal patients.
- Geriatric Depression Scale (GDS) – the Royal College of General Practitioners recommends this for people aged over 75 years. Depression is more common in older people.

Before starting the consultation, it is important to let the person know who you are and your role, and to give them the opportunity to explain about their problem.

During the consultation:

- Be aware of how the person conveys information, their behaviour, and appearance. For example:
  - Do they have good eye contact?
  - Have they showered?
  - Are they sweaty?
  - Are they speaking quite fast?
- Ask more specific questions about their mental state when reviewing depression and anxiety:
  - How are you feeling?
  - What's been on your mind recently?
  - Are you worried about anything?
- Consider using a specific tool (PHQ-9 for depression or GAD-7 for anxiety) to help support your findings.
- Find out about their expectations of medication prescribed. Ask:
  - What does it help with?
  - Do they think it is helping? (remember people often feel better on the medication and then think it is not working anymore and discontinue).
- Ask about adherence.
- Ask about recreational drug use (e.g. alcohol, tobacco use) and other prescribed/non-prescribed medications. See *Box 1.4* for medicines which can cause anxiety or depression.
- Ask about adverse effects – this is commonly a reason for discontinuation – feeling they are able to talk to someone about it can improve adherence.
- Find out a little about their life – what is a normal day for them like?
- Ask how their physical health is – are they able to engage with physical activity? This might be something as simple as a walking or gardening group, which may also help with the social aspects of their life.
- Consider asking about the future e.g. family planning.
- Ask about the socioeconomic or practical aspects of their life – in order to make sense of a person's story we need to start with the basics. If the person does not have their basic needs met it is going to be impossible for further higher order fulfilment. In other words, needs lower down in the hierarchy must be satisfied before individuals can attend to needs higher up. For example, if the patient presenting with symptoms of low mood is having difficulties with housing or finance it may be helpful to direct to them to services that can support them.

Box 1.4: Prescribed medicines that may cause depressive and anxiety symptoms

- Antibiotics (fluoroquinolones e.g. ciprofloxacin and levofloxacin)
- Anticonvulsants
- Antimalarial agents
- Barbiturates
- Caffeine
- Cardiovascular medication
- Chemotherapeutic agents
- Cimetidine
- Corticosteroids
- Isotretinoin
- Non-steroidal anti-inflammatory agents
- Opiates
- Oral contraceptives

Some questions for you to consider include:
- Is medication helpful for this patient or a hindrance?
- Do they have an understanding about their diagnosis?
- Is there stigma about the diagnosis?

If it is the first time you are meeting someone with depression or anxiety you may not know their premorbid personality. If you are having some ongoing contact the priority will be to build a therapeutic alliance. Try not to overwhelm them with too much information. Build a foundation of the basics such as:
- understanding the diagnosis/formulation
- how might medication help and what else might help
- asking about adherence.

As people with depression and anxiety may present with a range of physical symptoms and the medication can cause a wide range of unwanted effects, predicting management options can be unexpected often in the realm of uncertainty. This may test your ingenuity; often the best approach is to be pragmatic.

Assessing suicide risk (*Box 1.5*)

Antidepressant treatment has been associated with an increased risk of suicidal thoughts and acts particularly in adolescents and young adults. All antidepressants have been implicated, including those marketed for an indication other than depression (e.g. atomoxetine). It should be noted that:
- Although the relative risk may be elevated above placebo rates in some patient groups, the absolute risk remains very small.
- The most effective way to prevent suicidal thoughts and acts is to treat depression.
- Antidepressant medicines are most effective treatment currently available.[8]

For the most part, suicidality is greatly reduced by the use of antidepressants. Those who experience treatment emergent or worsening suicidal ideation with one antidepressant may be more likely to have a similar experience with subsequent treatments. Toxicity in overdose varies both between and within groups of antidepressants. Overdose risks with SSRIs are less than other antidepressants. Tricyclic antidepressants (TCAs), except for lofepramine, are associated with the greatest risk in overdose. Compared with other equally effective antidepressants recommended for routine use in primary care, venlafaxine is associated with a greater risk of death from overdose.

If a suicide risk exists, an antidepressant that is safe in overdose should be chosen or a small supply of mediation should be issued.

If you have a concern about risk of suicide it should be explored. Remember that for some people suicidal thoughts will be a chronic picture. All plans must be taken seriously and discussed with the patient. Importantly, make sure you have support in place to help process difficult feelings you may be left with as the clinician.

Questions to ask when exploring suicide include:
- How do you feel about the future?
- Have you ever felt that life isn't worth going on with?
- Have you ever had thoughts about taking your own life?
- Have you made any definite plans to do so and, if so, what are these plans and how recently have you considered carrying them out?
- What has stopped you from harming yourself so far?

If a person is assessed to be at risk of suicide:[7]

- Take into account toxicity in overdose if an antidepressant is prescribed or the person is taking other medication; if necessary, limit the amount of drug(s) available.
- Consider increasing the level of support, such as more frequent direct or telephone contacts. This will be more suitable for someone with closer direct clinical contact with the patient.
- Consider referral to specialist mental health services. Depending on urgency this may be A&E (immediate risk) or a mental health crisis team (can visit patient at home within 24 hours).

Box 1.5: Practice point: suicide

- Asking a patient about suicidal thoughts does not make suicide attempts more likely.
- Many patients deny thoughts about suicide – this should be thoroughly explored during a consultation.
- In the UK approximately 5,000 people commit suicide every year.
  - About 70% of all suicides are related to depressive illness.
- Of those who commit suicide, 70% consulted their GP in the previous 6-8 weeks, often complaining of symptoms other than depression.

The following are more at risk of suicide or self-harm:

- Recently widowed men
- Young men
- Those under 30, recently prescribed an SSRI antidepressant (in the previous week)

Stable on medication

If the patient is stable on their medication or further medication changes are unlikely to lead to significant improvements, it may be appropriate to think with them about anything further they would like to consider. This might include therapy, exercise, mindfulness and/or meaningful structure activities. If you are not sure, there will usually be a navigator service you can direct the patient to in your area which will be able to provide more information and options.

Possible relapse

If you find during your review the person is talking or behaving in a way that you have not observed before, they have active plans of suicide, or at risk to themselves or others, it is important to know who to contact. A crisis plan (see *Box 1.6* for an example) identifies potential triggers that could lead to a crisis, signs of becoming unwell, and strategies to manage such triggers, including importantly knowing where to seek help. Other possible signs of a relapse may be non-collection of medicines and apparent lack of self-care.

Box 1.6: An example of a crisis plan

Monday–Friday; 9am – 5pm. Should I feel unwell I will contact:
1. My family and friends
2. My GP
3. Secondary care mental health team

Signs that I am becoming unwell are:
- Increasingly low mood, tearfulness, increased anxiety
- Feeling like self-harm and planning acts to do so
- Feeling elated and too confident, experiencing things that others are not able to
- Having a generally odd physical malaise, feeling of unwellness or allergic reaction

Box 1.6: An example of a crisis plan (continued)

Contingency plan

Should I not be able to make contact with my usual supports above:

Help lines
- Mind Crisis Line: 020 7226 9415 between 5pm – 6.15 am
- The Samaritans helpline: 116 123, 24 hours a day, 7 days a week (free to call from home or mobile number, and won't show on phone bill)

Out of hours' doctor via the national NHS 111 call line

Crisis line (telephone numbers vary depending on location) – anyone can call this number 24 hours a day if they require urgent help for a mental health condition. People can also self-refer to the crisis resolution and home treatment teams via this number

Local hospitals and emergency services
- Emergency services by dialling 999 if it is an emergency or NHS 111 by dialling 111

Management

Managing adverse effects

Antidepressants are by far the most commonly prescribed class of drug for mental health disorders, and their use continues to rise with much debate.[19]

SSRIs have fewer adverse effects than tricyclic antidepressants. However, all medications can have unwanted effects. *Table 1.7* outlines some common adverse effects from antidepressants and suggestions on how they can be managed.

Managing hyperprolactinaemia

Long-standing increased plasma prolactin (with or without symptoms) is very occasionally seen with anti-depressant use. When it does occur, prolactin increases are usually small and short-lived and so symptoms are rare.

Routine monitoring is not recommended. If symptoms suggest the possibility of hyperprolactinaemia it is essential to the measure plasma prolactin.[8]

Managing hyponatraemia

Antidepressant-induced hyponatraemia is a particular risk with older adults. Consider hyponatraemia with antidepressants, especially serotonergic medicines – onset is usually within 30 days of starting treatment.

Symptoms include headache, dizziness, nausea, vomiting, confusion, malaise, restlessness, lethargy, cramps, disorientation and seizures. Risk factors include history of hyponatraemia, low body weight, extreme old age (>80 years) or female patients, low baseline sodium concentration, reduced renal function, warm weather, medical comorbidity (e.g. diabetes, COPD) and some medicines (e.g. NSAIDs, diuretics).[7]

Sodium levels should be measured if the patient has symptoms or is at high risk. The normal range for serum sodium is 135-145 mmol/L. If the serum sodium is >125 mmol/L, monitor sodium until normal; consider withdrawing the antidepressant. If the serum sodium is <125 mmol/L, refer to specialist medical care as there is an increased risk of seizures, coma and respiratory arrest; the antidepressant should be discontinued immediately.[20] Discontinuation symptoms may complicate the clinical picture.[8]

When restarting an antidepressant, consider an antidepressant from a different class, either a noradrenergic medicine such as lofepramine, mirtazapine, reversible monoamine oxidase inhibitor (moclobemide).[8] Nortriptyline or agomelatine are other options.[8]

Table 1.7: *Adverse effects of antidepressants and how to manage them*

Problem	Details	Management options
Treatment has stopped working	Placebo effects can occur at the start of treatment and are generally short lived	Consider optimising the dose Change medication if necessary
Feel more anxious	Anxiolytic effect takes some time to develop	Consider short-term cover with another anxiolytic such as diazepam Start with a low dose and build up to a therapeutic dose very gradually
Feel jittery	Parkinsonian adverse effects have occasionally been reported with SSRIs	An alternative medicine may be necessary
Sleep disturbances	Insomnia Too much sleep Sleeping at the wrong time Unusual happenings in the night (e.g. nightmares, night terrors, sleep-walking, leg movements)	Change timing of antidepressant Consider a sedating antidepressant (e.g. mirtazapine)
Headache and jaw pain on wakening	Could be nocturnal teeth grinding (fluoxetine is most commonly implicated)	An alternative medicine A mouth guard (see dentist) Muscle relaxation exercises Sleep hygiene CBT
Decreased libido/ erectile dysfunction	Sexual dysfunction is common in the general population. Baseline sexual functioning should be determined	Consider other causes (e.g. comorbidities) Likely to be fully reversible Advise them that functioning will return after treatment ends An alternative medicine (less common with mirtazapine, agomelatine, and vortioxetine)
Nausea	May vary from mild nausea to vomiting	Take medicine with food An alternative if severe symptoms
Sweating	As many as 20% of patients taking antidepressants experience excessive sweating[2]	Change medicine Seek specialist advice
Vivid dreams	May persist for some, but usually subside after a couple of weeks	Change timing of medicine to morning
Dry mouth	A common antimuscarinic side effect of antidepressant medication. It is when your salivary glands in your mouth do not make enough saliva to keep your mouth wet	Try using sugar-free gum
Tired	A common side effect of antidepressant medication which act on the H_1 histamine receptor. It can be useful to manage symptoms of poor sleep	Take most, if not all, of the daily dose at night just before going to sleep Non-sedating alternatives (e.g. if prescribed mirtazapine)
Constipation	A common antimuscarinic adverse effect of antidepressant medication. Antimuscarinic action can reduce GI secretions and interfere with the ability of the intestines to contract, which can result in constipation	Increased exercise, fluids and a diet high in fruit and fibre A stimulant laxative may be necessary in the long term
Diarrhoea	Less common than nausea and usually transient	An alternative medicine if it persists
Weight gain	Although the reactions to specific antidepressants vary between individuals, some antidepressant medications are more likely to lead to weight gain than others. It is not fully understood why antidepressants lead to weight gain in some people. One theory is that both metabolism and hunger levels may be affected. Also, depression itself may cause weight gain in some people and weight loss in others	Review diet Discuss exercise Change medicine (mirtazapine increases appetite and weight gain)

Monitoring requirements for agomelatine

People starting on agomelatine should have a liver function test before starting treatment. It should not be started if serum transaminases exceed three times the upper limit of normal. Once started, liver function should be monitored after 3, 6, 12, and 24 weeks, then regularly when clinically indicated or after a dose increase.[21]

Discontinue agomelatine if serum transaminases exceed three times the upper limit of normal, or if symptoms of liver disorder occur. Advise patients to seek immediate medical attention if symptoms such as dark urine, light coloured stool, jaundice, bruising, fatigue, abdominal pain or pruritus develop.

Note however that while it is licensed for depression, it is not listed on most formularies as the manufacturers failed to provide evidence for a NICE review.

Managing QT interval and cardiovascular disease risk

Non-tricyclic antidepressants generally have a low risk of inducing arrhythmias.[20] However, antidepressants should be used with caution in patients with risk factors for QT prolongation. Hypokalaemia and hypomagnesaemia should be corrected prior to treatment. For high risk patients (e.g. congenital long QT syndrome, bradycardia, ischaemic heart disease, myocarditis, myocardial infarction, left ventricular hypertrophy, a genetic predisposition, pre-existing QT prolongation, old age, female gender, hypokalaemia, hypomagnesaemia, hypocalcaemia, extreme physical exertion, stress or shock, anorexia nervosa and medicine interactions), ECG monitoring should be performed.

Consider stopping the antidepressant or reducing the dose if the QT interval is >500 ms or increases by 60 ms. A QT >500 ms or an increase of >60 ms during treatment confers a high risk of Torsades de Pointes.[22]

QT prolongation appears to be a class effect for all SSRIs and TCAs, and also occurs with venlafaxine. If QT prolongation or symptomatic arrhythmia occurs during antidepressant treatment, stop the antidepressant or reduce the dose and seek specialist advice.[22]

Citalopram and escitalopram are associated with a dose-dependent risk of QT prolongation. Citalopram is contraindicated with other medicines that prolong QTc, patients with known QT prolongation or congenital long QT syndrome. Careful consideration of the risk/benefit must be given before any decision to prescribe combination therapy with antipsychotics or if patients are prescribed other concurrent medicines that affect QTc.

Consider ECG monitoring for all patients prescribed:
- Doses towards the top of the licensed range
- Other medicines (e.g. diuretics) that through medicine interactions may add to the risk posed by the tricyclic antidepressant[6]

Depression itself may be a predisposing factor in the development of cardiovascular disease and myocardial infarction (MI)[23]. SSRIs, generally, are considered lower-risk agents when treating depression in those who have had an MI. Sertraline is the treatment of choice for patients with a recent MI[8] or unstable angina.[10] Other SSRIs and mirtazapine are likely to be safe.[8] The UK Medicines Information (UKMi) Specialist Pharmacy Service has a helpful summary of using antidepressants in cardiovascular disease.[24]

Avoiding serotonin syndrome

Serotonin syndrome (see *Figure 1.1* for symptoms) can occur with a single serotonergic drug at a therapeutic dose, or more frequently with a combination of serotonergic drugs or in overdose. Certain illegal drugs and dietary supplements also are associated with serotonin syndrome. Milder forms of serotonin syndrome may go away within a day of stopping the medications that cause symptoms. Severe serotonin syndrome can be fatal if not treated. If serotonin syndrome is suspected advise the patient to go to A&E.

Figure 1.1: *Symptoms of serotonin syndrome*[6]

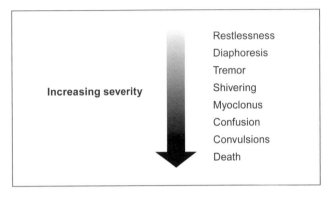

Drug interactions

St John's wort

This is not prescribable on the NHS, but people may choose to buy it. However, potential serious interactions with other drugs (including oral contraceptives, anticoagulants and anticonvulsants) may occur. People choosing to take St John's wort should be made aware of the risks of this preparation and supported to use it safely, or referred to their GP for review.

Selective serotonin reuptake inhibitors (SSRIs)

Fluoxetine, fluvoxamine and paroxetine are associated with a higher propensity for medicine interactions than other SSRIs.[2]

NSAIDs – SSRIs should not be normally offered to patients taking NSAIDs because of the increased risk of gastrointestinal bleeding. Offer an antidepressant with a lower propensity to cause this, such as mianserin, mirtazapine, moclobemide, reboxetine or trazodone. If there is no suitable alternative, gastroprotective medicines should be prescribed concurrently with the SSRI.[20]

Anticoagulants – SSRIs should not normally be offered to patients prescribed warfarin, aspirin or heparin because of their anti-platelet effect. Mirtazapine can be offered when taken with warfarin but note that the international normalised ratio (INR) may be increased slightly.[20]

If aspirin is used as a single agent, mirtazapine, mianserin, trazodone or reboxetine can also be offered. If there is no suitable alternative, a gastroprotective medicine should be prescribed concurrently.[20]

Triptans – SSRIs should not normally be offered to patients prescribed triptans (e.g. sumatriptan). Mianserin, mirtazapine or trazodone can be offered.

Atomoxetine – fluoxetine or paroxetine should not be offered to patients prescribed atomoxetine; a different SSRI can be offered.[5]

MAOB inhibitors (e.g. selegiline or rasagiline) – SSRIs should not be offered at the same time as a monoamine oxidase B inhibitor. Mirtazapine, mianserin, reboxetine, or trazodone can be offered.[20]

Other medicines – do not normally offer fluvoxamine to patients taking theophylline, clozapine, methadone or tizanidine. Offer a safer alternative such as sertraline or citalopram.[20]

Monoamine oxidase inhibitors (MAOIs)

All MAOIs (e.g. phenelzine, tranylcypromine, selegiline) have the potential to induce hypertensive crisis if foods containing tyramine (which is also metabolised by monoamine oxidase) are eaten, or medicines that increase monoamine neurotransmission are co-prescribed (e.g. alcohol, opioids, antidepressants, levodopa and buspirone).

These foods and medicines must be avoided for at least 14 days after discontinuing MAOIs. The reversible inhibitors of monoamine oxidase (e.g. moclobemide) have a much lower likelihood of causing a hypertensive crisis and dietary restrictions are usually not required.[20]

If swapping from an antidepressant to a monoamine oxidase inhibitor, the gap varies depending on the half-life of the antidepressant (usually two weeks). If swapped from fluoxetine, then the gap should be 5 to 6 weeks.[8]

Switching antidepressants

Deciding on medication changes in depression and anxiety can obfuscate the situation. However, a good question to consider is: if a change is made and there is an improvement in symptoms, what might it allow the patient to do to improve their situation? Remember a change in medication cannot change deprivation or housing issues. For example, if a patient explains their antidepressant is not working and they are at home watching TV with no structured activity. Will changing the antidepressant to improve their mood allow them to engage in some meaningful structured activity?

Switching antidepressants should be considered if:
- there are troublesome or dose-limiting adverse effects
- there has been no improvement.[4]

An antidepressant of a different class should be considered after more than one failure with a specific class. For example, venlafaxine should be considered after more than one failure with an SSRI. Switching between antidepressants should be done cautiously. Discontinuation symptoms, pharmacokinetic (e.g. elevation of tricyclic plasma levels by SSRIs) or pharmacodynamic interactions (e.g. serotonin syndrome) may be encountered during switching.

The speed of the cross-tapering should be judged by assessing patients' tolerability.[8] There are no set guidelines on how to cross taper – it is based on pharmacological principles (see *Table 1.8*).

Switching should be done cautiously and depends on the patient, the antidepressants used and the doses. In some cases cross-tapering may not be necessary (e.g. when switching from one serotonin reuptake inhibitor to another.[8]

Table 1.8: *Antidepressants: swapping and stopping[8]**

From	Agomelatine	Fluoxetine	Mirtazapine	Other SSRIs, vortioxetine	SNRIs duloxetine, venlafaxine	TCAs (except clomipramine)
Agomelatine		Stop agomelatine then start fluoxetine	Stop agomelatine then start mirtazapine	Stop agomelatine then start SSRI	Stop agomelatine then start SNRI	Stop agomelatine then start TCA
Fluoxetine	Cross-taper cautiously		Cross-taper cautiously	Stop fluoxetine. Wait 4-7 days then start low dose	Stop fluoxetine. Wait 4-7 daysnthen start SNRI	Stop fluoxetine. Wait 4-7 days then start low dose TCA
Mirtazapine	Cross-taper cautiously	Cross-taper cautiously		Cross-taper cautiously	Cross-taper cautiously	Cross-taper cautiously
Other SSRIs, vortioxetine	Cross-taper cautiously	Direct switch possible	Cross-taper cautiously	Direct switch possible	Direct switch possible	Cross-taper cautiously with low dose TCA
SNRIs duloxetine, venlafaxine,	Cross-taper cautiously	Direct switch possible	Cross-taper cautiously	Direct switch possible	Direct switch possible	Cross-taper cautiously with low dose TCA
TCAs (except clomipramine)	Cross-taper cautiously	Halve dose and add fluoxetine and then slow withdrawal	Cross-taper cautiously	Halve dose and add SSRI and then slow withdrawal	Cross-taper cautiously starting with low dose SNRI	Direct switch possible
Stopping	Can be stopped abruptly	At 20 mg/day just stop. At higher doses reduce over 2 weeks	Reduce over 4 weeks	Reduce over 4 weeks or longer if necessary	Reduce over 4 weeks or longer if necessary	Reduce over 4 weeks

*Adapted from The Maudsley Prescribing Guidelines in Psychiatry 13th Edition[8]

Stopping antidepressants

Stopping antidepressants can cause discontinuation symptoms.[25,26,27] A recent review estimated that an average of 56% of patients who stop or reduce antidepressant use experience withdrawal symptoms, with 46% of these reporting severe symptoms, and a significant proportion experiencing symptoms for several weeks, months, or longer.[28] While they can occur with all types,[4] there are differences between classes of antidepressant (e.g. symptoms are particularly marked on stopping paroxetine or venlafaxine).[26] These symptoms are a common reason why patients report mixed and negative experiences of taking and stopping antidepressants.[29,30,31]

It is important to emphasise that while antidepressants cause discontinuation symptoms, they are not dependence producing in the same way that alcohol, stimulants, opioids and benzodiazepines are. This does not however negate the reported patient experiences of more severe antidepressant withdrawal, but should provide reassurance that antidepressants do not share the addictive properties of known dependence-producing drugs.

Discontinuation of antidepressants should involve the dosage being tapered or slowly decreased to reduce the risk of distressing symptoms, which may occur over several months, and at a reduction rate that is tolerable for the patient. Whilst the withdrawal symptoms which arise on and after stopping antidepressants are often mild and self-limiting, there can be substantial variation in people's experience, with symptoms lasting much longer and being more severe for some patients. Ongoing monitoring is also needed to distinguish the features of antidepressant withdrawal from emerging symptoms which may indicate a relapse of depression.

The most common discontinuation symptoms reported with SSRIs are:

- dizziness, light headedness, vertigo, ataxia
- nausea, vomiting, diarrhoea
- lethargy, headache, tremor, sweating, anorexia
- paraesthesia, numbness, electric shock-like sensations
- irritability, anxiety, agitation, low mood.

The longer antidepressants have been used, the longer period of time treatment should be tapered. When a drug has only been used for a short period, has a long half-life (fluoxetine), or if there are serious side effects with the drug, more rapid withdrawal may be appropriate. However, a significant challenge for clinicians is the lack of a defined optimal rate of tapering to prevent discontinuation symptoms, and a lack of guidance and advice in this area.[25]

Current NICE guidance advises that this should normally be over a 4-week period, although acknowledges that some people may require longer periods.[7] As this advice is ambiguous, it is notable that the updated version of these guidelines (currently in draft form) propose that the dose be slowly reduced at a rate proportionate to the duration of treatment.

For example, this could be over some months if the person has been taking antidepressant medication for several years.[32] However, this is an area where patients and clinicians require ongoing support and would benefit from clear, evidence-based tapering recommendations.

Special groups

Older adults

There is no ideal antidepressant as all are associated with problems. SSRIs are better tolerated than TCAs, but they do have an increased risk of bleeds, particularly those with a history of bleeds or prescribed a non-steroidal medicine, aspirin, steroids or warfarin. If a non-steroidal medicine or aspirin is prescribed, a concurrent prescription for a gastroprotective agent should be considered.[7] The risk of haemorrhagic stroke may also be increased. Hyponatraemia, postural hypotension and falls (the consequence of which may be increased by serotonin reuptake inhibitor-induced osteopenia) are also a risk.[8]

Key points:

- An age appropriate dose should be prescribed taking into account general physical health and effect of concomitant medication on pharmacodynamics and pharmacokinetics.[7]
- In older people, response to antidepressants may take longer.[4] A minimum of 6 weeks treatment should be given before considering the treatment to be ineffective,[7] but it may be possible to identify non-responders as early as 4 weeks.[7]
- Antidepressants should be initiated at lower doses than used for younger adults.[4]
- The average older adult is more likely to be taking concurrent medicines[2] leading to a potential for medicines-medicine and medicines-disease interactions.
- Hyponatraemia is common in the elderly[4], and thus careful monitoring is advised in this patient group as older age is a risk factor.
- Depression in older adults with dementia should be prescribed according to the same principles as older adults, after a careful risk assessment. Antidepressants with anticholinergic side effects should be avoided where possible as they adversely affect cognition.[33]

Pregnancy

The use of antidepressants during pregnancy is common. In the UK, the large majority of women who are prescribed antidepressants stop taking them in very early pregnancy (<6 weeks gestation),[34] most likely because of concerns about teratogenicity. Patients who are already receiving antidepressants and are at high risk of relapse are best maintained on the same antidepressant during and after pregnancy.

Those who develop a moderate-severe or severe depressive illness during pregnancy should be treated with antidepressant drugs.

If initiating an antidepressant during pregnancy or for a woman considering pregnancy, previous response to treatment must be taken into account. The antidepressant that has previously proved to be effective should be considered. For previously untreated patients, sertraline may be considered. Paroxetine may be less safe than other SSRIs.

Screen for alcohol use and be vigilant for the development of hypertension and pre-eclampsia. Women who take SSRIs may be at increased risk of post-partum haemorrhage.

When taken in late pregnancy, SSRIs may increase the risk of persistent pulmonary hypertension of the newborn, but the absolute risk is very low. The neonate may experience discontinuation symptoms, which are usually mild, such as agitation and irritability, or rarely respiratory distress and convulsions (with SSRIs). The risk is assumed to be particularly high with short half-life drugs such as paroxetine and venlafaxine.

Continuing to breastfeed and then 'weaning' by switching to mixed (breast/bottle) feeding may help reduce the severity of reactions.

Before prescribing, refer to the individual drug entries for specific information and guidance.

Breastfeeding

It is usually advisable to continue the antidepressant prescribed during pregnancy. Switching drugs post-partum for the purpose of breastfeeding is usually not recommended. In each case previous response to treatment must be considered. When initiating an antidepressant post-partum, sertraline or mirtazapine may be considered. All infants should be monitored for drowsiness, poor feeding, irritability/restlessness. Before prescribing, refer to the individual drug entries for specific information and guidance.

People with epilepsy

Depression is the most common comorbidity in people with epilepsy (PWE) compared with the general population.[35,36] Rates vary from 3-9% in patients with well-controlled epilepsy to much higher (20-55%) in those with recurrent seizures and those treated at tertiary referral centres.[35,37,38]

The first consideration should always be to check the patients' anticonvulsant regimen for potential drug-induced depression. It may be that the patient would benefit from changing the anticonvulsant to another agent with a more favourable effect on mood rather than adding in an antidepressant. Non-pharmacological interventions such as CBT should be considered in people presenting with depression, in addition to the use of antidepressants. The risk of seizures with most antidepressants is low, but is probably not zero for any of them, and PWE should be made aware of this when prescribing. The risk of seizures increases with increasing doses. SSRIs are considered the first-line antidepressant option in PWE. Sertraline may be considered the better option due to low reported incidence of seizures and reduced interaction potential with the anticonvulsants. Fluvoxamine and fluoxetine may not be the best choices due to an increased risk of drug interactions.

Information and advice

Sleep hygiene and behavioural intervention

Consider suggesting these practices and habits which help promote good sleep:

- Sleep environment
  - Use the bed only for sleeping. Avoid other activities such as eating, work, reading and internet/chat on the bed.
  - Quieter bedroom, comfortable temperature and a well-made bed are more conductive to sleeping.
  - Bright light and light of shorter wavelength (green and blue light) suppress melatonin secretion. A less bright bedroom and lights of longer wavelength (red and orange lights) can aid sleep.
- Sleep schedule
  - Try to have a regular bed and wake-up time, including the weekend. Most importantly, getting up at the same time each morning – regardless of how poor the previous night's sleep was.
  - Sleep when feeling tired and sleepy, rather than spending too much time in the bed awake.
  - If no sleep after 20-30 min in the bed, get out of bed and do something calming (e.g. reading a boring book until sleepy). Avoid doing anything too stimulating or interesting.
- Sleep habits and rituals
  - Having a simple bedtime routine helps to unwind (e.g. story time, reading, music).
  - Avoid naps during the day. However, naps are important for young children and preferably in the early afternoon.
- Food, drinks and drugs
  - Hunger causes restless sleep. A heavy meal before bed can interrupt sleep.
  - A light snack (low protein, high carbohydrate) can help. Foods containing melatonin (e.g. rice, corn and oats) or its precursor tryptophan (e.g. warm milk, nuts) can act as a natural sleep inducer.
  - Avoid caffeine (e.g. tea, coffee, colas, chocolate), nicotine and alcohol (this fragments and reduces total sleep time) for at least 4-6 hours before going to bed.
  - Certain medications can adversely affect sleep directly (e.g. stimulants) or by interfering with melatonin synthesis (e.g. NSAIDS – aspirin, ibuprofen).
- Exercise
  - Regular exercise aids good sleep.
  - Gentle exercise before bed can help to feel relaxed; strenuous exercise before bedtime is not advisable.
  - Having a warm bath 1-2 hours before bedtime can be useful. This raises the body temperature and makes people feel sleepy as the body temperature drops again.

Useful resources

General resources for patients and healthcare professionals

- Mind provides advice and support to empower anyone experiencing a mental health problem – www.mind.org.uk
- The Samaritans provides 24-hour, confidential, emotional support for anyone feeling distressed or in despair – www.samaritans.org
- The British Association for Behavioural and Cognitive Psychotherapies maintains a database of cognitive behavioural therapy specialists who are accredited in the UK and Ireland – www.babcp.com
  - Other accredited websites to find a therapist – www.psychotherapy.org.uk, www.bpc.org.uk

- Choice and Medication provides reliable, up-to-date and straightforward information and advice about the medicines used in mental illness – www.choiceandmedication.org.uk (access usually available for patients via their mental health service)
- Find Psychological therapies (IAPT) services – www.nhs.uk/Service-Search/Psychological%20 therapies%20(IAPT)/LocationSearch/10008
- Books on Prescription helps you to understand and manage your health and wellbeing using self-help reading. The books are chosen by health experts and people living with the conditions covered – www.reading-well.org.uk/books/books-on-prescription

Resources for patients and healthcare professionals for anxiety
- Anxiety UK – www.anxietyuk.org.uk
- No Panic – www.nopanic.org.uk

Recommended reading for depression
- Veale D, Willson R. Manage Your Mood: How to Use Behavioural Activation Techniques to Overcome Depression
- Roslyn R. Defeating Depression: How to use the people in your life to open the door to recovery
- Greenberger D. Mind Over Mood, Second Edition: Change How You Feel by Changing the Way You Think

Recommended reading for anxiety
- Kennerley H. Overcoming anxiety: a self-help guide using cognitive behavioural techniques
- Williams C. Overcoming Anxiety, Stress and Panic: A Five Areas Approach
- Veale D, Willson R. Overcoming Health Anxiety: a self-help guide using cognitive behavioural techniques

Resources for patients and healthcare professionals
- Depression UK – a self-help organisation made up of individuals and local groups – www.depressionuk.org
- Cruse Bereavement Care – charity providing information and support after someone you know has died – www.cruse.org.uk
- NHS Choices Mood Zone – provides self-help and support strategies, audio guides and videos – www.nhs.uk/conditions/stress-anxiety-depression/pages/low-mood-stress-anxiety.aspx
- Pharmacist Support – an independent charity working for pharmacists and their families, former pharmacists and pharmacy students to provide help and support in times of need – www.pharmacistsupport.org
- Campaign Against Living Miserably (CALM) – male suicide awareness charity that operates web-chat and telephone advice 5pm to 12am, 7 days a week, 365 days a year – www.thecalmzone.net

References

1. American Psychiatric Association (2000). *Diagnostic and statistical manual of mental disorder*, 4th edition, text rev. Washington, DC: Author.
2. Lamers F *et al*. Comorbidity patterns of anxiety and depressive disorders in a large cohort study: the Netherlands study of depression and anxiety (NESDA). *J Clin Psychiatry* 2011; 72: 341.
3. Alonso J *et al*. Prevalence of mental disorders in Europe: results from the European study of the epidemiology of mental disorders (ESEMeD) project. *Acta Psychiatr Scand Suppl.* 2004; 420: 21-7.
4. Cleare A *et al*. Evidence-based guidelines for treating depressive disorders with antidepressants: A revision of the 2008 British Association for Psychopharmacology guidelines. *Journal of Psychopharmacology* 2015; 29(5): 459-525.
5. Office for National Statistics (2018). Deaths registered in England and Wales (series DR): 2017. www.ons.gov.uk/peoplepopulationand community/birthsdeathsandmarriages/deaths/bulletins/deathsregisteredinenglandandwalesseriesdr/2017

6. Cowen P *et al. Shorter Oxford Textbook of Psychiatry*, 7 edition ed. Oxford: Oxford University Press, 2017.

7. National Institute for Health and Care Excellence (2009). Depression: The NICE guideline on the treatment and management of depression in adults. www.nice.org.uk/guidance/cg90

8. Taylor D *et al. The Maudsley Prescribing Guidelines in Psychiatry*, 13th Edition. London: Wiley Blackwell, 2018.

9. Bazire S. *Psychotropic Drug Directory* 2016. Stratford Upon Avon: Lloyd-Reinhold Publications, 2016.

10. Wittchen HU, Jacobi F. Size and burden of mental disorders in Europe – a critical review and appraisal of 27 studies. *European Psychopharmacology* 2005; 15: 357-76.

11. Baldwin D *et al.* Evidence-based guideline for the pharmacological treatment of anxiety disorders, post-traumatic stress disorder and obsessive-compulsive disorder: a revision of the 2005 guidelines from the British Association for Psychopharmacology. *Journal of Psychopharmacology* 2014; 28(5): 1-37.

12. Roy-Byrne P *et al.* Anxiety disorders and comorbid medical illness. *General Hospital Psychiatry* 2008; 30(3): 208-25.

13. Guaiana G *et al.* Hydroxyzine for generalised anxiety disorder. *Cochrane Database of Systematic Reviews*, issue 12. Chichester: John Wiley & Sons Ltd.

14. Hofmann S, Smits J. Cognitive-behavioural therapy for adult anxiety disorders: a meta-analysis of randomised placebo-controlled trials. *Journal of Clinical Psychiatry* 2008; 69: 621-32.

15. Meltzer H *et al.* The reluctance to seek treatment for neurotic disorders. *J Ment Health* 2009; 319-327.

16. Shepard N, Parker C. Depression in adults: recognition and management. *Clinical Pharmacist* April 2017; 9(4).

17. Morrissey J, Callaghan P. *Communication skills for mental health nurses: an introduction.* Open University Press, 2011.

18. Kai J, Crosland A. Perspectives of people with enduring mental ill health from a community-based qualitative study. *British Journal of General Practice* 2001; 51: 730-737.

19. Ilyas S, Moncrieff J. Trends in prescriptions and costs of drugs for mental disorders in England 1998–2010. *Br J Psychiatry* 2012; 200(5): 393-8.

20. National Institute for Health and Care Excellence (2010). Depression in adults with a chronic physical health problem. www.nice.org.uk/guidance/cg91/evidence/full-guideline-243876061

21. British National Formulary. Number 78. London. BMJ Group and Pharmaceutical Press. 2019.

22. Medsafe (2013). QT prolongation with antidepressants. www.medsafe.govt.nz/profs/PUArticles/December2013QTProlongationAndAntidepressants.htm

23. Dickens C *et al.* New onset depression following myocardial infarction predicts cardiac mortality. *Psychosom Med* 2008; 70: 450-455.

24. Specialist Pharmacy Service (2018). What is the antidepressant of choice in coronary heart disease (CHD)? www.sps.nhs.uk/articles/what-is-the-antidepressant-of-choice-in-coronary-heart-disease-chd/

25. Wilson E, Lader M. A review of the management of antidepressant discontinuation symptoms. *Therapeutic Advances in Psychopharmacology* 2015; 05(6): 357-68.

26. Fava G *et al.* Withdrawal Symptoms after Selective Serotonin Reuptake Inhibitor Discontinuation: A Systematic Review. *Psychotherapy and Psychosomatics* 2015; 84(2): 72-81.

27. Horowitz M, Taylor D (2019). Tapering of SSRI treatment to mitigate withdrawal symptoms. *The Lancet Psychiatry* 2019; 6(6): 538-546.

28. Davies J, Read J. A systematic review into the incidence, severity and duration of antidepressant withdrawal effects: Are guidelines evidence-based? *Addictive Behaviors* 2019; 97: 111-121.

29. Gibson K *et al.* 'In my life antidepressants have been…': a qualitative analysis of users' diverse experiences with antidepressants. *BMC Psychiatry* 2016; 16(1).

30. Read J, Williams J. Adverse effects of antidepressants reported by a large international cohort: Emotional blunting, suicidality, and withdrawal effects. *Current Drug Safety* 2018; 13(3): 176-86.

31. Cartwright C *et al.* Long-term antidepressant use: patient perspectives of benefits and adverse effects. *Patient Preference and Adherence* 2016; (10): 1401-07.

32. National Institute for Health and Care Excellence (2018). Consultation draft. Depression in adults: treatment and management. www.nice.org.uk/guidance/gid-cgwave0725/documents/full-guideline-updated

33. National Institute for Health and Care Excellence (2016). Dementia: assessment, management and support for people living with dementia and their carers. www.nice.org.uk/guidance/ng97

34. Petersen I *et al.* Pregnancy as a major determinant for discontinuation of antidepressants: an analysis of data from The Health Improvement Network. *J Clin Psychiatry* 2011; 72: 979-985.

35. Ojong M, Allen SN. Treatment of depression in patients with epilepsy. *US Pharmacist* 2012; 37(11): 29-32.

36. Cardamone L *et al.* Antidepressant therapy in epilepsy: can treating the comorbidities affect the underlying disorder? *Br J Pharmacol* 2013; 168: 1531-1554.

37. Muzerengi S, Moor CC. What do we know about depression in people with epilepsy? *Prog Neurol Psychiatry* 2013; March/April:20-24.

38. Scottish Intercollegiate Guidelines Network (2018). Diagnosis and management of epilepsy in adults. www.sign.ac.uk/media/1079/sign143_2018.pdf

Case studies

Case study 1

You are a specialist mental health pharmacist working in a GP practice. John, aged 25 years, is a student and has a diagnosis of depression. He wants to see a clinician to discuss his medication, paroxetine, as he no longer wishes to take it.

Points to consider

- How would you approach this issue, and what questions would you ask?

You speak with John and listen sensitively to his concerns and he tells you that while paroxetine has helped significantly with his mood, it has reduced his libido and there is a delay in orgasm, and he is mostly unable to climax which is causing problems in his relationship.

Points to consider

- Are these likely to be adverse effects of paroxetine?
- What would you ask John to gain further insight into the issue?

You are aware that adverse effects can be unpleasant and can affect the quality of life in many patients. Sexual dysfunction is a common problem in depression and is also a common problem with antidepressant medication.

You ask John when the issues started, enquire about his lifestyle and look at his medical record. John explains the sexual dysfunction occurred soon after starting the paroxetine. Besides being overweight, there are no other contributing causes such as recreational drug use, diabetes, alcohol misuse or cardiac disease that you are aware of.

Points to consider

- What management options would you consider to help resolve the issue?

John has tried citalopram in the past and you discuss non-pharmacological treatment strategies, however you feel it would be most appropriate to try an antidepressant with a lower risk of sexual dysfunction.

Points to consider

- Which antidepressants would be appropriate options for John?

Mirtazapine is your first choice, but due to possible, unacceptable weight gain and sedation for the patient you decide that vortioxetine would be a better option.

Case study 2

You are a practice-based pharmacist working in a GP surgery. You are seeing Lucy, aged 55 years, who is a stay-at-home mum. You have seen Lucy before with her partner, Kelly, after her dose of antidepressant was increased. Kelly is very concerned about Lucy as her mood has deteriorated – she says Lucy has always had depression but it has never been this bad.

Lucy is sobbing, dry retching, unable to put her thoughts together and no longer thinks she can go on. She describes a 'chatter of voices' in her head, but says that these are her own thoughts rather than external voices. They are saying 'everything will get worse' and 'it's the end of everything' – her thoughts have been at this intensity for the past week.

Kelly is afraid to go out for any length of time as she is afraid of what Lucy may do to herself and what she may find when she gets home. This is a very different presentation to when you saw Lucy in the past. Lucy is currently the carer for her mother, aged 84 years, who lives in a care home – this seems to have triggered her current depression. She confides she has not been taking her medication for the past week and storing it to take an overdose. She previously took an overdose three years ago.

> **Points to consider**
> * What concerns do you have?
> * How would you approach this situation?

You tell Lucy and Kelly you are very concerned and they need urgent additional support. You discuss with one of your senior colleagues at the practice and decide the best way forward would be to send her to A&E to have a review with the specialist mental health services team. Lucy and Kelly agree; Kelly feels she is able to take Lucy to A&E. You arrange transport to A&E and call ahead to let the mental health liaison team know the patient is attending.

Case study 3

You are a practice pharmacist working in a GP surgery. You see James, aged 28 years, an American student who is currently taking bupropion for his depression. He started bupropion in America six months ago for a severe episode of depression.

He tells you he is here for the next year but has run out of medication. He has helpfully brought along his last clinic letter from his psychiatrist which confirms the medication prescribed and the dose. He wants to continue bupropion as it has significantly helped with his depression. He is also in the process of finding a private therapist.

> **Points to consider**
> * What are your initial thoughts on this therapy?

You explain to James that while bupropion is licensed in America for depression, it is not licensed for depression in the UK. It is also not on the usual CCG formulary.

> **Points to consider**
> * How would you manage this situation?

You contact the specialist mental health team for their thoughts. They let you know it is on the trust formulary as a third-line antidepressant, and if the patient is benefitting, to continue the medication for the time being if the GP feels comfortable prescribing it. They also send you a helpful patient leaflet from the choice and medication website on unlicensed medications.

> **Points to consider**
> * What important information do you need to tell James about this treatment?

You explain the off-label nature of the medication with James and ensure that he is aware of the risks, and you document this in his patient record. The GP is willing to continue the bupropion prescription.

Case study 4

You are a practice-based pharmacist working in a busy GP surgery. Jane, aged 40 years, is sitting in the doctor's surgery wringing her hands and crossing and uncrossing her legs.

She has a diagnosis of generalised anxiety disorder and attends the GP practice complaining of upper epigastric pain which persists despite her trying every antacid on the chemist's shelves. She has had several endoscopies, none of which revealed any abnormality. She also has lower back pain and numerous headaches which do not seem to respond to the common analgesics. She is a frequent visitor to the doctor who can never find anything wrong with her.

She says she is worried about the future, but cannot explain exactly why. Every time she thinks about it her heart races and she breaks out in a cold sweat. Sometimes she thinks she is going to have a heart attack. She has booked in an appointment to see you because she wants to change her medication. She is prescribed citalopram and has tried fluoxetine in the past.

Points to consider

- What are your initial thoughts and concerns about Jane and her treatment?

During your appointment it becomes clear Jane has only taken the medication for a few days, taking regular starting doses before noticing her anxiety getting much worse. She does not want to take the medication she has tried in the past.

Points to consider

- What information and advice would you provide?
- How would you manage this situation?

You explain the medication might have caused some initial exacerbation of her symptoms and that it may be helpful to start a different antidepressant at half the normal starting dose and consider a short course of diazepam when required. You suggest starting another SSRI such as sertraline at 25 mg once a day and increase by 25 mg every one to two weeks with a review in three weeks' time. You also recommend diazepam – 7 tablets of 2 mg to the GP.

During the consultation you find she feels very lonely since the death of her mother a few years ago. She previously enjoyed gardening but has had to move to a different property without a garden. Jane explains that she does not want to have therapy because she has tried it before and it wasn't helpful.

Points to consider

- What non-pharmacological interventions might be useful for Jane?

You look up a gardening group nearby that she can attend, which she finds daunting but would like to try, and provide her with the details to get in touch.

Case study 5

You are a community pharmacist. Tim, a man in his 50's, comes for another emergency supply of his antidepressant medication for his anxiety disorder. He is also on antiepileptic medication levetiracetam 1500 mg twice a day and lacosamide 150 mg twice a day.

He has been stressed at work about a big project and in his distress sometimes he has been doubling his dose of antidepressant medication, citalopram, in the hope it might reduce his anxiety. He is prescribed the maximum dose of 40 mg/day by his GP, which means sometimes he is taking twice the maximum BNF dose.

Points to consider

- How would you respond to Tim?

You explain to Tim that doubling his dose of citalopram is dangerous, puts him at increased risk of unwanted effects, and erratic use of the medication will not reduce his anxiety symptoms. He should take the medication as prescribed.

Points to consider

- What other aspects of Tim's health would you enquire about?

You ask Tim about his seizure control and he mentions he had a brief seizure last week which is unusual.

Points to consider

- What may have contributed to this seizure?

You explain to Tim that you are concerned that citalopram at the high dose may be reducing his seizure threshold, meaning he is more likely to have a seizure.

Points to consider

- How would you manage this situation?

You advise Tim to book an appointment with his GP to try to manage his anxiety symptoms better. You provide him with an emergency supply of citalopram as you do not want him to experience discontinuation symptoms, and he has agreed not to take more citalopram than prescribed.

Points to consider

- What non-pharmacological interventions might be useful for Tim?

He may also benefit from non-pharmacological therapy. You discuss mindfulness, which he thinks is a good idea and will follow up on.

CHAPTER 2

Asthma

Toby Capstick and Lynn Elsey

Overview

Asthma is a common chronic condition that affects 5.4 million people in the UK, including 1.1 million children,[1] and 1 in 5 of these suffer from severe asthma. It contributes to a large burden on the NHS, including 77,124 UK hospital admissions in 2016/17,[2] (75% of which are thought to be avoidable),[3] and 1,484 deaths in 2017[1] (two-thirds of which are thought to be preventable).[1,2]

Asthma is a reversible obstruction of the airways characterised by intermittent inflammation that causes narrowing of the airways and limits airflow. Asthma also causes damage to the nerve endings in the airways making them more hypersensitive and easily irritated.[4] People with asthma typically experience periods of chest tightness, shortness of breath and wheeze in between periods of normal lung function.

Asthma attacks may occur at random with no obvious precipitating factors or may be caused by poor adherence to treatment, or a trigger such as exposure to allergens (i.e. house dust mites, animal fur, pollen), tobacco smoke, pollution, cold air, exercise, or viruses such as cold or influenza.

Risk factors for developing asthma include having a family history of asthma, a history of atopy, severe respiratory infection as a child, or occupational exposure to causative agents (e.g. isocyanates, flour and grain dust, colophony and fluxes, latex, animals, aldehydes and wood dust).

Asthma is a lifelong condition that, if treated appropriately, can be controlled to achieve a resolution of asthma symptoms, normal lung function and no limitation of normal activities.

Diagnosis

A diagnosis of asthma is essentially a clinical diagnosis, with no gold standard diagnostic criteria. It is made based on symptoms of wheeze, breathlessness, chest tightness and cough, with evidence of variable lung function (see *Box 2.1*).

In both adults and children, the presence of characteristic symptoms of asthma are neither sensitive nor specific in isolation to confirm a diagnosis of asthma, but the presence of the episodic nature of symptoms (e.g. diurnal variation, acute asthma attacks) may improve the predictive value.

Most children with asthma have intermittent cough, wheeze and exercise-induced symptoms, but only about a quarter of children with these symptoms have asthma.[4] Objective tests that can increase the probability of a diagnosis of asthma (rather than confirm it definitively) include those that measure variable lung function or the presence of airway inflammation.[4]

As symptoms alone are not diagnostic, any patient with suspected asthma should be asked about their clinical history to identify features that increase the probability of a diagnosis of asthma. These include:
- current symptoms (daytime and nighttime)
- pattern of symptoms (over a day, week and year)
- precipitating or aggravating factors
- relieving factors
- impact on work and lifestyle
- home and work environment
- smoking history

- history of allergies including atopic dermatitis
- family history of atopic/allergic diseases.

Peak flow charting

It can be useful for patients to chart their peak expiratory flows (PEF) twice a day as this can give an idea of peak flow variability, and therefore the likelihood of asthma. The patient should monitor their PEF for two to four weeks, allowing the mean variability to be calculated. One study concluded that the number of days with diurnal variation was more accurate than calculating the mean variation.[4]

Spirometry

Lung function tests can be used to confirm the presence of airflow obstruction, with this being demonstrated by an FEV_1/FVC ratio of less than 70%. However, more than half of patients being investigated, who have normal spirometry, will have asthma (i.e. false negatives), particularly when they are asymptomatic with well-controlled asthma.[4]

Bronchodilator reversibility tests compare a patient's FEV_1 before and after a dose of a $beta_2$-agonist bronchodilator, and a positive test in the context of airflow obstruction increases the probability of asthma. In adults, an improvement in FEV_1 of ≥12% and ≥200 mL is a positive test for reversibility, although this can also be positive in COPD, but a larger improvement in FEV_1 of at least 400 mL strongly supports a diagnosis of asthma. In children, an improvement in FEV_1 of ≥12% is regarded as a positive test.

At least one in three people with a negative bronchodilator reversibility test will have asthma, and other tests are required to confirm a diagnosis in patients where a diagnosis of asthma is suspected.

Challenge tests

Challenge tests are used to measure airway hyperresponsiveness and airway response to inhalation of a substance that provokes bronchospasm in people with asthma. Lung function is measured and then the patient is exposed to progressively increasing amounts of histamine, methacholine or mannitol. If the patients FEV_1 drops by 20% (histamine or methacholine), or 15% (mannitol), it can indicate that they have reactive airways.[4]

Challenge tests are a good indicator for those without a definitive diagnosis of asthma already but if it is suspected based upon clinical judgment, signs and symptoms and response to anti-asthma therapy, but spirometric testing has not shown airflow obstruction.

Exhaled nitric oxide

Nitric oxide is produced in the lungs as a result of eosinophilic airway inflammation and is present in the breath. It is associated with a pathophysiology of airways disease such as asthma. In eosinophilic asthma there is a rise in exhaled nitric oxide and the measurement can indicate an increase in inflammation and loss of asthma control.

Fractional expiratory nitric oxide (FeNO) can be measured using portable nitric oxide monitors to assess the current inflammation in a patient's airway. In adults, a FeNO level of 40 ppb or more is regarded as a positive test, whilst in children, a level of 35 ppb or more is positive.

It can also be a good indicator of a patient's adherence or response to inhaled corticosteroids (ICS), because patients with poor adherence to ICS may have a raised FeNO, and can be shown to reduce significantly with good adherence.

In severe asthma clinics, FeNO suppression tests are used in practice to identify whether a raised FeNO is due to poor adherence to ICS treatment, or non-steroid responsive disease. Patients are given daily direct or indirect (facilitated by a 'breath-actuated dose counter') observation of ICS/LABA dosing, and FeNO is measured at days 0, 1, 2 and 7. A positive FeNO suppression test indicating poor adherence is confirmed by a reduction in FeNO of at least 42%.

Approximately one in five adults with a positive FeNO test will not have asthma (i.e. false positives) and one in five adults with a negative FeNO test will have asthma (i.e. false negatives). The latter is particularly the case in people who smoke since this causes a decrease in exhaled nitric oxide and can, therefore, give a false negative test.

Blood eosinophils

Eosinophils are associated with inflammation in the airways, and elevated blood eosinophils may indicate that the patient is likely to be responsive to inhaled corticosteroids. However, they could be affected by parasitic infection or drugs such as antidepressants.

Immunoglobulin E (IgE)

Measuring total and allergen-specific IgE levels is useful to demonstrate an atopic status and identify potential triggers for worsening asthma. A raised allergen-specific IgE >0.35 kU/L in adults or a total IgE in adults >100 kU/L demonstrates atopy and increases the probability of a diagnosis of asthma, although a positive result is poorly predictive. In contrast, a normal IgE result substantially reduces the probability of asthma.[4]

Skin-prick testing

This can be used to identify allergies and confirm an atopic status; however, there are relatively few standardised allergens commercially available. The results are read 15 minutes after administration of the test, and a positive test (wheal ≥3 mm) in adults or children demonstrates an atopic phenotype but is poorly predictive of a diagnosis of asthma.[4]

Box 2.1: Practice point: diagnosis

- Diagnosis of asthma is made based on symptoms of wheeze, breathlessness, chest tightness and cough, with evidence of variable lung function.
- Peak flow charting can demonstrate peak flow variability and therefore the likelihood of asthma.
- Lung function tests can be used to confirm the presence of airflow obstruction.
- A rise in exhaled nitric oxide can indicate an increase in inflammation and loss of asthma control.
- Elevated blood eosinophils may indicate that airway inflammation may respond to inhaled corticosteroids.
- Total and allergen-specific IgE levels are useful to demonstrate an atopic status and identify potential triggers for asthma.

Phenotypes

Diagnostic difficulties are one of the most challenging and complex issues in the management of difficult asthma today. There is increasing research supporting the concept that difficult asthma has a number of different phenotypes, with different mechanisms driving symptoms, which could respond differently to different classes of medicines.

Asthma is often regarded as an allergic airway inflammatory condition mediated by eosinophils and T_H2 immune pathways, which is responsive to corticosteroids. More recently, alternative asthma phenotypes based on clinical characteristics, non-T_H2 asthma inflammatory processes and triggers have been proposed such as obesity-associated, smoking-associated and neutrophilic asthma, which are less responsive to conventional asthma medicines such as ICS.[5]

Whilst the current understanding of asthma phenotyping and effective therapies is insufficient to allow individualised treatment in present-day practice, this principle is likely to become increasingly important in the future management of difficult asthma.

Pharmacy input

Pharmacists in all sectors have opportunities to provide education for people with asthma, and furthermore, may be able to identify those with poor asthma control. Possible roles include:

1. Referral when patients present at community pharmacy with potential symptoms of asthma
2. Regular assessment of inhaler technique for new or ongoing inhaled therapies
3. Adherence monitoring, through monitoring of repeat prescriptions of preventative therapies, and excessive use of reliever inhalers
4. Highlight loss of control through overuse of reliever inhalers
5. Educate patients on the aims of the different treatments used for asthma

Pharmacists can play multiple roles in the diagnosis and treatment of asthma. Patients may present at a community pharmacy seeking treatment for themselves or a child who is displaying early signs of asthma such as nighttime cough. At this point, history taking is vital to identify risk factors such as eczema or family history of asthma. All patients presenting with these symptoms must be referred for further assessment.

Pharmacists should undertake a structured clinical assessment to assess the initial probability of asthma. This should be based on:

- a history of recurrent episodes (attacks) of symptoms, ideally corroborated by variable peak flows when symptomatic and asymptomatic
- symptoms of wheeze, cough, breathlessness and chest tightness that vary over time
- recorded observation of wheeze heard by a healthcare professional
- personal/family history of other atopic conditions (in particular, atopic eczema/dermatitis, allergic rhinitis)
- no symptoms/signs to suggest alternative diagnoses.

Pharmacists may assess patients within the GP surgery monitoring prescription collection of preventative inhalers or overuse of reliever inhalers. They can also escalate or de-escalate treatments in line with the patient's current symptoms. GP pharmacists can undertake annual asthma reviews to optimise the patient's asthma treatment, ensure that the patient has an up-to-date asthma treatment plan and escalate patients with difficult or severe asthma.

Hospital pharmacists may interact with asthma patients at a variety of stages. At admission, the pharmacist can assess patients' inhaler technique and check the patient's adherence to their current medications. They may also refer up to the specialist asthma team. Throughout the patient's stay in hospital, the pharmacist must ensure that the patient is receiving the appropriate treatment and counsel the patient on any new treatments started. At discharge, a final check of inhaler technique will help to ensure that the patient is using the treatment correctly at home. Within the outpatient setting, patients may be reviewed by specialist asthma pharmacists who may alter their asthma prescription and escalate those with severe asthma to biologic therapy.

Pharmacy review

Regular review of people with asthma offers the opportunity to monitor current symptom control and the impact asthma is having on daily activities and quality of life, to assess the risk of future asthma attacks, and to link these to management options.

Asthma is best monitored by routine clinical review on at least an annual basis by a healthcare professional with appropriate training in asthma management. The review can be undertaken in primary and/or secondary care according to clinical need and local service arrangements. The suggested components of a review are listed in *Table 2.1*, focusing on current symptoms, risk of asthma attacks, management strategies, and self-management.

Table 2.1: *Components of an asthma review (adapted from BTS/SIGN asthma guidelines, 2019)[4]*

Parameter	Suggested assessment
Current symptom control	• Bronchodilator use • Validated symptom score • Time off work/school due to asthma
Risk of future attacks	• Past history of asthma attacks • Oral corticosteroid use • Prescription data: frequent SABA and infrequent ICS • Exposure to tobacco smoke
Tests/investigations	• Lung function (spirometry or PEF) • Growth (height and weight centile) in children
Management	• Inhaler technique • Adherence (self-report, prescription refill frequency) • Non-pharmacological management (trigger avoidance, breathing exercises) • Pharmacological management (consider multimorbidity and polypharmacy)
Supported self-management	• Education/discussion about self-management • Provision/revision of a written personalised asthma action plan

Pharmacists assessing patients with asthma should determine their asthma control using specific questions, such as the Royal College of Physicians (RCP) '3 Questions' (See *Box 2.2*), as well as asking about adherence to their preventer inhaler, use of reliever inhaler (whether this has increased in recent days or weeks), how many course of oral corticosteroids they've required, and use of a PEF meter.

Box 2.2: RCP '3 Questions'

In the last week/month:
• Have you had difficulty sleeping because of your asthma symptoms (including cough)?
• Have you had your usual asthma symptoms during the day (cough, wheeze, chest tightness or breathlessness)?
• Has your asthma interfered with your usual activities (e.g. housework, work/school etc.)?
If the patient answers yes to any question, further assessment should be made.

During an asthma consultation, inhaler technique should be assessed and optimised using either the person's inhalers or placebo devices. If necessary, their inspiratory effort should be checked (e.g. with an In-Check DIAL G16 inspiratory flow meter) to ensure that they can inhale through their prescribed inhaler device at the correct speed. PEF can also be measured to determine or compare to their best PEF as a measure of asthma control and allow severity of any asthma attack.

In specialist asthma centres, exhaled nitric oxide may also be measured as a marker of active eosinophilic inflammation and response to ICS treatment if a FeNO machine is available, although currently the routine use of FeNO testing to monitor asthma in adults or children is not recommended.[4] Signs and symptoms that asthma is not well controlled include:
• chest tightness/wheeze
• increased nighttime wakening with wheeze cough
• inability to speak in full sentences
• reduced ability to carry out usual daily activities

- increased use of reliever inhaler
- reduced PEF, especially if reduced below 75% of best
- raised FENO above 30 ppb, suggesting poor adherence or response to ICS.

Information and advice

For asthma to be adequately controlled, patients must be given sufficient information to understand what asthma is and how it is treated. The intermittent nature of asthma can mean that some patients do not realise that treatment is lifelong, and inhaled corticosteroid inhalers should continue to be used regularly, even when the condition is quiescent.

Patient education is essential to ensure they understand these issues and how to self-care. As front-line healthcare professionals, pharmacists can provide this education and support. This includes signposting to patient resources for further information such as the Asthma UK website (www.asthma.org.uk) which includes inhaler technique videos (www.asthma.org.uk/advice/inhaler-videos), smartphone apps such as RightBreathe (www.rightbreathe.com), which allows patients to set reminders to use their inhalers, and every patient should be provided with a personalised asthma action plan. Education around the different medications in their device is important to ensure the patient understands the importance of regular use of their preventative inhaler and the risks of overuse of their reliever inhaler. Pharmacists can also provide information on the different types of asthma treatments.

Patients should be advised on important non-pharmacological strategies to aid symptom control and reduce the risk of asthma attacks, including smoking cessation advice, breathing exercises and trigger avoidance strategies. Reducing exposure to tobacco smoke can improve asthma symptom control, and providing very brief advice alongside referral to local stop smoking services will maximise the opportunity to successfully stop smoking. Pharmacists may wish to undertake online training on smoking cessation advice from the National Centre for Smoking Cessation Training (www.ncsct.co.uk). Very brief advice consists of three simple components:

- ASK and record smoking status, and whether they live with a smoker.
- ADVISE patient of health benefits of quitting, and inform them that the best way to quit is with a combination of trained support and medication.
- ACT on patient's response and refer smokers who want to quit to their local NHS stop smoking service.

Patients with confirmed triggers for worsening asthma symptoms or asthma attacks should be advised about how to avoid these. For example, patients with pollen allergies should be advised to keep windows closed on days when there is a high pollen count. There is, however, limited evidence that single strategies to remove exposure to indoor allergies, such as house dust mite or pets, have a positive impact on asthma control.

Patients should be advised to exercise regularly to maintain good physical and cardiovascular health and reduce the chance of breathlessness from deconditioning being mistaken as worsening asthma. Weight reduction strategies should be advised in obese patients as this can improve asthma control and quality of life.

Interventions

If a patient develops an acute viral or bacterial illness, this may impact their asthma control. Patients should be educated on how to monitor their symptoms and peak flow. An asthma action plan should be developed to allow patients to recognise a loss of asthma control, improve self-management of their symptoms and highlight when a patient needs to seek medical attention (see the asthma action plan section). Antibiotics should only be prescribed where there is clear evidence of a bacterial infection.

Inhaler technique

Pharmacists should assess inhaler technique regularly and following an asthma attack. Improving a patient's inhaler technique can have a large impact on their symptoms. Ensuring a patient understands the seven steps of inhaler technique is vital:[6]

1. Prepare the device (i.e. take the cap off etc.).
2. Prepare/load the dose (i.e. shake the device etc.).
3. Breathe out fully and gently away from the device.
4. Place the device in your mouth, ensuring a tight seal around the mouthpiece.
5. Breathe in slow and steady for pressurised metered-dose inhaler (pMDI), or quick and deep for a dry powder inhaler (DPI).
6. Remove the device and hold breath for up to 10 seconds.
7. Wait for a few seconds and repeat if necessary.

   The patient's technique can be assessed as either:

- Optimal – perfect technique
- Satisfactory – some minor, but no critical errors
- Unsatisfactory – at least one critical error (one that significantly reduces the delivered dose to the lungs, such as not removing the cap from an MDI)

SABA usage

Excessive usage of SABA inhalers in asthma (more than one canister each month) is associated with a three-fold increased risk of attendance at emergency departments, and hospitalisation.[7] Good asthma control is characterised by using a SABA reliever inhaler no more than twice a week, so a 200-dose salbutamol pMDI should be expected to last 50 weeks.

Whilst ideally every patient using more than this should be reviewed urgently to identify and manage potentially worsening control, this is unlikely to be achievable due to the large numbers of patients on each GP practice register.

Pragmatically, patients should be asked about their SABA usage at every annual asthma review, and practice asthma registers should be interrogated to identify patients at highest risk. Many practices and CCGs aim to identify patients collecting more than six to 12 SABA inhalers each year who require an urgent review to discuss the risks of overuse of SABA and how this can indicate poor control.

Asthma action plan

Completing an asthma action plan for patients can help them to understand what their symptoms mean, what the aim is of their different treatments and when to seek help. The action plan can be based on the patient's PEF measurements and/or symptoms.

There is no set format to an asthma action plan, but these can include specific advice about recognising loss of asthma control, assessed by symptoms and/or peak flows, actions to take if asthma deteriorates, including seeking emergency help, increasing the ICS dose, or starting oral steroids. For example, action plans should recommend to commence a rescue course of oral corticosteroids if the PEF falls below 75% of the patient's best or predicted value, or to seek immediate medical assistance if the PEF drops below 50% of the patient's best or predicted value. You can download a copy of an asthma action plan from the asthma UK website (www.asthma.org.uk).

Adherence

The average adherence rate to medications in chronic conditions such as asthma is 50%. In asthma, it is estimated that only 30-70% of patients will be adherent. Non-adherence to preventative therapies can lead to poor control, overuse of reliever therapies and may lead to a life-threatening asthma attack. The National Review of Asthma Deaths[8] report highlighted the need for regular electronic surveillance of repeat prescriptions for preventer inhalers.

Community and GP practice-based pharmacists are in an ideal situation to monitor this and must highlight where adherence is poor. Improving adherence to ICS treatment can have significant benefits in asthma, with one meta-analysis concluding that achieving a 25% increase in adherence results in an approximate 10% reduction in severe exacerbations.[9]

When asking patients about their adherence, it is important to phrase questions in a non-threatening manner, and then explore reasons for non-adherence. Unintentional poor adherence may occur due:

- the price of prescription charges
- poor inhaler technique
- poor memory
- lack of understanding.

Intentional poor adherence may occur due to:

- patients' beliefs about the necessity
- concerns they have about their medication.

Improving adherence can be difficult, but ultimately rewarding and requires good communication skills and involving the patient as a partner in shared decision making to address their concerns and personal goals, and agreeing to an appropriate treatment regimen.

Different techniques can be used to improve adherence depending on whether it is intentional or unintentional. See *Box 2.3* for some examples of intentional and non-intentional non-adherence and how to help manage them.

Box 2.3: Examples of intentional and unintentional non-adherence and how to manage them

- Intentional non-adherence due to fear of adverse effects from steroids.
  - Educate the patient around the risk of adverse effects of inhaled steroids in comparison to oral steroids.
- Intentional non-adherence due to belief that asthma is well controlled.
  - Educate patient on the benefits of preventer therapy and the necessity for continued use despite current asthma control. It can be useful to show the patient diagrams of inflamed asthma airways to demonstrate where the preventer inhaler is acting.
- Unintentional non-adherence due to issues with paying for prescriptions.
  - Signpost the patient to the website for setting up a pre-payment certificate to assist with paying.
- Unintentional non-adherence due to a busy life.
  - Rationalise their treatment considering a once a day preventer of MART regime to increase the likelihood of them remembering their preventer therapy.

Medication

There are currently two national guidelines for the treatment of asthma in the UK, the BTS/SIGN asthma guidelines (2019),[4] and the NICE asthma guidelines.[10] Whilst there are many similarities, there are also differences in stepwise treatment recommendations. In this chapter, we will mainly consider the BTS/SIGN asthma guidelines (2019) as it is the more established UK guideline. It should be noted, however, that these organisations plan to collaborate to develop a single guideline.

The aim of asthma management is to control the disease. Complete control of asthma is defined[4] as:

- no daytime symptoms
- no nighttime awakening due to asthma
- no need for rescue medication
- no asthma attacks
- no limitations on activity, including exercise
- normal lung function (in practical terms FEV_1 and/or PEF >80% predicted or best)
- minimal adverse effects from medication.

A phased approach aims to abolish symptoms as soon as possible and to optimise peak flow by starting treatment at the level most likely to achieve this. The objective of treatment is to achieve early control and to maintain it by increasing treatment as necessary and decreasing treatment when control is good. Patients should start treatment at the level most appropriate to the initial severity of their asthma.

Before initiating a new drug in patients who have uncontrolled asthma, it is important their adherence with existing therapies is confirmed, inhaler technique is checked, and any trigger factors eliminated.

Inhaler devices

The mainstay of asthma treatment is inhaled therapy. Consequently, it is essential that patients and healthcare professionals know how to use inhalers correctly. Patients should only be prescribed inhalers after they have received training in the use of the device and have demonstrated satisfactory technique. It is good practice to only prescribe inhalers by brand name to ensure that patients are dispensed familiar inhaler devices that they can use properly.

In children, a pMDI and spacer is the preferred method of delivering a SABA and ICS, as young children may be unable to produce the inspiratory effort required to use higher resistance dry powder inhalers. A face mask is required until the child can breathe reproducibly using the spacer mouthpiece.

Intermittent reliever therapy

A short-acting bronchodilator (usually a SABA) should be prescribed to relieve symptoms in adults and children. For those with infrequent short-lived wheeze, occasional use of reliever therapy may be the only treatment required. However, where there is a confirmed diagnosis of asthma, an ICS preventer inhaler should be prescribed for all patients as this treats and controls asthma, whilst a SABA merely relieves symptoms. SABA inhalers should only be used on an as required basis for the relief of symptoms, and it is important that patients understand this.

If patients achieve good control of their asthma, they should have little or no need to use their SABA inhaler, and certainly should not need to use it more than twice a week. Patients who use one or more SABA inhalers a month (or more than 12 a year) are at risk of poor asthma outcomes (e.g. asthma attacks) and require an urgent review to identify why they are requiring so much SABA and to take measures to improve control.

Adverse effects of SABA treatment are not common with occasional use, but larger doses in patients with poorly controlled or severe asthma include tremor or palpitations, and may signal the need to review overall asthma management and counsel the patient to avoid unnecessary overuse of their reliever inhaler.

Preventer treatment

Inhaled corticosteroids (ICS) are the most effective medicines used to treat and control asthma in both adults and children. They are recommended for adults and children who meet any of the following criteria:
- Asthma attack in the past 2 years
- Using inhaled SABA three times a week or more
- Symptomatic three times a week or more
- Waking one night a week with asthma symptoms

Many non-atopic children under five with recurrent episodes of viral-induced wheezing do not go on to have chronic atopic asthma and the majority do not require treatment with regular ICS.

Patients should start at a dose of ICS appropriate to the severity of their disease; this should usually be a low dose for adults (see *Table 2.2*), or a very low dose for children. In mild-to-moderate asthma, the use of initially high ICS doses of ICS before stepping down confers no benefit.

Table 2.2: *Adult doses of inhaled corticosteroids (adapted from BTS/SIGN asthma guidelines, 2019)*[4]

ICS	Dose		
	Low dose	Medium dose	High dose*
Aerosol inhalers			
Beclometasone dipropionate			
Non-proprietary	100 micrograms two puffs twice a day	200 micrograms two puffs twice a day	200 micrograms four puffs twice a day
Clenil Modulite MDI	100 micrograms two puffs twice a day	200 micrograms two puffs twice a day	250 micrograms two puffs twice a day
Kelhale (extrafine) MDI	50 micrograms two puffs twice a day	100 micrograms two puffs twice a day	100 micrograms four puffs twice a day
Qvar (extrafine) MDI, Autohaler, Easi-Breathe	50 micrograms two puffs twice a day 100 micrograms one puff twice a day	100 micrograms two puffs twice a day	100 micrograms four puffs twice a day
Soprobec MDI	100 micrograms two puffs twice a day	200 micrograms two puffs twice a day	250 micrograms two puffs twice a day
Ciclesonide			
Alvesco MDI	80 micrograms two puffs once a day	160 micrograms two puffs once a day	160 micrograms two puffs twice a day
Fluticasone propionate			
Flixotide MDI	50 micrograms two puffs twice a day	125 micrograms two puffs twice a day	250 micrograms two puffs twice a day
Dry powder inhalers			
Beclometasone			
Easyhaler	200 micrograms one puff twice a day 400 micrograms one puff once a day	200 micrograms two puffs twice a day	n/a
Budesonide			
Non-proprietary Easyhaler	100 micrograms two puffs twice a day	200 micrograms two puffs twice a day	400 micrograms two puffs twice a day
Budelin Novolizer	n/a	200 micrograms two puffs twice a day	200 micrograms four puffs twice a day
Pulmicort Turbohaler	100 micrograms two puffs twice a day 200 micrograms one puff twice a day	200 micrograms two puffs twice a day 400 micrograms one puff twice a day	400 micrograms two puffs twice a day
Fluticasone propionate			
Flixotide Accuhaler	100 micrograms one puff twice a day	250 micrograms one puff twice a day	500 micrograms one puff twice a day
Mometasone			
Asmanex Twisthaler	200 micrograms one puff twice a day	400 micrograms one puff twice a day	n/a

*High doses should only be used after referring the patient to specialist care.

At low doses, the most common adverse effects of ICSs are due to oropharyngeal drug deposition and include oral candidiasis and dysphonia (hoarseness and difficulty in speaking). These can often be prevented by rinsing the mouth after use or using a spacer; if oral thrush does develop it should be treated with antifungal therapy such as nystatin liquid.

High doses of ICS are more likely to cause systemic adverse effects including diabetes, skin thinning, easy bruising, cataracts, and adrenal suppression. Any patient displaying these symptoms should be referred for a medical review. Patients prescribed high dose ICS for prolonged periods should have a morning cortisol level checked for evidence of adrenal suppression. If adrenal suppression is suspected, a sudden drop in steroid exposure could lead to adrenal crisis; the patient must be counselled on the risk of missing doses of their steroid inhaler.

Explaining the safety of ICS to patients is vital to maintain good adherence to treatment. Each patient should be assessed for the risks and benefits of treatment, and all other topical steroids (such as intranasal corticosteroids) should be taken into consideration.

Patients on high dose ICS should be given a steroid warning card, but the warnings could adversely affect adherence and so patients should be reassured about the safety of treatment. There is little evidence that low doses of ICS cause any short-term detrimental effects apart from the local adverse effects. In fact, the ability of ICS to reduce the need for multiple oral courses of steroids outweighs any associated adverse effect.

Children treated with medium or high dose ICS should have their height and weight monitored, as systemic adverse effects may include growth failure and adrenal suppression. The dose or duration of ICS treatment required to place a child at risk of clinical adrenal insufficiency is unknown but is likely to occur at or above medium ICS doses (see *Table 2.2*). Adrenal insufficiency should be considered a possibility in any child taking these doses of ICS who present with shock or a decreased level of consciousness. In such circumstances, serum biochemistry and blood glucose levels should be checked urgently, and intramuscular hydrocortisone may also be required. Consequently, children prescribed medium doses of ICS should be under the care of a specialist paediatrician.

Initial add-on therapy

In patients who are uncontrolled on low dose (adults) or very low dose (children) ICS, options for stepping-up treatment include either increasing the ICS dose or the addition of a long-acting beta$_2$-agonist (LABA) or a leukotriene receptor antagonist (LTRA).

Compared to increasing the ICS dose, the addition of a LABA achieves a similar reduction in the risk of exacerbations, but produces greater improvements in lung function, with an increased number of symptom-free days, and lower requirement for rescue short-acting beta$_2$-agonist therapy. The addition of LTRA to low dose ICS is effective in preventing asthma attacks and has a similar effect on asthma control as high dose ICS as single therapy.

Recommendations in the current BTS/SIGN[4] and NICE[10] asthma guidelines differ in that the former recommends using LABA as initial add-on therapy, whilst the latter recommends LTRA. While both guidelines agree that LABA add-on therapy produces small but greater improvement in morning and evening PEF and quality of life, a significant reduction in rescue medicine use and an increase in the proportion of symptom-free days,[11] NICE recommends LTRA because the low price of generic montelukast means that LTRA is more cost-effective than LABA.

When a LABA is used in asthma, it should be prescribed in a combination ICS/LABA inhaler to ensure adherence to both drugs and to prevent patients from only using their LABA inhaler and not their ICS. LABA monotherapy in asthma has been associated with an increase in asthma deaths, but this is not seen when used in combination with an ICS. Otherwise, LABA drugs are well tolerated, with the most common adverse effects including tremor, palpitations and muscle cramps.

LTRAs such as montelukast are generally well tolerated, with the most common adverse effects including headache and sleep disturbance with vivid dreams. If the patient develops any of these adverse effects they should be trialled off the leukotriene receptor to assess if the symptoms resolve. Recently, the Medicines and Healthcare products Regulatory Agency (MHRA) highlighted the risks of neuropsychiatric reactions with montelukast, and patients should be advised to stop treatment and seek medical advice immediately should they occur.[12]

Where asthma remains uncontrolled despite low dose ICS with LABA, before stepping up treatment, it is essential to confirm the diagnosis and to check adherence and inhaler technique.

Options for increasing treatment include increasing the ICS dose in adults from low dose to medium dose (or in children from very low dose to low dose) or to add in an LTRA. See *Table 2.3* for details of low, medium and high doses of combination inhalers.

Table 2.3: *Adult doses of ICS/LABA combination inhalers (adapted from BTS/SIGN asthma guidelines, 2019)*[4]

ICS	Dose		
	Low dose	Medium dose	High dose*
Combination inhalers			
Beclometasone dipropionate (extrafine) with formoterol			
Fostair MDI	100/6 one puff twice a day	100/6 two puffs twice a day	200/6 two puffs twice a day
Fostair NEXThaler	100/6 one puff twice a day	100/6 two puffs twice a day	200/6 two puffs twice a day
Budesonide with formoterol			
DuoResp Spiromex	160/4.5 one puff twice a day	160/4.5 two puffs twice a day 320/9 one puff twice a day	320/9 two puffs twice a day
Symbicort Turbohaler	100/6 two puffs twice a day 200/6 one puff twice a day	200/6 two puffs twice a day 400/12 one puff twice a day	400/12 two puffs twice a day
Fobumix Easyhaler	80/4.5 two puffs twice a day 160/4.5 one puff twice a day	160/4.5 two puffs twice a day 320/9 one puff twice a day	320/9 two puffs twice a day
Fluticasone propionate with formoterol			
Flutiform MDI	50/5 two puffs twice a day	125/5 two puffs twice a day	250/10 two puffs twice a day
Flutiform K-haler	50/5 two puffs twice a day	125/5 two puffs twice a day	n/a
Fluticasone propionate with salmeterol			
Seretide Accuhaler	100/50 one puff twice a day	250/50 one puff twice a day	500/50 one puff twice a day
AirFluSal Forspiro	n/a	n/a	500/50 one puff twice a day
Seretide Evohaler	50/25 two puffs twice a day	125/25 two puffs twice a day	250/25 two puffs twice a day
AirFluSal MDI	n/a	125/25 two puffs twice a day	250/25 two puffs twice a day
Aloflute MDI	n/a	125/25 two puffs twice a day	250/25 two puffs twice a day
Combisal MDI	50/25 two puffs twice a day	125/25 two puffs twice a day	250/25 two puffs twice a day
Fusacomb Easyhaler	n/a	250/50 one puff twice a day	500/50 one puff twice a day
Sereflo MDI	n/a	125/25 two puffs twice a day	250/25 two puffs twice a day
Sirdupla MDI	n/a	125/25 two puffs twice a day	250/25 two puffs twice a day
Stalpex DPI (Orbicel)	n/a	n/a	500/50 one puff twice a day
Seretide Accuhaler	100/50 one puff twice a day	250/50 one puff twice a day	500/50 one puff twice a day
Fluticasone furoate with vilanterol			
Relvar Ellipta	n/a	92/22 one puff once a day	184/22 one puff once a day

*High doses should only be used after referring the patient to specialist care.

Single combination inhaler for maintenance and reliever therapy (MART)

The use of a single ICS/LABA combination inhaler for maintenance and reliever therapy (MART) is an alternative approach to using fixed-dose ICS/LABA inhaler in addition to a separate SABA reliever inhaler. At present, MART regimen is only licenced for use with budesonide/formoterol (DuoResp Spiromex, Fobumix Easyhaler or Symbicort Turbohaler) or beclometasone/formoterol (Fostair MDI or NEXThaler) inhalers.

In this regimen, the ICS/LABA inhaler is used regularly once or twice a day, with an extra dose used as necessary to provide fast relief of symptoms due to the rapid onset of reliever effect of the LABA formoterol. This additional PRN (as required) dose gives the patient an extra dose of ICS to reduce any early airway inflammation. This ensures that, as the need for a reliever increases, the dose of preventer medication is also increased, with the aim to increase overall asthma treatment early in deteriorating asthma control and preventing a full asthma attack.

It is important that this MART regimen is underpinned by a self-management plan to enable patients to self-monitor their asthma symptoms and understand when it is appropriate to use an extra dose of their ICS/LABA inhaler. There is evidence that by using this regime there may be a reduction in the overall steroid dose needed to treat an exacerbation.

If patients are switched from regular fixed dose ICS/LABA to a MART regimen, the total regular dose of daily ICS should not be decreased. Patients taking rescue doses of their combination inhaler once a day or more regularly should have their treatment reviewed, as this suggests poor asthma control. Careful education of patients about the specific issues around this management strategy is required to ensure the appropriate use of their inhaler and avoid overuse.

Specialist therapies

It should be expected that only a small proportion of patients will continue to have suboptimal control on low to medium dose ICS with LABA and or LTRA (or very low to low dose ICS in children). In these situations, patients should be referred to specialist asthma services.

Treatment options in these patients include increasing ICS dose in adults to high doses (see *Table 2.3*), or sequential trials of additional controller medicines including tiotropium, theophylline or LTRA if not already trialled.

In adults with severe asthma, the addition of tiotropium to high dose ICS/LABA may have additional benefits in reducing the need for rescue oral corticosteroids, and small improvements in lung function and asthma control.[13] The addition of theophylline may have some beneficial effects but is often limited by significant adverse effects including nausea, indigestion, headaches, arrhythmias, and seizures requiring 6 to 12 monthly therapeutic drug monitoring.

Continuous oral corticosteroids are rarely recommended but may be required under specialist care in patients with confirmed asthma who remain uncontrolled despite adequate trials of high dose ICS and all other add-on therapies. Such patients should be monitored closely for systemic adverse effects, including monitoring blood pressure, blood sugar and lipids, bone mineral density, growth in children, cataracts and glaucoma.

Patients who are adherent to optimal top step therapy but remain poorly controlled requiring repeated courses of oral steroids and/or hospital admissions can be classified as having severe asthma. These patients require referral to a severe asthma centre for review and may be eligible for monoclonal antibody treatment.

Treatment options include omalizumab (Xolair®) as add-on anti-IgE therapy for severe allergic asthma; mepolizumab (Nucala®), resliuzmab (Cinqaero®) and benralizumab (Fasenra®) as add-on anti-IL5 or anti-IL5 receptor therapy for severe eosinophilic asthma; and dupilumab (Dupixent®) as add-on anti-IL4/anti-IL13 therapy for severe eosinophilic asthma.

Patients should be reviewed regularly, and once asthma control has been achieved, consideration should be made to step down treatment to use the lowest effective doses to avoid adverse effects. Stepping down treatment is recommended every three weeks in patients whose asthma is stable. Which drug is reduced or stopped at each review depends on patient preference, response, adverse effects and severity of asthma. When the ICS dose is reduced, this should be reduced by 25% to 50% at each step.[4]

Inhaled corticosteroids exhibit a dose-response curve for clinical efficacy, but this starts to plateau at around 100-200 micrograms per day and peaks by 500 micrograms per day.[14] This suggests the majority of adults with asthma would be unlikely to achieve any significant clinical benefits from increasing ICS doses above medium doses. Consequently, the use of high doses in adults (see *Table 2.2* and *Table 2.3*) should be reserved for specialist care only.

It is important to note that the efficacy of ICS may be reduced by current or past smoking - this may be overcome by increasing the dose. However, the most effective therapy is smoking cessation and all patients should be offered advice and support.

In primary care, pharmacists should closely monitor severe asthmatics particularly to ensure continued adherence to their preventative therapies. Good communication between primary care, community pharmacist and the severe asthma service is essential to ensure patients remain on the correct therapies, and that any changes in adherence or control (increased SABA use or additional courses of oral steroids) are highlighted early to the specialist centre. This will enable the specialist centre to correctly assess the severity of the patient's asthma. Any change in treatment should be advised by the specialist centre.

Drug interactions

Drug interactions can occur between the treatments commonly used in asthma. Severe asthma patients are at an increased risk due to the additional medications they may be on such as azoles. The list below is not exhaustive, and any new medications should be checked against the patients current treatments for interactions.

- Theophylline and antibiotics – if a patient is on regular oral theophylline and is started on ciprofloxacin or clarithromycin, a reduction in their theophylline dose should be considered. Generally, halving the dose is sufficient. The patient's levels should be closely monitored and the dose needs to be increased to the previous dose once the course of antibiotics is finished. The patient should be counselled on possible signs of toxicity (e.g. headache, nausea, palpitations).
- Inhaled steroids and azoles – azoles such as itraconazole can increase blood steroid levels following inhaled steroids. A reduction in inhaled corticosteroid dose will be required. The dose may need to be halved. It is important to increase the inhaled corticosteroids if the azole is stopped.

Box 2.4: Practice point: asthma management

- Patients should start treatment at the level most appropriate to the initial severity of their asthma.
- Before initiating a new drug in patients, it is important to check their adherence and inhaler technique and eliminate trigger factors.
- Patients who use one or more SABA inhalers a month (or more than 12 a year) are at risk of poor asthma outcomes.
- Patients should be referred to specialist asthma services if they are not controlled on low to medium dose ICS with LABA and or LTRA.

Special groups

Paediatrics

A clear diagnosis of asthma can be difficult in children. Infants may not be able to carry out tests such as FENO and spirometry. A thorough family and symptom history are essential. A trial of an inhaled corticosteroid may be required, but this should be started at the lowest possible dose and regularly reviewed. Children should always be supplied with an appropriate spacer to improve their inhaler technique.

Pregnancy

Women should be advised of the importance of maintaining good control of their asthma during pregnancy to avoid problems for both mother and baby. It is important to always counsel women with asthma regarding the importance and safety of continuing their asthma medications during pregnancy to ensure good asthma control. It is the advice of obstetricians that the risk of stopping any of the patient's regular asthma treatments may put them at risk of an asthma attack which could lead to hypoxia in the baby.

Box 2.5: Practice point: special groups

- Children should always be supplied with an appropriate spacer to improve inhaler technique.
- Pregnant women should always be counselled on the importance and safety of continuing their asthma medication during pregnancy to ensure good asthma control.
- Continuing asthma medication in pregnancy reduces the risk of an asthma attack and hypoxia in the baby.

Follow-up

Most people with asthma should have an annual asthma review with their GP or healthcare professional to determine their current and recent asthma control, assess their risk of future exacerbations and optimise (stepping up or down) medication and reinforce self-management education.[4] Pharmacists can provide this service in primary care.

Patients should also have a follow-up review with their GP within two working days after treatment or discharge from hospital following an asthma attack.[4] This is to ensure that recovery from the acute event is complete, to determine the reasons for the asthma attack and to explore strategies to avoid these in the future. Inhaler technique should be re-checked and the importance of maintaining good adherence to treatment reinforced.

Referral

Pharmacists should ensure they are aware of the multidisciplinary team and local services available to help support people with asthma in the community. Physiotherapists can provide education on breathing exercises and dysfunctional breathing reduction techniques, which can improve symptoms and quality of life. Psychological disorders such as anxiety and depression are more prevalent in people with asthma and are associated with worse asthma control and increased risk of asthma attacks. Patients should be referred to mental health services for psychological interventions such as cognitive behavioural therapy.

Patients should be referred to specialist asthma services if they have severe asthma requiring treatment with high dose ICS or frequent exacerbations, or at high risk of asthma death. These patients can be assessed by specialist multidisciplinary teams to review their diagnosis, optimise comorbidities and consider treatment with biologic therapies. This can avoid the need for continuous maintenance oral corticosteroids and the risk of associated systemic adverse effects.

Useful resources

- GINA guidelines – www.ginasthma.org/wp-content/uploads/2019/04/GINA-2019-main-Pocket-Guide-wms.pdf
- NICE Clinical Knowledge Summary – www.cks.nice.org.uk/asthma
- NICE guidelines – www.nice.org.uk/guidance/ng80
- BTS/SIGN guidelines – www.brit-thoracic.org.uk/quality-improvement/guidelines/asthma
- Asthma Treatment Plans – www.asthma.org.uk/for-professionals/professionals
- National Centre for Smoking Cessation Training – www.ncsct.co.uk
- Inhaler technique videos – www.asthma.org.uk/advice/inhaler-videos
- RightBreathe – www.rightbreathe.com

References

1. Asthma UK (2014). www.asthma.org.uk/asthma-facts-and-statistics

2. Royal College of Physicians (2014). Why asthma still kills: The National Review of Asthma Deaths (NRAD). www.rcplondon.ac.uk/projects/outputs/why-asthma-still-kills

3. Asthma UK. Time to Take Action. 2014. Available at: www.asthma.org.uk/globalassets/campaigns/compare-your-care-2014.pdf

4. British Thoracic Society and Scottish Intercollegiate Guidelines Network (2019). British guideline on the management of asthma. www.brit-thoracic.org.uk/quality-improvement/guidelines/asthma/

5. Wenzel SE. Asthma phenotypes: the evolution from clinical to molecular approaches. *Nat Med* 2012; 18: 716-725.

6. UK Inhaler Group. Inhaler Standards and Competency Document. 2016. Available at: www.respiratoryfutures.org.uk/media/69775/ukig-inhaler-standards-january-2017.pdf

7. Silver HS *et al.* Quarterly assessment of short-acting beta(2)-adrenergic agonist use as a predictor of subsequent health care use for asthmatic patients in the United States. *J Asthma* 2010; 47: 660-6.

8. Engelkes M *et al.* Medication adherence and the risk of severe asthma exacerbations: a systematic review. *Eur Respir J* 2015; 45: 396-407.

9. Medicines and Healthcare products Regulatory Agency (2019). Montelukast (Singulair): reminder of the risk of neuropsychiatric reactions. www.gov.uk/drug-safety-update/montelukast-singulair-reminder-of-the-risk-of-neuropsychiatric-reactions

10. National Institute for Health and Care Excellence (2017). Asthma diagnosis and management. www.nice.org.uk/guidance/ng80

11. Chauhan BF, Ducharme FM. Addition to inhaled corticosteroids of long-acting beta2-agonists versus anti-leukotrienes for chronic asthma. *Cochrane Database of Systematic Reviews*, issue 1. John Wiley & Sons Ltd, 2014.

12. Pearson MG, Bucknall CE, editors. Measuring clinical outcome in asthma: a patient-focused approach London: Royal College of Physicians of London; 1999.

13. Kew KM, Dahri K. Long-acting muscarinic antagonists (LAMA) added to combination long-acting beta$_2$-agonists and inhaled corticosteroids (LABA/ICS) versus LABA/ICS for adults with asthma. *Cochrane Database of Systematic Reviews*, issue 1. John Wiley & Sons Ltd, 2016.

14. Holt S *et al.* Dose-response relation of inhaled fluticasone propionate in adolescents and adults with asthma: meta-analysis. *BMJ* 2001; 323: 253-256.

Case studies

Case study 1

Ellen attends her community pharmacy to request an emergency supply of a salbutamol inhaler. She explains that she has finished the inhaler issued to her two weeks ago and is still feeling wheezy and cannot get to see her GP.

Points to consider

- How many salbutamol inhalers is she using each month?
- Is she using a preventer inhaler?
- What are her current symptoms?
- Ask the 3 RCP questions.
- Is she acutely unwell?
- Is Ellen under a specialist asthma team?
- Does she have an asthma action plan?
- How many courses of oral corticosteroids has she received in the last 12 months?

When you check Ellen's records you find that she has received 15 salbutamol inhalers from the pharmacy in the last 12 months. She is also on a Fostair 100/6 NEXThaler, 2 puffs twice a day, but has only received six of these from the pharmacy in that period. You ask her about her inhalers and she admits that she does not always take her Fostair inhaler as she does not feel it works well.

Points to consider

- Can the patient use her inhaler correctly?
- Does the patient understand the difference between the reliever and preventer inhaler?
- Are there any other reasons for her non-adherence to her preventer inhaler?

Ellen explains that she finds it difficult to afford both the salbutamol and the Fostair inhaler. She tends to get her salbutamol more regularly as she feels this gives her the quickest relief from her symptoms. Her inhaler technique is fair with her NEXThaler.

Points to consider

- What steps could be taken to reduce the cost of her inhalers?
- What counselling should be given on her inhaler technique?

You contact Ellen's GP and discuss her symptoms and non-adherence. The decision is made to switch her to Fostair maintenance and reliever therapy (MART). After explaining this regimen and counselling her on her inhaler technique she demonstrates good technique with the NEXThaler. She returns later that day with a prescription for a new Fostair inhaler. She now has an asthma action plan and you discuss this with her.

Points to consider

- What are the benefits of MART for Ellen?
- Which education resources could you signpost Ellen to?
- When should she be reviewed again?

Case study 2

Marie is admitted to the accident and emergency department with an exacerbation of her asthma. Her peak expiratory flow (PEFR) is 200, which is 50% of her best PEFR of 400. Her SpO_2 is 95%, respiratory rate is 28 breaths per minute, her pulse is 115 beats/min and she is struggling to speak in sentences. She has been prescribed:

- Prednisolone 40 mg once a day
- Salbutamol nebuliser 5 mg four times daily
- Ipratropium 500 micrograms four times daily

Points to consider

- Is this prescription appropriate?
- What monitoring should be done?

You are a pharmacist working on medical admission unit (MAU) where she has been transferred to. You speak to Marie about her medication before admission to complete her medicines reconciliation and she gives you permission to access her Summary Care Record (SCR).

Her current repeat medication list is:

- Qvar 100 micrograms MDI 2 puff twice a day
- Salbutamol 100 micrograms MDI 2 puffs when required
- She has listed allergies/adverse events to NSAIDS (wheeze).

Points to consider

- What stage of the BTS/SIGN asthma treatment guidelines is Marie on?
- What other information would it be important to gather about Marie's medicines?

You confirm with Marie's community pharmacy that she is collecting her medication regularly – they highlight that they have been concerned that Marie has been collecting salbutamol every month. Looking at her acute prescription records you see that Marie has had three courses of oral steroids over the last 12 months.

Points to consider

- How would you optimise Marie's asthma treatment?
- Would referral to a specialist severe asthma centre be appropriate for Marie?

Marie is initiated on a Flutiform MDI 125/5, two puffs twice a day. She has also been started on montelukast 10 mg at night.

Points to consider

- Do you think it is appropriate to start both of these treatments?
- Is the strength of the inhaler appropriate?
- What reference source would you consult?

On your ward round you ask Marie to show you how she is using her new inhaler. She is breathing in very fast and struggling to coordinate the use of the inhaler. She tells you that she is struggling to breathe more slowly and to push down the inhaler.

Points to consider

- What devices are available to help you assess Marie's inhaler technique?
- What changes could be made to her device to improve her technique?

It appears that Marie finds it easier to use a dry powder inhaler and she has good technique with an Ellipta device, so she is initiated on a Relvar Ellipta 92/22 micrograms, one puff daily.

Marie is discharged home to complete two more days of prednisolone tablets. The doctor has also prescribed salbutamol and ipratropium nebulisers.

Points to consider

- Do you think this prescription is appropriate?
- What counselling should the patient have on discharge?
- What could be implemented to help Marie self-manage her asthma at home?

You develop an asthma treatment plan with Marie.

Points to consider

- What advice should the plan include?

CHAPTER 3

Atrial fibrillation

Helen Williams

Overview

Atrial fibrillation (AF) is the most common cardiac arrhythmia, with an estimated prevalence of 2.5% in the general population in England,[1] with men more commonly affected than women.[2] The risk of developing AF increases dramatically with age, with a prevalence of over 10% in people aged over 80 years.[3]

Many predict a doubling in the prevalence of AF over the next 25 years in line with ageing of the population. AF is one of the 10 most common causes of hospital admission in the UK and is associated with a significant cost.

AF is characterised by a breakdown of the coordinated electrical activity in the upper chambers of the heart – 'the atria' – which causes them to fibrillate, rather than to contract. The disordered electrical activity leads to unpredictable conduction of impulses to the ventricles resulting in an irregular cardiac rhythm, which may also be rapid. The typical symptoms of AF include palpitations, breathlessness, dizziness or lightheadedness and chest pain.

AF is categorised as:

- Paroxysmal – episodes of AF that terminate spontaneously or with intervention in less than seven days. In many cases, paroxysmal AF will self-terminate within minutes, and this presents a significant challenge for diagnosis.
- Persistent – AF that occurs for longer than seven days and ends spontaneously or with treatment, such as pharmacological or electrical cardioversion. Cardioversion is a procedure by which AF or other cardiac arrhythmia is restored to normal sinus rhythm by the prescription of specific anti-arrhythmic drugs or the application of controlled electric shocks.
- Permanent – sometimes termed 'accepted' AF, this refers to AF that persists despite attempts to restore normal sinus rhythm or that is no longer treated with the aim of restoring sinus rhythm.

AF is commonly considered to be a progressive disease starting with paroxysmal, self-terminating AF, through persistent AF and eventually to permanent AF as a result of on-going electrical and structural remodelling of the atria. Typical risk factors for the development of AF include coronary heart disease, hypertension, heart failure, hyperthyroidism, obesity and heart valve disease.

AF can have devastating consequences – the failure of the atria to pump efficiently allows blood to pool, leading to the formation of blood clots, which can move from the heart to the brain and cause strokes. The presence of AF increases the risk of stroke five-fold,[4] with AF-related strokes associated with higher mortality and greater disability than non-AF related strokes.[5] All forms of AF carry an increased risk of stroke, and stroke prevention is a major element of AF management.

Stroke care represents a significant financial burden to the NHS and social care, with a recent analysis of the Sentinel Stroke National Audit Project (SSNAP) database concluding that the cost of each stroke is £22,429 in the first year and £46,039 over five years.[6] As AF-related strokes carry a higher risk of longer-term disability than non-AF related strokes, the average cost of an AF stroke over 5 years is likely to be higher than reported by SSNAP.

Despite the availability of vitamin K antagonist oral anticoagulants and direct oral anticoagulants (DOACs), people are still experiencing preventable AF-related strokes due to suboptimal care. For example, in England in 2016/17 there were 15,785 strokes in people with known AF prior to hospital admission; of these 7,483 were not prescribed anticoagulant therapy at the time of their stroke. The outcome for many of these untreated AF patients was poor, with 26% dying and a further 45% left with moderate to severe disability.[7]

Diagnosis

Currently, of the expected 1.41 million people in England with AF, only 1.174 million are aware of their condition.[8] Some patients with AF will present with some or all of the classic symptoms of AF (breathlessness/dyspnoea, palpitations, lightheadedness or dizziness and chest discomfort). Coupled with an irregular pulse, these should lead the clinician to consider AF as a diagnosis.

However, up to 40% of people with AF are asymptomatic,[9] completely unaware that they have an irregular heartbeat, and are therefore untreated and at risk of stroke. Evidence has shown that at least a proportion of these patients can be identified through opportunistic case finding using simple pulse checks, which should be embedded in routine clinical practice, particularly for those aged over 65 years, as well as those with long-term conditions such as ischaemic heart disease, diabetes, hypertension, chronic kidney disease, prior stroke or chronic obstructive pulmonary disease (COPD).

While pulse checks are a simple way to identify people with possible AF, new technologies have been introduced in recent years to support the detection of AF with higher sensitivity and specificity. The Microlife Watch BP Home A is a blood pressure device with a built-in AF detection algorithm and was recommended by NICE as a tool for detecting AF during routine blood pressure checks in 2014.[10] The Kardia mobile ECG sits on the back of a smartphone or tablet and can generate and analyse a single lead ECG rhythm strip recorded through the user's fingertips.[11] Meta-analysis has demonstrated that screening devices with built-in AF algorithms are more accurate than manual pulse checks.[12]

Box 3.1: Practice point: how to check a pulse manually

- Ask the patient to sit down for 5 minutes.
- Check they have not recently smoked or consumed caffeine.
- Hold the patient's hand with the palm facing up and elbow slightly bent.
- Place your index and middle finger at the base of the thumb (between the wrist and the tendon attached to the thumb).
- Count the number of beats for 30 seconds, and then double that to calculate the heart rate in beats per minute.
- Assess whether the pulse rhythm is regular or irregular.

At rest, a normal heart rate should be 60 to 100 beats per minute.

An irregular pulse rhythm indicates possible AF and warrants further investigation. In AF, the heart rate can be normal but may also be considerably higher than 100 beats per minute.

Pharmacy input

Community pharmacists and those based in GP practices can check pulses, manually or via mobile technology to identify those with possible AF. Targeted case finding focusing on those aged over 65 years, for example at the time of flu vaccination, or in those known to have chronic conditions is a practical approach.

Pharmacists must ensure the local GP practices are aware and have pathways in place to accept referrals for patients with irregular pulses to ensure timely diagnosis. There are examples of pathways where community pharmacists can refer directly to a one-stop AF clinic to confirm the diagnosis and, if necessary, initiate treatment (such as CAPTURE-AF[13] and CareCity One Stop Shop Atrial Fibrillation pathway[14]) which have been shown to minimise delays.

Where AF is suspected, the diagnosis is usually confirmed by 12 lead ECG, which will show the characteristic absence of p-waves (which in sinus rhythm are present and indicate coordinated electrical activity in the atria) and an irregular ventricular rhythm. Sometimes a fibrillation wave can be seen along the baseline between QRS complexes.

Where paroxysmal AF is suspected but the 12 lead ECG shows sinus rhythm, a longer duration of ECG monitoring of 24 hours or more may be required to capture the paroxysms and confirm the diagnosis using a

Holter monitor or patch ECG recorder. In some cases, implantable loop recorders may be required to confirm the diagnosis where symptomatic episodes are very infrequent.

Pharmacists also have significant roles in caring for people once they have been diagnosed with AF to ensure they receive the right treatment and are monitored appropriately.

Pharmacy review

The assessment of patients with a diagnosis of AF should focus on two key issues:
- Preventing AF-related stroke
- Controlling heart rate and/or rhythm

Preventing AF-related stroke

Practice-based pharmacists can help ensure that stroke risk is appropriately assessed in patients with AF, but this can also be undertaken by community pharmacists conducting medication reviews, and those working in acute settings. All patients with AF who are not currently prescribed anticoagulation should have their stroke risk assessed at least annually.

Stroke risk should be evaluated using the CHA_2DS_2VASc score (see *Figure 3.1*), which should be calculated for all patients with paroxysmal, persistent or permanent AF and even those who have converted back to sinus rhythm but are at risk of arrhythmia recurrence (e.g. following ablation therapy). In order to calculate the CHA_2DS_2VASc score, a full medical history should be established to identify the relevant risk factors.

All patients with CHA_2DS_2VASc of two or more should be offered oral anticoagulation. In addition, NICE advises that anticoagulant therapy should be considered for men with a CHA_2DS_2VASc of one.[15] In people with AF not currently receiving anticoagulant therapy, CHA_2DS_2VASc should be recalculated annually, as the score will change over time.

Figure 3.1: *CHA_2DS_2VASc risk calculator and annual risk of stroke (www.chadsvasc.org)*

CHA_2DS_2VASc risk factors

Risk factors	Score
Congestive heart failure	1
Hypertension	1
Age ≥ 75	2
Age 65-74	1
Diabetes mellitus	1
Stroke/TIA/thrombo-embolism	2
Vascular disease	1
Sex female	1
Your score	0

View results

CHA_2DS_2VASc clinical risk estimation

CHA_2DS_2VASc score	Patients (n = 7329)	Adjusted stroke rate (% year)
0	1	0%
1	422	1,3%
2	1230	2,2%
3	1730	3,2%
4	1718	4,0%
5	1159	6,7%
6	679	9,8%
7	294	9,6%
8	82	6,7%
9	14	15,2%

Bleeding risk is commonly cited as a reason for not offering anticoagulation. Bleeding risk can be assessed using the HAS-BLED score (see *Figure 3.2*) – any modifiable risk factors for bleeding should be identified and addressed, such as uncontrolled hypertension, concomitant use of medicines such as NSAIDs or aspirin, and excess alcohol intake.

Figure 3.2: *HAS-BLED bleeding risk score (www.chadsvasc.org)*

HAS-BLED clinical characteristic

Clinical characteristic	Points awarded
Hypertension	1
Abnormal liver function	1
Abnormal renal function	1
Stroke	1
Bleeding	1
Labile INRs	1
Elderly (age >65)	1
Drugs	1
Alcohol	1
Your score	0

View results

HAS-BLED clinical risk estimation

HAS-BLED score	Number of patients	Number of bleeding	Bleeds per 100 patient years
0	798	9	1,13
1	1286	13	1,02
2	744	14	1,88
3	187	7	3,74
4	46	4	8,70
5	8	1	12,50
6	2	0	0
7	-	-	-
8	-	-	-
9	-	-	-
Total	798	9	1,13

People with HAS-BLED scores ≥3 should not be excluded from receiving anticoagulant therapy to prevent AF-related stroke but may need closer monitoring, for example, earlier and more regular follow-up to assess for any signs of bleeding, and checking FBC one month after initiation and thereafter as clinically indicated. Similarly, risk of falls should not be used as a reason not to prescribe anticoagulant therapy.

Anticoagulant choice

Anticoagulation with warfarin reduces the risk of AF-related stroke by 64%,[16] and the direct oral anticoagulants (DOACs) are at least as effective as warfarin in reducing stroke risk. NICE endorses the use of warfarin or a DOAC for the prevention of AF-related stroke.[15]

Some international guidelines, however, endorse DOACs first line in view of the lower risk of potentially devastating intracranial haemorrhage with DOACs when compared with warfarin. The choice of drug should be based on the person's clinical features and preferences. Many clinicians and patients favour DOACs as they do not need the regular monitoring of the international normalisation ratio (INR), that is a requirement of warfarin therapy. However, it is important to note that DOACs do need ongoing monitoring throughout therapy, particularly of renal function, the burden of which largely falls to general practice.

Box 3.2: Practice point: the international normalised ratio (INR)

- The INR is a laboratory measurement of how long it takes blood to form a clot. It is used to determine the effects of oral anticoagulants on the clotting system.
- In AF, patients on warfarin are dosed to achieve a target INR of 2.5; with the target INR range of 2-3.

As there are a number of treatment options, pharmacists should ensure that patients requiring anticoagulant therapy for stroke prevention in AF are supported to make a shared decision regarding their treatment. Decision aids are available to inform the discussion with patients regarding the benefits and risks of anticoagulant therapy for stroke prevention in AF including:

- NICE 2014: Patient Decision Aid. Atrial fibrillation: medicines to help reduce your risk of a stroke – what are the options? www.nice.org.uk/guidance/cg180/resources/atrial-fibrillation-medicines-to-help-reduce-your-risk-of-a-stroke-what-are-the-options-patient-decision-aid-pdf-243734797
- Don't wait to anticoagulate. www.dontwaittoanticoagulate.com/clinician/calculator
- A simple tool, developed by a GP in the Midlands, Dr Yassir Javaid (see *Table 3.1*).

Table 3.1: *The benefits and risks of anticoagulant therapy*

CHA_2DS_2VASc	Number of events per 1000 AF patients per year		HAS-BLED score
	AF-related strokes prevented by anticoagulation	Major bleeds caused by anticoagulation	
1	4	4	1
2	17	12	2
3	25	15	3
4	38	21	4
5	57		

This table was produced by Dr Yassir Javid (adapted from NICE: patient decision. Aid-atrial fibrillation: medicines to help reduce your risk of a stroke – what are the options? June 2014) and is based on the likely risk/benefit of warfarin in AF patients. The NOACs have been shown to be at least non-inferior to warfarin in terms of reducing ischaemic stroke in AF patients. Dabigatran 150 mg twice daily has been shown to be superior to warfarin in reducing ischaemic stroke.

The NOACs are not more significantly hazardous than warfarin in terms of causing major bleeds in AF patients. Dabigatran 110 mg, apixaban 5 mg and edoxaban have actually been shown to be associated with significantly fewer major bleeds than warfarin.

Warfarin

Whether managed in a centralised anticoagulation service, in GP practice, in a community pharmacy or if the patient undertakes self-testing at home, monitoring the INR for patients on warfarin is essential.

Patients with AF treated with warfarin to prevent stroke should be dosed to achieve an INR between 2 and 3. The INR should be monitored regularly (at least once every 12 weeks once the INR is stable) and achieve a time in therapeutic range (TTR) of 65% or more.

Before issuing a prescription for warfarin the prescriber and community pharmacist dispensing the warfarin should confirm that appropriate monitoring is in place – this could be through accessing local lab results through a shared patient record, or by reviewing the patients 'yellow book' to assess the INR.

If a pharmacist has concerns regarding the INR monitoring, for example, due to out of range results or missed or infrequent tests, they should seek advice from the anticoagulant clinic or the patient's GP.

In patients where the TTR is less than 65% or the patient has had one INR above 8, two INRs above 5 or two INRs less than 1.5 in a six-month period – anticoagulant therapy should be reassessed, taking into account cognitive function, adherence to therapy, illness or interacting drug therapies and any lifestyle factors which may have affected INR control.[15] If INR control cannot be improved, alternative anticoagulation strategies should be considered.

For all patients prescribed warfarin, pharmacists should address the following issues:

- Check the most recent INR and the date of the next check. Ensure that the patient is aware of the importance of INR monitoring.
- Assess adherence – ask non-threatening questions about drug adherence and offer counselling to support improved adherence where necessary and address any specific underlying issues or concerns the patient may have.
- Assess bleeding risk – ask patients if they have experienced any episodes of bleeding. Patients should be reassured if they experience 'nuisance bleeding' such as infrequent self-limiting nose bleeds, bleeding gums when brushing teeth or unusual bruising, or minor bleeds such as single episodes of haematuria (blood in the urine), haematemesis (blood in vomit) or haemoptysis (coughing up blood).
- Advise the patient that, should they experience frequent or severe bleeding (significant blood loss, or bleeding that will not stop despite pressure) they should seek advice from their GP, anticoagulant clinic or urgent care.
- Assess for other adverse effects of warfarin – these are outlined in *Box 3.3*.
  - Depending on the severity of adverse effects, these may require drug withdrawal and substitution for an alternative anticoagulant, such as a DOAC or low molecular weight heparin.
- Assess for any important drug interactions – both prescribed and OTC medication should be reviewed (see *Box 3.6*).
  - Specific drugs can increase the effect of warfarin resulting in an increase in the INR, whilst other drugs can cause a reduction in the effect of warfarin, resulting in a reduction in INR. INR should be monitored closely when a drug affecting warfarin is initiated or following a change in dose to allow the warfarin dose to be adjusted.
- Advise on interaction with foods and food supplements including avoiding cranberry juice (increased INR). Grapefruit juice may cause a modest rise in INR in some patients taking warfarin. Some foods such as liver, broccoli, brussels sprouts and green leafy vegetables, which contain large amounts of vitamin K can reduce the INR. Sudden changes in diet can potentially affect control of anticoagulation. Advise patients to maintain a consistent dietary intake.
- Patients should be advised to moderate their alcohol intake and avoid binge drinking.
- Check blood pressure – hypertension is a major cause of intracranial haemorrhage (ICH) on anticoagulant therapy. If systolic BP is raised above 160 mmHg, this should be addressed through the escalation of antihypertensive therapies. Patients should be aware that sudden onset severe headache or dizziness could indicate ICH and they should seek urgent medical advice.
- Educate the patient on the benefits and risks of anticoagulant therapy and address any outstanding concerns.

Box 3.3: Important prescribing information for warfarin

Contraindications:
- Recent haemorrhagic stroke
- Clinically significant bleeding
- Within 72 hours of major surgery with risk of severe bleeding
- Within 48 hours postpartum
- Pregnancy (first and third trimesters)

Cautions:
- Drugs where interactions may lead to a significantly increased risk of bleeding (see *Box 3.6*)
- Thrombophilia: people with protein C deficiency are at risk of developing skin necrosis when starting warfarin treatment
- High risk of bleeding: warfarin should be given with caution to patients where there is a risk of serious haemorrhage (e.g. concomitant NSAID use, recent ischaemic stroke, bacterial endocarditis, previous gastrointestinal bleeding)
- Surgery
  - Where there is no risk of severe bleeding, surgery can be performed with an INR of <2.5
  - Where there is a risk of severe bleeding, warfarin should be stopped 3 days prior to surgery. Bridging therapy should be considered
- Active peptic ulceration: due to a high risk of bleeding, people with active peptic ulcers should be treated with caution
- Thyroid disorders: the rate of warfarin metabolism depends on thyroid status. People with hyper- or hypothyroidism should be closely monitored on starting warfarin therapy
- The following may exaggerate the effect of warfarin tablets, and require the dose to be reduced:
  - Weight loss
  - Acute illness
  - Smoking cessation
- The following may reduce the effect of warfarin tablets, and require the dosage to be increased:
  - Weight gain
  - Diarrhoea
  - Vomiting

Common adverse effects:
- Sudden onset severe headache/dizziness – possible intracranial headache
- Bleeding including bleeding gums, haematuria, haematemesis, haemoptysis, melaena, heavy menstrual bleeding, continuous bleeding from cuts/grazes
- Diarrhoea and/or nausea and vomiting
- Jaundice, liver dysfunction
- Pancreatitis
- Skin disorders such as rash, alopecia, purpura, 'purple toes' syndrome, skin necrosis
- Calciphylaxis

Direct oral anticoagulants (DOACs)

In the UK, the prescribing of DOACs has grown year-on-year since their introduction and now accounts for more than 50% of all oral anticoagulant prescribing. DOACs are particularly suited to initiation and monitoring in primary care. More advanced prescribing pharmacists may be involved in the initiation of DOACs (see *Box 3.4*).

Safe initiation of DOACs relies on a number of factors, often referred to as the 'ABCD':

- Age – some DOACs require dose reduction with increasing age.
- Bodyweight – some DOACs require dose reduction in low bodyweight.
- Creatinine clearance – must be calculated to accurately determine an appropriate dose.
- Drug interactions – DOACs have a number of drug interactions which affect dosing.

Box 3.4: Practice point: switching to DOACs in patients already taking warfarin[17]

1. Check clinical system for recent urea and electrolytes (U&Es), liver function tests (LFTs) and full blood count (FBC) (within last 3 months).
2. At next INR visit – check INR, record weight, take bloods if not already available or if they are unstable.
3. Calculate creatinine clearance (CrCl).
4. Prescribe DOAC at appropriate dose and advise them to obtain supplies.
5. Advise when to stop warfarin in relation to starting DOAC (INR should be <2.5 when DOAC is started).
6. Provide written instructions and involve family members/carers where possible to minimise the risk of patients taking both warfarin and the DOAC concurrently. Particular care should be taken where patients are using medication compliance aids to minimise the risk of incorrect dosing.
7. Provide an up-to-date Anticoagulant Alert card.
8. Where the switch to a DOAC is undertaken outside the GP practice, provide accurate information relating to indication, baseline tests and monitoring requirements to allow primary care to safely take over prescribing responsibility.
9. Inform community nursing teams if they have been monitoring INR or administering warfarin.

Renal function, assessed using the Cockcroft-Gault equation (see *Figure 3.3*) to calculate the creatinine clearance (CrCl), is essential to determine an appropriate dose – estimated glomerular filtration rate (eGFR) must not be used to guide dosing. All DOACs are contraindicated when CrCl falls below 15 mL/min. For more important prescribing information for DOACs, see *Box 3.5*.

Figure 3.3*: Cockcroft-Gault equation to calculate creatinine clearance (CrCl)*

Creatinine clearance (CrCl) =

(140-age[years]) × ideal body weight or actual if less (kg) × constant

---

Serum creatinine (µmol/L)

Constant = 1.23 for men; 1.04 for women

Specialist input, including checking DOAC levels, should be considered for extremes of bodyweight (50 kg and 120 kg). There is little data to support the use of DOACs in patients >160 kg and therefore warfarin may be appropriate in this cohort. Other patients in whom specialist advice may be sought prior to initiation are people:

- with gastrointestinal or genitourinary bleeding within three months, intracranial haemorrhage within the last six months, severe menorrhagia or known bleeding disorders
- on dual antiplatelet therapy
- on renal dialysis
- with abnormal blood results:
  - bilirubin >1.5 × upper limit of normal (ULN)
  - liver function tests (LFTs) >2 × ULN
  - platelets <100
- with an abnormal clotting screen
- with low haemoglobin with no identifiable cause

- who have had transcatheter aortic valve replacement, mitral valve replacement or repair within the last three months
- who have active cancer
- who are pregnant, planning a pregnancy or breastfeeding.

Box 3.5: Important prescribing information for DOACs

Contraindications:
- Known hypersensitivity to ingredients
- Clinically significant active bleeding
- Mechanical valve in situ
- Renal impairment (drug specific)
- Hepatic disease
- Recent high-risk bleeding lesion (e.g. intracranial haemorrhage in last <6 months)
- Pregnancy or breastfeeding
- Recent stroke, surgery, GI bleed, ulcers
- Recent fibrinolytic surgery (less than 10 days ago)
- Concomitant warfarin therapy

Cautions:
- People on phenytoin, carbamazepine and other P-glycoprotein and CYP344 inhibitors
- People on P-glycoprotein and CYP344 inducers
- Renal dysfunction (CrCL 30 <30 mL/min)
- Concomitant antiplatelets
- Adherence issues identified

Common adverse effects:
- Dizziness
- Headache
- Symptomatic bradycardia
- Worsening of heart failure symptoms
- Coldness or numbness in the extremities
- Hypotension, especially in patients with heart failure
- Nausea, vomiting, diarrhoea, constipation
- Fatigue

Modifiable risk factors for bleeding should be identified and addressed where possible before anticoagulant therapy is initiated.

Key modifiable risk factors for bleeding include:
- Systolic blood pressure >160 mmHg – escalate antihypertensive therapy
- Reduced renal or liver function – review nephrotoxic or hepatotoxic drug therapy
- Concomitant drug therapy such as aspirin, NSAIDs, high dose steroids or SSRIs – review and stop or minimise dose where possible
- Excess alcohol intake – advise no more than 8 units per week

Pharmacists in all settings can play a part in monitoring DOACs by being aware of the required dose adjustments (see *Table 3.2*) and assessing the appropriateness of the drug and dose for the patient based on age, weight, renal function (if available) and drug interactions.

Table 3.2: *DOAC dosing in atrial fibrillation*

	Apixaban	Edoxaban	Rivaroxaban	Dabigatran
Standard dose	5 mg twice daily	60 mg once daily	20 mg once daily (with food)	150 mg twice daily
Reduced dose	2.5 mg twice daily	30 mg once daily	15 mg once daily (with food)	110 mg twice daily
Criteria for reduced dose	Two or more of: • Age ≥ 80 years • Weight ≤60 kg • Serum creatinine ≥133 micromol/L OR CrCl 15-29 mL/min	One or more of: • Weight ≤60 kg • CrCl 15-50 mL/min • Concurrent treatment with ciclosporin, dronedarone, erythromycin, or ketoconazole	CrCl 15-49 mL/min	• Age ≥80 years • Concurrent treatment with verapamil • Consider reducing dose for: — reflux/gastritis — age 75-80 years — CrCl 30-50 mL/min — high bleed risk
Contraindicated	CrCl <15 mL/min			CrCl <30 mL/min

Patients should be asked if they are having regular renal checks – most patients should have at least annual checks but in the frail elderly, renal function (with calculation of CrCl) should be undertaken at least every 6 months or more frequently if the CrCl falls below 30 mL/min.[18]

Beyond the monitoring of renal function, pharmacists should:

- Assess adherence – ask non-threatening questions about drug adherence, offer counselling to support improved adherence where necessary and address any specific underlying issues or concerns the patient may have.
- Assess bleeding risk – ask patients if they have experienced any episodes of bleeding. Patients should be reassured if they experience 'nuisance bleeding' such as infrequent self-limiting nose bleeds, bleeding gums when brushing teeth or unusual bruising, or minor bleeds such as single episodes of haematuria (blood in the urine), haematemesis (blood in vomit) or haemoptysis (coughing up blood).
  - If bleeding is frequent or severe (significant blood loss, or bleeding that will not stop despite pressure) advise patients to seek advice from their GP, anticoagulant clinic or urgent care.
- Assess for other adverse effects of DOACs – these are rare but include anaemia, dizziness and headache, gastrointestinal disturbance including dyspepsia, nausea, constipation, diarrhoea, pruritis and fatigue.
  - In most circumstances, if the patient experiences these adverse effects, the most sensible strategy is to try a different DOAC.
- Assess for any important drug interactions – both prescribed and OTC medication should be reviewed (see *Box 3.6*).
- Check blood pressure – hypertension is a major cause of intracranial haemorrhage (ICH) on anticoagulant therapy. If systolic BP is raised above 160 mmHg, this should be addressed through the escalation of antihypertensive therapies. Patients should be aware that sudden onset severe headache or dizziness could indicate ICH and they should seek urgent medical advice.
- Educate the patient on the benefits and risks of anticoagulant therapy and address any outstanding concerns.

Box 3.6: Drug interactions for anticoagulants

Key drug interactions for warfarin
Drugs which potentiate the effects of warfarin
- Allopurinol, capecitabine, erlotinib, disulfiram, azole antifungals (e.g. ketoconazole, fluconazole)
- Omeprazole, paracetamol (prolonged regular use) propafenone, amiodarone, tamoxifen methylphenidate
- Zafirlukast, fibrates, statins
- Erythromycin sulfamethoxazole metronidazole

Drugs which antagonise the effects of warfarin
- Barbiturates, primidone, carbamazepine, griseofulvin, oral contraceptives, rifampicin, azathioprine, phenytoin

Drugs with variable effect
- Corticosteroids, nevirapine, ritonavir

Other drug interactions
- Broad spectrum antibiotics may potentiate the effect of warfarin by reducing the gut flora which produce vitamin K
- Orlistat may reduce absorption of vitamin K
- Cholestyramine and sucralfate potentially decrease absorption of warfarin
- Increased INR has been reported in patients taking glucosamine and warfarin
- Herbal preparations containing St John's wort (*Hypericum perforatum*) must not be used whilst taking warfarin due to a proven risk of decreased plasma concentrations and reduced clinical effects of warfarin
- Many other herbal products have a theoretical effect on warfarin, however, most of these interactions are not proven
  - Patients should generally avoid taking any herbal medicines or food supplements whilst taking warfarin and should be told to advise their doctor if they are taking any, as more frequent monitoring is advisable

Key drug interactions for DOACs
Drug interactions are drug specific, but common interactions to look out for include:
- Strong P-glycoprotein inhibitors – e.g. ketoconazole, itraconazole, cyclosporin, dronedarone, ritonavir, indinavir, clarithromycin
- Other P-glycoprotein inhibitors – e.g. verapamil, amiodarone, quinidine, pozaconazole
- Inducers of CYP3A4 and P-glycoprotein – e.g. rifampicin, carbamazepine, phenytoin, St John's wort
Specific advice on managing drug interactions can be found in the manufacturers' summaries of product characteristics (SPCs) for the individual agents.

Myths and misconceptions

There are many reasons why patients have not been offered anticoagulation in routine clinical practice, many of which are based on misconceptions based on bleeding risk which need to be challenged.

Frailty, extremes of age, history of falls, cognitive dysfunction and prior bleeds are not contraindications to anticoagulant therapy. NICE guidance is very clear that aspirin monotherapy should not be used to reduce stroke risk in AF.[15] Where anticoagulation is contraindicated or not tolerated a left atrial appendage closure device may be considered, this blocks the atrial appendage which is often the location of blood clot formation in AF.[15]

Practice-based pharmacists should undertake an annual systematic review of all patients with AF who are not currently anticoagulated to:
- check CHA_2DS_2VASc score has been calculated accurately and modifiable bleeding risk factors have been addressed
- review all patients prescribed aspirin monotherapy for stroke prevention in AF and offer anticoagulation

- identify why patients with $CHA_2DS_2VASc \geq 2$ are not prescribed anticoagulants and assess if anticoagulation has been withheld inappropriately
- identify patients with $CHA_2DS_2VASc \geq 2$ who have declined anticoagulation previously and revisit this with a face-to-face discussion using a shared decision-making approach
- identify patients with $CHA_2DS_2VASc \geq 2$ who have a contraindication to anticoagulation, who should be referred for consideration of a left atrial appendage occlusion device.

Community pharmacists may also identify individuals with AF who are not currently anticoagulated and should refer them back to their GP practice for review unless they are very low risk (i.e. young with no additional CHA_2DS_2VASc risk factors).

Control of rate and rhythm in atrial fibrillation

All patients with AF should have a pulse check at least annually to assess heart rate. A raised heart rate in AF (>120 beats per minute) can result in the development of tachycardia-induced cardiomyopathy.

Patients should also be asked about the occurrence, frequency and severity of symptoms of AF – breathlessness/dyspnoea, palpitations, lightheadedness or dizziness and chest discomfort.

Rate and rhythm control are used to manage the symptoms of AF and prevent adverse remodelling in the heart. A standard beta blocker (such as bisoprolol) or a rate-controlling calcium channel blocker (such as diltiazem or verapamil) are the first-line rate-control options for the majority of people with AF.[15]

Digoxin may be considered for rate control in sedentary patients with persistent or permanent AF (it should not be used in paroxysmal AF). The initial aim of rate control strategies is to attain a resting heart rate of less than 110 beats per minute and assess whether symptoms have resolved. If symptoms persist, resting heart rate should be lowered further with a higher dose of the initial therapy or combination therapy, aiming to achieve a resting heart rate between 60-100 beats per minute.

Rhythm control should be considered as a first-line strategy:

- in people where the AF has a reversible cause
- in people who have heart failure thought to be primarily caused by AF
- in people with new-onset atrial fibrillation and in those with atrial flutter whose condition is considered suitable for an ablation strategy to restore sinus rhythm
- where rhythm control is considered more suitable based on clinical judgement.

Rhythm control should also be considered where an initial rate control strategy has failed to control symptoms. Rhythm control strategies include electrical or pharmacological cardioversion, long-term drug therapy to maintain sinus rhythm and ablation of the electrical pathways underlying the AF.

The first-line drug used for rhythm control is a standard beta blocker, such as bisoprolol. If this is unsuitable or ineffective, amiodarone may be considered particularly in the presence of left ventricular impairment or heart failure. A 'pill in the pocket' strategy using flecainide or sotalol may be considered for people with infrequent paroxysms and few symptoms, or where symptoms are induced by known precipitants (such as alcohol or caffeine) to allow the patient to manage episodes as they occur and avoid the long-term toxic effects of anti-arrhythmic drug therapy.

If drug treatment fails, radiofrequency catheter ablation may be used to 'break' the abnormal circuits in the heart and destroy areas of the heart muscle which are triggering the AF.

Pharmacists can identify patients requiring rate or rhythm control intervention by checking their pulse and asking if they experience any symptoms related to AF, such as breathlessness/dyspnoea, palpitations, lightheadedness or dizziness and chest discomfort. If symptoms are present, the assessment should cover the severity of symptoms and the frequency with which they occur. If patients experience regular or severe symptoms then escalation of rate-controlling strategies or consideration of rhythm control strategies may be required. A pulse check may reveal a fast resting heart rate – patients with resting heart rates of more than 110 bpm, should have their rate control reviewed.

For important prescribing information for beta blockers, see *Box 3.7*.

Box 3.7: Beta blocker therapy

Contraindications:
- Acute heart failure, or during episodes of heart failure decompensation requiring IV inotropic therapy, or cardiogenic shock
- Second or third degree AV block, sick sinus syndrome or sinoatrial block
- Symptomatic hypotension
- Severe unstable asthma
- Severe forms of peripheral arterial occlusive disease or severe forms of Raynaud's syndrome
- Untreated phaeochromocytoma
- Metabolic acidosis

Cautions:
- Bronchospasm (bronchial asthma, obstructive airways diseases)
- Diabetes mellitus with large fluctuations in blood glucose values – symptoms of hypoglycaemia (e.g. tachycardia, palpitations, sweating) can be masked.
- Strict fasting
- During ongoing desensitisation therapy. As with other beta blockers, bisoprolol may increase both the sensitivity towards allergens and the severity of anaphylactic reactions. Epinephrine treatment may not always yield the expected therapeutic effect
- First degree AV block
- Prinzmetal's angina
- Peripheral arterial occlusive disease. Aggravation of symptoms may occur especially when starting therapy
- Patients with psoriasis or with a history of psoriasis should only be given beta blockers (e.g. bisoprolol) after a careful balancing of benefits against risks

Common adverse effects:
- Dizziness – consider alternative rate controlling agent if not tolerated
- Headache – consider alternative rate controlling agent if not tolerated
- Symptomatic bradycardia – if heart rate falls below 50 beats per minute consider dose reduction
- Worsening of heart failure symptoms – reduce dose by one increment and seek advice from specialist heart failure team
- Coldness or numbness in the extremities – consider alternative rate controlling agent if not tolerated
- Hypotension, especially in patients with heart failure – reduce dose by one increment and seek advice from specialist heart failure team
- Nausea, vomiting, diarrhoea, constipation – consider alternative rate controlling agent if not tolerated
- Fatigue – consider alternative rate controlling agent if not tolerated

Advice for patients

When initiating anticoagulant treatment patients will need some information and advice and this is useful to reinforce at regular reviews. See *Box 3.8* for a checklist of counselling points to cover.

Box 3.8: Practice point: counselling points

- **Explanation of an anticoagulant** (increases clotting time and reduces risk of clot formation) and explanation of indication for therapy (AF and stroke risk reduction/DVT/PE)
- **Differences between DOAC and warfarin** (if applicable for patients converting from warfarin to DOAC therapy or offering choice of anticoagulation agent)
  - No routine INR monitoring
  - Fixed dosing
  - No dietary restrictions and alcohol intake permitted (within national guidelines)
  - Fewer drug interactions
- **Name of drug:** generic & brand name.
- **Explanation of dose:** strength & frequency
- **INR monitoring:** need for regular INR monitoring on warfarin to guide dose, which may change depending on the INR result
- **Duration of therapy:** lifelong for AF or explain course length for DVT/PE treatment or prevention
- **To take with food (dabigatran and rivaroxaban)** – not required for apixaban, edoxaban or warfarin
- **If doses are missed:**
  - Apixaban and dabigatran can be taken within 6 hours of missed dose, otherwise omit the missed dose
  - Edoxaban and rivaroxaban can be taken within 12 hours of missed dose, otherwise omit the missed dose
  - Warfarin can be taken within 12 hours of a missed dose. If there are less than 12 hours until the next dose, skip the missed dose and continue as prescribed when the next dose is due
- **If extra doses are taken:** obtain advice immediately from pharmacist/GP/NHS Direct (111)
- **Importance of adherence:** particularly with the DOACs due to the short half-life. Increase risk of stroke and/or thrombosis if non-compliant with prescribed therapy
- **Common and serious adverse effects and who/when to refer:** symptoms of bleeding/unexplained bruising (provide advice about avoidance of contact sports)
  - Single/self-terminating bleeding episode – routine appointment with GP/pharmacist
  - Prolonged/recurrent/severe bleeding/head injury – A&E
  - Major bleeds managed/reversed by supportive measures, prothrombin complex concentrate (PCC), and availability of antidote
- **Drug interactions and concomitant medication:** avoid NSAIDs. Always check with a pharmacist regarding OTC/herbal/complimentary medicines
- **Inform all healthcare professionals of anticoagulant therapy:** GP, nurse, dentist, pharmacist
- **Pregnancy and breastfeeding:** potential risk to fetus – obtain medical advice as soon as possible if pregnant/considering pregnancy. Avoid in breastfeeding
- **Storage:** dabigatran must be kept in original packaging – moisture sensitive. All other DOACs are suitable for standard medication compliance aids/dosette boxes if required. Warfarin is not generally suitable for use in a medicine compliance aid due to the variable dose based on INR
- **Follow-up appointments, blood tests, and repeat prescriptions:** where and when
- **Issue relevant patient information AF booklet/leaflet and anticoagulant patient alert card**
- **Give person the opportunity to ask questions** and encourage follow up with community pharmacist

Useful resources

- The AHSN Network 2020. AF Toolkit – www.aftoolkit.co.uk/af-dataCPPE
- Anticoagulation – www.cppe.ac.uk/gateway/anticoag
- NES Scotland. Pharmaceutical Care of People with Atrial fibrillation – www.nes.scot.nhs.uk
- NICE 2014. Atrial fibrillation: management – www.nice.org.uk/guidance/cg180
- Royal Pharmaceutical Society – Guidance for the safe switching of warfarin to direct oral anticoagulants (DOACs) for patients with non-valvular AF and venous thromboembolism (DVT / PE) during the coronavirus pandemic.

References

1. National Cardiovascular Intelligence Network. Atrial fibrillation prevalence estimates for local populations. London: National Cardiovascular Intelligence Network; 2015. www.gov.uk/government/publications/atrial-fibrillation-prevalence-estimates-for-local-populations

2. Magnussen C *et al.* Sex differences and similarities in atrial fibrillation epidemiology, risk factors, and mortality in community cohorts. *Circulation* 2017; 136: 1588-1597.

3. Go AS *et al.* Prevalence of diagnosed atrial fibrillation in adults: national implications for rhythm management and stroke prevention: the anticoagulation and risk factors in atrial fibrillation (ATRIA) study. *JAMA* 2001; 285(18): 2370-2375.

4. Wolf PA, Abbott RD, Kannel WB. Atrial fibrillation as an independent risk factor for stroke: the Framingham Study. *Stroke* 1991; 22: 983-988.

5. Ali AN *et al.* Clinical and economic implications of AF related stroke. *J Atr Fibrillation* 2016 Feb-Mar; 8(5): 1279.

6. Xu XM *et al.* The economic burden of stroke care in England, Wales and Northern Ireland: using a national stroke register to estimate and report patient-level health economic outcomes in stroke. *European Stroke Journal* 2018; 3(1): 82-91.

7. Stroke Association. AF: how can we do better? London: Stroke Association; 2018. www.stroke.org.uk/sites/default/files/af-data_2018_england_eng_2.pdf

8. NHS Digital. Quality and Outcomes Framework, achievement, prevalence and exceptions data 2018-19. London: NHS Digital; 2019. www.digital.nhs.uk/data-and-information/publications/statistical/quality-and-outcomes-framework-achievement-prevalence-and-exceptions-data/2018-19-pas

9. Ballatore A *et al.* 2019 Subclinical and asymptomatic atrial fibrillation: current evidence and unsolved questions in clinical practice. *Medicina (Kaunas)* 2019; 55(8): 497.

10. National Institute for Health and Care Excellence (NICE). MTG13: WatchBP Home A for opportunistically detecting atrial fibrillation during diagnosis and monitoring of hypertension. London: NICE; 2013. www.nice.org.uk/guidance/MTG13

11. National Institute for Health and Care Excellence (NICE). MIB35: AliveCor Heart Monitor and AliveECG app (Kardia Mobile) for detecting atrial fibrillation. London: NICE; 2015. www.nice.org.uk/advice/mib35

12. Taggar JS, Coleman T, Lewis S *et al.* Accuracy of methods for detecting an irregular pulse and suspected atrial fibrillation: a systematic review and meta-analysis. *Eur J Prev Cardiol* 2016; 23(12): 1330-1338.

13. Royal Brompton & Harefield NHS Foundation Trust. CAPTURE-AF [online]. London: Royal Brompton & Harefield NHS Foundation Trust. www.rbht.nhs.uk/our-services/heart/heart-rhythm/capture-af

14. Care City. One stop shop atrial fibrillation pathway. London: Care City; 2018. www.carecity.london/publications/blueprints/1-care-city-af-blueprint-v3

15. National Institute for Health and Care Excellence (NICE). CG180: Atrial fibrillation management. London: NICE; 2014. www.nice.org.uk/guidance/cg180

16. Hart RG *et al.* Meta-analysis: antithrombotic therapy to prevent stroke in patients who have nonvalvular atrial fibrillation. *Ann Intern Med* 2007; 146: 857-67.

17. Royal Pharmaceutical Society (RPS). Guidance for the safe switching of warfarin to direct oral anticoagulants (DOACs) for patients with non-valvular AF and venous thromboembolism (DVT/PE) during the coronavirus pandemic. London: RPS; 2020. www.rpharms.com/Portals/0/RPS%20document%20library/Open%20access/Coronavirus/FINAL%20Guidance%20on%20safe%20switching%20of%20warfarin%20to%20DOAC%20COVID-19%20Mar%202020.pdf?ver=2020-03-26-180945-627

18. Steffel J. The 2018 European Heart Rhythm Association practical guide on the use of non-vitamin K antagonist oral anticoagulants in patients with atrial fibrillation. *European Heart Journal* 2018; 39(16): 1330-1393.

Case studies

Case study 1

Peter, aged 66 years, has hypertension and type 2 diabetes. He is currently prescribed amlodipine 10 mg daily, ramipril 5 mg daily and metformin 500 mg twice daily. You review him in your diabetes clinic and note that he has an irregular pulse on manual palpation with a pulse rate of 78 bpm.

Points to consider

- What investigations, if any, would you consider at this stage?

You request an ECG which confirms atrial fibrillation (AF) and, following discussion with the GP, you call the patient back to discuss this new diagnosis.

Points to consider

- What tool would you use to calculate Peter's risk of stroke?
- What tool would you use to calculate Peter's bleeding risk due to anticoagulation?

Peter has a CHA_2DS_2VASc score of 3, which equates to a 3.2% risk of stroke per annum, and a HAS-BLED score of 1, which equates to a risk of 1 bleed per 100 patient-years.

Points to consider

- How would you describe atrial fibrillation to Peter?
- What would you say about anticoagulant therapy?

You explain to Peter that the irregular heart rhythm that you picked up at his last visit is AF and that this puts him at a higher risk of having a stroke. You also highlight that AF-related strokes are associated with a higher risk of dying or being left with long-term disability than non-AF related strokes. You explain that treatment with an anticoagulant drug reduces the risk of stroke substantially and use the following chart to explain the benefits of anticoagulation in terms of stroke prevention and the risks in terms of bleeding.

	Number of events per 1000 AF patients per year		
CHA_2DS_2VASc	AF-related strokes prevented by anticoagulation	Major bleeds caused by anticoagulation	HAS-BLED score
1	4	4	1
2	17	12	2
3	25	15	3
4	38	21	4
5	57		

Peter indicates that he is not keen to take warfarin as he understands that there is a lot of monitoring involved – he has a disabled wife who requires 24-hour care at home and he does not want to have to attend regularly for blood tests.

You reassure Peter that there are other options now which do not require such rigorous monitoring and offer him a DOAC which he agrees to take.

Points to consider

- What would you check before starting anticoagulation with a DOAC?

You check his most recent bloods which were taken for his diabetes check and calculate his creatinine clearance as 62 mL/min using the Cockcroft-Gault equation and his body weight.

Points to consider

- Which DOACs are suitable for Peter?

Based on his age, body weight, creatinine clearance and lack of interacting drugs he could take any of the DOACs; but in line with local prescribing guidance, you initiate rivaroxaban 20 mg daily.

Points to consider

- What information about DOAC treatment would you give Peter?

You counsel Peter on the key elements of DOAC therapy including:
- Drug, dose, frequency, and duration of therapy
- Taking rivaroxaban with food to aid absorption
- Importance of taking regularly at the same time each day to prevent stroke
- How to manage missed doses
- How to manage any adverse effects particularly bleeding
- Drug interactions: avoid NSAIDs. The need to check with a pharmacist regarding OTC/herbal/complementary medicines
- Importance of informing other healthcare professionals whilst on DOAC therapy
- Follow-up appointments, blood tests, and obtaining repeat prescriptions

You also provide written information to support the discussion including an AF booklet and anticoagulant patient alert card and ask Peter if he has any further questions. He does not have specific questions now, but you remind him that if he has any concerns he should seek advice from the GP practice or the community pharmacy.

Points to consider

- When should Peter be invited for a review?

You arrange to give him a call in three weeks to see how he is getting on with the new tablet. After Peter leaves, you ensure the AF is correctly coded on the GP system and add a recall for bloods in 12 months to recheck the creatinine clearance.

Case study 2

Julie, aged 84 years, has known atrial fibrillation (2001), as well as hypertension (1984), heart failure (2008), depression (2007) and prior stroke (2013). She was recently admitted to hospital due to acute decompensation and has been discharged on the following regimen:

- Indapamide 2.5 mg daily
- Apixaban 5 mg twice daily (previously on warfarin 3 mg daily; but low INR control noted on admission)
- Ramipril 5 mg daily
- Bisoprolol 3.75 mg twice daily
- Furosemide 80 mg twice daily
- Clopidogrel 75 mg daily
- Atorvastatin 40 mg daily
- Escitalopram 10 mg daily

Her discharge summary indicates creatinine of 124 micromol/L.

You review her 10 days post-discharge. From a heart failure perspective, you note that she is being seen by the community HF nurses who have reduced her furosemide to 40 mg daily; she has been weighing herself daily and now weighs 58 kg, which is her dry weight. Her BP is 124/60 mmHg, pulse rate is 92 bpm. You order repeat bloods but they are not available at the review.

Points to consider

- What are Julie's CHA_2DS_2VASc and HAS-BLED scores?
- What are the implications for her treatment?

You note that her anticoagulant therapy was changed from warfarin to a DOAC whilst she was in hospital and calculate that her CHA_2DS_2VASc score is 7 (age, female, hypertension, heart failure and prior stroke), so she has an annual stroke risk of approximately 10%, with a HAS-BLED of 3-3.74% risk of major bleed.

Points to consider

- How can the HAS-BLED risk be reduced?
- What information is relevant when you consider how to change her treatment?

You know that the HAS-BLED score could be reduced to 2 by stopping the clopidogrel (1.88% risk of major bleeds), so you review her notes and hospital letters and exclude any recent cardiovascular events in the last year.

She is at very high risk of an AF-related stroke, so you discuss with her the ongoing need for anticoagulation and ask her if she has any concerns. She asks why she has been switched from warfarin, which she had been on for many years, and asks what she needs to know about this new drug.

Points to consider

- How would you respond to Julie's question?

You reassure Julie that there is good evidence that apixaban is at least as good as warfarin in protecting her from AF-related strokes; it is associated with a lower rate of bleeding, it is also more predictable in its effects and therefore she will need less regular monitoring – you point out that the hospital clinicians may have been concerned about her low INR on admission to hospital.

You go through the DOAC counselling checklist to reinforce her understanding of the new drug and discuss with her that you want to stop the clopidogrel, which is no longer required, and stopping the drug will reduce the risk of bleeding in the future – Julie agrees and you delete the drug from the repeat prescribing list and advise her to stop taking this from now on. You check Julie's creatinine clearance which is 27 mL/min.

Points to consider

- Are there any other adjustments to treatment required?

Based on her creatinine clearance, as well as her age (≥80 years) plus her weight (≤60 kg), Julie is on the wrong dose of apixaban. She should be prescribed apixaban 2.5 mg twice daily and you therefore reduce her dose immediately, with a view to rechecking her creatinine clearance when her up-to-date bloods are returned.

Points to consider

- What follow-up is required for Julie?

Due to her poor renal function, she will need regular renal function checks (every three months) to assess any fluctuations. You arrange to check in with Julie remotely in two weeks to see how she is getting on with the apixaban, make a note to follow up her blood results and recheck her creatinine clearance once available, update her repeat prescription list to remove the warfarin on the GP system and order bloods for three months.

CHAPTER 4

Bipolar disorder

Georgina Ell

Overview

Bipolar disorder is a common mental health condition thought to affect between 0.4% and 1% of the adult population.[1] Onset usually occurs around age 15-19 years, however, diagnosis is often postponed due to delay in contact with mental health services.[1] The prevalence of bipolar disease is equal across the sexes, although it is recognised that woman are more likely to suffer from more depressive episodes than their male counterparts.[2]

When bipolar symptoms are most severe, patients can put themselves at risk of harm; it can damage relationships; patients may partake in risky behaviours, and in some situations they can pose a risk to others. In patients with bipolar, life expectancy is often reduced. Patients with bipolar have a 10-15% lifelong risk of suicide – this is a 10-20 times higher risk than in the general population.[1,2]

Bipolar is a lifelong condition and patients can have periods of stability which are sandwiched between periods of relapse.[1] Most patients should continue to take medication long term in order to stabilise their mental state and prolong the periods of remission. As well as taking medication, psychological therapies are an option, and patients should aim to reduce risky behaviour, such as using illicit substances, to keep themselves stable.[2,3] The cause of bipolar is unknown, but there is thought to be a genetic element, although the mechanism or specific gene has not been identified. This hypothesis is reinforced by the fact that prevalence increases to 1 in 3 when there is a family history of bipolar and from results of twin and family studies.[3,4] There are other theories about the aetiology of bipolar, including biochemical, endocrine and electrolyte disturbances. However, it is not known what causes the symptoms of depression and mania.[3,4]

Diagnosis

Bipolar is diagnosed by a specialist in mental health. They take a thorough history, collateral history from friends or family, as well as completing a mental state examination.[4] Geeky medics (an online resource) has an OSCE preparation which demonstrates the different aspects of a mental state examination.[5] In order to receive a diagnosis of bipolar, patients have to have experienced two separate periods of depression and mania or hypomania separated by a period of remission.[6]

Bipolar disorder is characterised by fluctuating episodes of mania (severe functional impairment lasting at least 7 days, abnormally elevated mood), hypomania (reduced function for 4 or more days) and depressed episodes (abnormally low mood).[3,4]

There are two different manifestations of the condition:[1,6]

- Bipolar I – Mania. Episodes of mania, in some people (but not all) there may also be episodes of depression
- Bipolar II – Bipolar depression. Episodes of depression and symptoms of hypomania, but not all people experience episodes of mania

Patients can also experience rapid cycling bipolar; this is when they experience four or more episodes of mania or depression within 12 months.[6] *Table 4.1* outlines the symptoms that can be seen in the different stages of bipolar.

Table 4.1: *Bipolar symptoms*

Depressive symptoms	Manic symptoms
Low mood	Grandiose ideas
Thoughts of self-harm/suicidal thoughts	Pressure of speech (talking fast, unable to interrupt)
Lack of sleep/disturbed sleep	Increased sex drive
Lack of desire	Inappropriate behaviour (e.g. gambling, increased spending)
Lack of appetite	Psychotic symptoms

Treatment

The main aim of treatment is to maintain the patient in remission for as long as possible to enable them to lead normal lives.[1] If maintained on appropriate treatment, most patients can function normally, however, it is estimated that they will only remain completely symptom-free for approximately 50% of the time.[2]

There are two treatment aims for patients with bipolar:[4]

- To treat the acute phase, whether this is mania or depression
- To lengthen the periods of remission and prevent further episodes (prophylaxis)

Treatment should take into account patients' individual preferences – if patients are allowed to make informed decisions about their treatment and care, they are more likely to be compliant with the treatment plan.[7] Information provided should also be tailored to the needs of the individual and it is important to include their family or carers in any discussion or decisions around treatment and care if the patient is happy to do so.[3,4]

All patients with bipolar (regardless of the subtype) should be offered evidence-based psychological intervention known to be effective for bipolar disorder. The benefits and risks of a psychological intervention should be discussed with the patient.[4]

Patients with acute mania nearly always require admission to hospital.[4] This is usually under section 2 or 3 of the Mental Health Act 1983.[8] In an acute stage, it is difficult to treat a patient in the community as they often require urgent treatment to settle their mental state. In a manic stage, they may require medication to rapidly sedate or control aggressive symptoms.[2,3,4] In this stage antipsychotics and benzodiazepines are often used – the benzodiazepines can be reduced and withdrawn when symptoms improve, but it is recommended to continue the antipsychotics for prophylaxis.[2,4]

The second-generation antipsychotics (atypical), have shown efficacy in both treatment of mania and prophylaxis and demonstrate antimania and mood stabilising properties. The first-generation antipsychotics (typical) are useful in treating mania but they are often required to be used alongside a mood stabiliser in prophylaxis phase. NICE guidelines[4] recommend starting an antipsychotic or sodium valproate due to their fast antimanic effects. (Note: antipsychotics will not be covered in this chapter as they will be covered in **Chapter 15**).

In acute manic episodes, consideration must be given to medicines which may precipitate a manic episode and if the patient presents as manic, these medicines should be discontinued.[2] These can include antidepressants, stimulants and other non-psychotropic medicines, including steroids and some antiretrovirals.[9]

In acute depressive episodes, patients may require an antidepressant. If prescribed it should be alongside a mood stabiliser to prevent switch to mania.[2,4] (Note: antidepressants are not covered in this chapter as they are covered in **Chapter 1**).

The mode of action of mood stabilisers is not fully understood, but it is thought their effects on gamma aminobutyric acid (GABA), serotonin and dopaminergic are responsible for their efficacy.[10,11]

Pharmacy input

Pharmacists as frontline healthcare professionals and experts in medicines, so can support patients living with bipolar disorder by providing advice about medicines, recognising early signs of toxicity, warning signs of relapse, or instability and directing them to the correct setting to obtain help.

In addition, pharmacists can be a link between the psychiatrist, GP and patients to ensure that medication changes are communicated between the different teams, as well as ensuring continuity of care across all settings. They can counsel patients on medication compliance, and with access to patients' medication records they can monitor polypharmacy, provide advice on potential drug interactions and how to optimise medicines, as well as simplifying medication regimens and arrange compliance aids if necessary.[7]

Patients will have regular contact with the community pharmacist when they are collecting their repeat prescriptions. Mood stabilisers are the main treatment for this condition; they require special monitoring and the patient should be counselled on their adverse effects. The pharmacist has an important role to play in ensuring the patient is educated on these matters – if the patient is aware of adverse effects and monitoring, and how to manage these it could help them to take control of their condition. This would mean the patient is more likely to be compliant with their medication.[7]

Pharmacists working in secondary care have an important role to play in obtaining an accurate medication history including over-the-counter (OTC) medicines and illicit drugs when patients are admitted to hospital, or attend their clinic.[7] It is important as part of the medication history to review the patient's compliance. There is an important role for pharmacists to play in providing appropriate medication strategies and recommendations on pharmaceutical therapeutic drug monitoring and appropriate physical health monitoring, which is required for the mood stabilisers.[4]

During hospital admissions, pharmacists can ensure all medicines prescribed for bipolar are optimised, that drug levels are monitored when appropriate, and doses adjusted according to these levels, patient response, and tolerance. It is important for pharmacists to be aware of the adverse effects of mood stabilisers so they are able to identify if the presenting complaint could be attributed to the mood stabiliser.

Pharmacy review

Preventing and recognising relapse

Patients with bipolar will experience relapses at some point as the disease progresses, these can occur even if the patient is compliant with their medication. Being aware of the initial warning signs can help identify early relapse and prevent this from progressing to a full relapse episode. *Table 4.2* lists some common triggers for relapse.[12]

It may not be possible for people with bipolar to avoid all of these potential triggers, but being aware of them and how to react can go some way to help prevent serious relapse. It is not always easy for someone with a manic episode to recognise the early signs and that is why it is important for friends and family to be aware of these symptoms.

Patients are at higher risk of relapse if they still experience some symptoms of bipolar despite being on treatment – these patients are the ones who would benefit from a full medication review and optimisation of medicines.[2] Whilst each patient is individual and may, therefore, experience different relapse symptoms, it may be useful to have an idea of general early warning signs.[13] If someone with bipolar disorder is acting in an unusual manner, it is important to voice your concerns as early identification can result in early treatment, faster resolution of symptoms and a shorter episode. Warning signs are changes in the way a patient behaves, thinks or feels and any of these could indicate they are becoming unwell.[14] *Table 4.3* lists early warning signs for the different types of bipolar.

Table 4.2: *Common triggers for relapse*

Potential trigger	Example
Stressful life events	Birth, death, losing a job, getting a promotion, end of a relationship, moving house
Disruption to sleep pattern	Jet lag, birth of a baby, social events
Disruption to routine	Change in sleeping pattern, change in eating habits, changes in social activity/regular activity
Excessive stimulation from external stimuli	Social activities, work deadlines, traffic, light, crowds
Excessive internal stimulation	Over stimulation from excitement and activity, stimulating substances (e.g. caffeine, nicotine)
Abuse of illicit drugs	Alcohol, cannabis and other illegal drugs
Conflict and stressful interactions	Fighting or conflicts at work, or with family members
Untreated or unmanaged illness	Hypothyroidism, infections
Prescription medicines	Steroids, antiretrovirals, antidepressants

Table 4.3: *Early warning signs*

Early warning signs of mania/ hypomania	Early warning signs of depression	Early warning signs for mixed episode
Lack of sleep	Loss of interest	Agitated or restless
Rapid speech	Lack of energy	Easily distracted
Increased energy	Feeling tired	Weight loss
Irritable	Anxiety	Feeling tired
Racing thought	Self-neglect	Engages in dangerous behaviour
Poor judgement	Physical pains/illnesses	Sleep problems
Risky behaviour	Feeling sad	Rapid speech
Heightened senses	Self-isolation	Loss of interest
Increased sex drive	Decreased sex drive	Increased activities
Changes in appearance – dying hair, bright clothes, inappropriate clothes	Forgetfulness	Typical signs of depression or mania

Being aware of a patient's condition and what is normal for them will help identify relapses and ensure they get the help and treatment they need to prevent these.[13] It can also ensure that if they are becoming unwell, they get timely treatment which could prevent a full relapse.

Table 4.4 outlines the input that pharmacists within different settings and with different skill levels can have with patients with bipolar.

Table 4.4: *Input from pharmacists in different setting*

Pharmacist role	Interventions
All pharmacists, irrelevant of setting	• Be aware of main medications used to treat bipolar and their main adverse effects • Be aware of the signs and symptoms of lithium toxicity • Assess patient's compliance and offer advice to help with this • Discuss adverse effect and physical health monitoring with patient • Be aware of drug interactions of bipolar medicines • Ensure adequate communication between care settings • Be aware of early signs of relapse and where to refer patient if you suspect these
Community pharmacist	• Notice non-compliance (if patient fails to collect repeat prescriptions) flag up to GP/mental health team • Notice early warning signs of relapse – discuss with patient and/or GP • Identify drug interactions with bipolar medicine, over-the-counter medicines and other prescribed medicines • Provide advice on adverse effects and toxicity from bipolar medicines and refer if appropriate • Provide advice and ensure patient has attended for physical health monitoring • Remind GP about physical health monitoring for mood stabilisers • Refer patient to useful website and support • Offer stop smoking advice (higher risk of smoking in patients with mental health) • Refer to dietician if weight is a problem • Ensure adequate supply of medicine and discuss barriers to compliance • Check purple lithium book prior to dispensing lithium
Pharmacist working in GP practice	• Ensure GP's knowledge is up-to-date on monitoring requirements for mood stabilisers • Ensure monitoring is carried out of patients with bipolar within the practice – ensure GP has a register of patients prescribed mood stabilisers • Review plasma levels and provide advice to GPs on dose adjustments • Meet with patients and review medications – advise on adverse effect management • Provide advice on compliance with medicines • Review patient's physical health assessments (e.g. bloods, ECG and weight and offer advice to patient if there are abnormalities) • Ensure summary care records (SCR) and GP records are up-to-date with all patient's physical and mental health medicines • Advise GPs on cost effective medications and ensure adequate reviews • If women of childbearing age prescribed sodium valproate, ensure there is an annual review
Pharmacist working in secondary care clinic or ward	• Ensure you take an accurate medication history, including mental health medicines prescribed by mental health team • Identify if bipolar medicines are responsible for admission – be able to identify signs of toxicity • Advise team on when to take plasma level and be able to interpret and advise on result • Identify and advise on possible drug interaction and provide advice on alternative medicines if appropriate • Be aware of signs and symptoms of relapse and know where to refer patient • Be aware of monitoring for bipolar medicines, ensure this is done and be able to interpret results and offer advice if any abnormalities • Counsel patients on medicines they are prescribed and compliance • Ensure patient has adequate supply of medicine • On discharge liaise with community mental health team and GP to ensure smooth transition of care
Independent prescriber working within hospital/clinic	• Ensure you take an accurate medication history • Be aware of potential drug interactions and how to manage them • Discuss compliance and adverse effects and toxicity of bipolar drugs • Be aware of signs and symptoms of toxicity and where to refer if needed • Be aware of contact for patient's community mental health team and ensure documentation of your review is sent to them as well as patient's GP • Be able to identify if presenting complaint is maybe an adverse effect of mood stabiliser • Be aware of signs of relapse and know where to refer if you suspect these • Discuss healthy eating and lifestyle, provide advice on alcohol and smoking cessation

Table 4.4: *Input from pharmacists in different setting (continued)*

Pharmacist role	Interventions
Specialist mental health pharmacist	• Meet with patient to review past medicines and response and assess for adverse effects • Identify and be aware of drug interactions and provide advice on how to manage them • Provide advice on how to manage adverse effects and provide advice to psychiatrist about alternative treatments if adverse effects are severe or not tolerable • Identify potential barriers to compliance and advise psychiatrist how to manage these • Identify possible relapse indicators and refer to psychiatrist • Liaise with GP and community pharmacy about medication issues
Independent prescriber with mental health within their scope of practice	• Review patient's mental state and adverse effects and prescribe medication as appropriate • Ensure accurate medication history is taken prior to prescribing • Liaise with GP and other HCP to communicate your prescribing • Assess patient's compliance and barriers to compliance and use this to help guide your prescribing • Request patient's physical health monitoring and review results to guide your prescribing • If abnormalities identified in the results, provide advice or refer to specialist for further input

Medicines

When reviewing a patient with bipolar, consider their current prescribed medication and symptoms, as well as potential adverse effects. Ask about their current mood as this could help identify early relapse features or unresolved symptoms.

If the patient's mood is low, they may be isolating themselves; consider a depressive relapse – early detection and a medical review could help prevent a long-term problem. If their mood is elevated, they may appear erratic and chaotic; consider a manic relapse – again, early detection may help prevent a long-term or severe episode and avoid hospital admission.[13]

Ask about compliance – you may suspect non-compliance (e.g. if they are not collecting prescriptions regularly). This may need escalating as compliance plays a vital role in ensuring the patient's condition is managed.[15] There may be many reasons for non-compliance and it is important to explore this with your patient during their review.[7] With lithium, sodium valproate and carbamazepine you can determine compliance by taking plasma levels.[2] With other medicines, where plasma levels are not available, then an honest discussion is needed to determine compliance.[3]

While compliance can be a difficult subject to raise, there are also other difficult but important areas to discuss during a review. These are listed in *Table 4.5*.

Pharmacists have an important role in ensuring patients are aware of the main adverse effects of their medicines and the monitoring requirements. Particularly with mood stabilisers, awareness of adverse effects can prevent toxicity and ensure the patient seeks advice when required, enabling them to access suitable care. Ensuring patients are aware of the available treatment options will help them to become compliant with medication – increasing compliance is one of the greatest ways to prevent relapse in patients with bipolar.[3]

Patients prescribed lithium should be issued with a purple book (available from MHRA).[16] This provides information about adverse effects and monitoring, and is also a place to record any physical health monitoring.[16] It is important to ensure all monitoring has been completed before any additional lithium is given to the patient. It can help prompt discussion with them about the monitoring requirements and when this was last carried out. The book should be used by pharmacists to ensure it is safe and appropriate to dispense lithium.

Patients with mental health problems have poorer physical health than their counterparts, and the medicines which they are prescribed can also impact on their physical health.[17,18] It is therefore important to ensure patients are aware of the physical health monitoring that is required when they are taking these medicines and that they keep up-to-date with the monitoring.[3]

- For community pharmacists, this would include liaising with the patient and their GP to ensure that the required monitoring has been carried out prior to dispensing of repeat prescriptions.
- For pharmacists working within the CCG or GP practices, this would include ensuring GPs are aware of monitoring requirements for psychotropic medications and checking these are carried out as part of audit, as well as part of patient medication reviews.
- For pharmacists working within secondary care setting, this would include ensuring blood tests and monitoring are completed when patients are under their care, reviewing these results and advising the prescribers on the outcome.
- For independent prescribing pharmacists, this may include requesting bloods and sending patients for these tests, as well as discussing the results with the patient and providing advice on the results.

Table 4.5: *Review questions and how to ask them*

Topic	Reason for asking this	Example of how to ask	Action required
Compliance	<ul><li>To check if they are taking medication, as non-compliance could result in relapse</li><li>To determine reasons for non-compliance (e.g. adverse effects)</li></ul>	<ul><li>Do you have any problems taking your medicines?</li><li>Do you take all your medicines every day?</li><li>Are there some medicines you sometimes miss?</li></ul>	<ul><li>Have an honest and open discussion about compliance</li><li>Explain benefits of taking medication</li><li>Refer to discuss changes to medicines if experiencing adverse effects</li></ul>
Assessment of mental state	<ul><li>To ensure patient is stable</li><li>To check that patient is not relapsing</li></ul>	<ul><li>How would you describe your mood?</li><li>Do you feel well?</li><li>Do you feel like you did when you became unwell in the past?</li><li>Is anything troubling you?</li></ul>	<ul><li>If relapse or deterioration is suspected, you may need to inform the mental health team</li><li>If patient doing well, acknowledge this and explore what has been helpful</li></ul>
Assessment of risk	<ul><li>If you suspect patient is unwell, are they at risk of harm to themselves or other?</li></ul>	<ul><li>Consider using a phrase like: I know these questions may be difficult to answer but I have to ask them.<ul><li>Have you had any thoughts about harming yourself?</li><li>Do you have any thoughts about harming others?</li><li>Do you have any plans to end your life?</li></ul></li></ul>	<ul><li>Answers will determine the urgency of referral</li><li>You may need to ask more questions about plans and intentions and protective factors if someone has plans for suicide</li></ul>
Drug and alcohol use	<ul><li>These may affect medication, and/or mental state</li></ul>	<ul><li>Do you use any illegal drugs?</li><li>Do you drink alcohol? (ask about quantity and strengths)</li></ul>	<ul><li>For risk management you need to determine what and how much</li><li>You can use tools to help (e.g. audit for alcohol)</li><li>Think about risks of withdrawal</li></ul>
Physical health	<ul><li>Physical health conditions may affect mood</li><li>Physical health may affect medicines</li></ul>	<ul><li>Do you have any other health problems?</li><li>Do you see any other specialists?</li></ul> Medication history may be useful here	<ul><li>You may need to make GP or specialists aware of other conditions that may affect prescribing and choice of drug</li><li>You may need to ensure they have had regular health checks</li></ul>

Lithium

Lithium is the treatment of choice for prophylaxis of bipolar – it lessens frequency, duration and severity of episodes and so is considered the most effective agent for prophylaxis.[2,4] Lithium has demonstrated efficacy in the acute phase, however, its use in this phase is limited by the fact that it requires a slower titration and it often takes 10-14 days before its effects are seen.[19,20] In acutely unwell patients, it is usually initiated after the initial antipsychotics which are beneficial in the manic stage because of their sedating effects.[4,19] Lithium should be considered the first choice for monotherapy as it has best empirical evidence and is recommended by NICE.[4]

The narrow therapeutic range and complex adverse effects often limits the use of lithium. There is a clear correlation between plasma levels and efficacy, as well as toxicity.[20]

The monitoring requirements for lithium are outlined in *Table 4.6*.

Table 4.6: *Monitoring requirements for lithium*[3,4,19]

Monitoring	Baseline level required	Frequency	Purpose
Lithium level	5-7 days after initiation (time to steady state)	Every 2 weeks until stable, then 3-6 monthly If adverse effects experienced After dose changes	Monitor for efficacy and toxicity (see *Box 4.1*) Acute phase or repeat relapse 0.8-1.0 mmol/L Prophylactic 0.4-0.8 mmol/L
Renal: urea & electrolytes (U&Es)	Yes	Every 3-6 months If renal damage suspected	Check for transient polyuria, diabetes insipidus or Kidney damage
Thyroid levels	Yes	Every 6 months	T4 may be reduced TSH may be increased
Calcium levels	Yes	Every 6 months	Calcium levels may be increased. This may be more prominent in the first 4 weeks
Heart: ECG	Yes	Every 6 months	There may be reversible T wave changes
Weight/BMI	Yes	Every 6 months	Weight gain is a common adverse effect

When monitoring lithium levels:[20]
- Serum lithium levels should be taken 12 hours post-dose. This is taken as a venous blood sample and can be processed by local laboratories, so the results are usually available within 24 hours.
- For patients on twice daily dosing, the level should be taken immediately before the next dose is due.
- For patients on once daily dosing, the lithium is usually taken at night and the plasma level taken in the morning.[20]
- It takes 5-7 days for lithium to reach steady state, so plasma levels should be taken 5-7 days following dose changes or changes to formulation or lithium brand, due to differences in bioavailability.

Box 4.1: Lithium toxicity[3,19]

- Levels above 1.5 mmol/L are regarded as toxic, and if not treated, this toxicity can lead to weakness, acute renal failure, seizures, coma and death.
- Toxic levels can be initiated by renal failure, overdose, dehydration, reduced salt intake or drug interactions.
- Signs and symptoms of toxicity include course tremor, sedation, diarrhoea and vomiting, tinnitus, worsening of other adverse effects, vertigo and feeling cold.

Most of the lithium is excreted unchanged in the urine, and in a healthy adult, the half-life is normally between 10-24 hours.[20] Due to the long half-life, prolonged release preparations are not required. However, they are preferable as their slower absorption results in a reduced risk of high peak plasma levels which helps reduce adverse effects.[10,20]

Valproate

Depakote (semisodium valproate) is currently the only licensed form of valproate in the UK for management of mania associated with bipolar, as well as continuation when there is an initial response.[2,21] Semisodium valproate is the prodrug of sodium valproate – there are only minor differences in the pharmacokinetics of semisodium valproate and sodium valproate. In the plasma, both drugs are converted into valproic acid which is what is measured by therapeutic drug monitoring.[2]

Sodium valproate is teratogenic and is associated with significant birth defects and developmental disorders in children who are born to women who take valproate whilst pregnant. In the UK, prescribing valproate to women of childbearing age is contraindicated unless there is no alternative and the woman is on the pregnancy prevention programme.[22]

If lithium is ineffective as monotherapy then considerations should be given to adding valproate to current therapy; if lithium is not tolerated or inappropriate, then valproate can be used first line.[4,23] The monitoring requirements for valproate are outlined in *Table 4.7*.

Table 4.7: *Valproate monitoring*[3,4,23]

Monitoring	Baseline level required	Frequency	Purpose
Valproic acid level	No	As indicated if non-compliance and toxicity suspected	In bipolar only it is indicative of compliance and toxicity, not efficacy Aim for 50-100 mg/L
Liver function tests (LFTs)	Yes	6-12 months	Check for hepatic failure and severe liver damage (rare)
Full blood count (FBC)	Yes	Annually	Check for agranulocytosis and thrombocytopenia (rare)
Pregnancy test	Yes for women	Women signed up to PPP	Valproate is teratogenic
Weight/BMI	Yes	Repeat when necessary	Weight gain is a common adverse effect

Valproate levels are not routinely required; however, they may be useful if non-compliance, infectiveness or toxicity is suspected. Valproate reaches steady state after 2-3 days, the level should be taken at the trough, so 12 hours post-dose or prior to next dose if twice daily dosing.[24]

Lamotrigine

Lamotrigine appears to be useful in depressive aspects of the illness;[2,4] it has a licence in the UK for prophylaxis for patients with predominant episodes of depression in bipolar I.[21] In bipolar I, lamotrigine should be used in combination with another antimanic medication, but it should not be used in acute mania as it is not effective for this indication,[2] and the requirements for its slow titration mean it will take a number of weeks to reach therapeutic doses. However, it can be used as monotherapy in bipolar II.[25]

Lamotrigine should be slowly titrated over 6 weeks to a maintenance dose to avoid dermatological problems. The patient should be advised to report any rash during initiation and maintenance treatment. Its use is also limited by headaches, dizziness and visual problems.[3,25] The monitoring requirements for lamotrigine are outlined in *Table 4.8*.

Table 4.8: *Lamotrigine monitoring*[24]

Monitoring	Baseline	Frequency	Purpose
Lamotrigine levels	No		
LFTs	Yes	Annually	Check for hepatic failure and severe liver damage (rare)
FBC	Yes	Annually Repeat FBC if sign and symptoms of blood dyscrasia	Check for blood dyscrasia (rare)
Weight/BMI	Yes	Aged <18 years: monthly for 6 months then every 6 months Not required in over 18s	Weight gain is an uncommon adverse effect
U&Es	Yes	Annually	Check for renal impairment (dose adjustments necessary)
Rashes	Advise patient to be aware of skin reactions/rash	Ongoing review	Severe rashes are a common adverse effect – more common at start of treatment

Carbamazepine

Carbamazepine is also not recommended within the current NICE guidelines for treatment of bipolar.[4] The evidence for efficacy is poor; it is probably only effective in preventing manic relapses.[19] Moreover, it is an enzyme-inducing drug causing numerous drug interactions and so is unsuitable for many patients.[2,26]

Carbamazepine has however been used for many years for prophylaxis of bipolar disorder. Clinical experience suggests its efficacy is similar to lithium, but with superiority in treating rapid cycling bipolar,[2] although this is not endorsed by NICE.[4] It is effective in the acute phase or prophylactically, and can be used alone when lithium is not effective or tolerated, or in combination with lithium or antipsychotics.[2,3]

It is recommended to start at a low dose and increase gradually to avoid the adverse effects of dizziness and nausea which can be problematic when starting therapy.[26] Like lamotrigine, there is a risk of a rash which must be monitored as it could indicate leukopenia or Stevens-Johnson syndrome which limits its use.[26]

Other treatments

Gabapentin and topiramate are not recommended by NICE[4] to treat bipolar disorder due to a lack of robust evidence for efficacy.

Medication changes

Adverse effects

Details on the common adverse effects of drugs used to treat bipolar and how to manage them are outlined in *Table 4.9*.

Table 4.9: *Adverse effects of mood stabilisers and how to manage them*[19,23,24,25]

Medication	Adverse effect	Treatment options
Lithium	Tremor	Mild: not dangerous — consider prescribing propranolol/atenolol if appropriate Severe: could be an indication of toxicity. Patient would require lithium levels measured and lithium withheld until levels reviewed
	GI disturbance Mild: nausea, pain Severe: diarrhoea, vomiting	Mild: should be transient, prescribe symptomatic medicines Severe: could indicate toxicity, patient would require a lithium level measured and lithium withheld until levels reviewed
	Polydipsia	Advise patients to drink water, suck or chew sugar-free gum or sweets Arrange blood tests if severe
	Weight gain	Advise patients to control diet and exercise. Signpost patient to dietician and NHS websites
Sodium valproate	Increased appetite, weight gain	Advise patients to control diet and exercise, and signpost to dietician and NHS websites
	GI disturbance	Advise patients to take with or after food. Consider using a modified release (MR) formulation which may reduce peaks in plasma levels
	Hair loss	This can be distressing. Advise patients that usually hair regrows, although it can return curly
	Sleepiness	Change the timing of dose to night, measure levels and reduce dose if possible
Lamotrigine	Sleepiness	Change timing of the dose to night or take larger dose at night
	Dizziness	Advise patient that this is normally transient and to stand up slowly
	Rash	Serious adverse effect. Stop medication and contact prescriber. As an independent prescriber you would need to refer back to consultant for alternative medication and review
	Increased bruising/bleeding	Could be bone marrow suppression, which is a serious adverse effect – arrange blood test; if confirmed, stop medication and contact prescriber. If independent prescriber, may need to refer back to consultant
Carbamazepine	Sleepiness	Change timing of the dose or try the modified release preparation
	Dizziness	Advise patient that this is normally transient and to stand up slowly
	Rash	Serious adverse effect – stop carbamazepine and contact prescriber
	Sore throat/bruising	Could be agranulocytosis/thrombocytopenia, which is a serious adverse effect – arrange a blood test; if confirmed, stop medication and contact prescriber. If independent prescriber, may require referral back to consultant

Relapse prevention

The British Association of Psychopharmacology[2] advises that if an identified stressor is present or imminent, or if the patient is displaying early signs of relapse, then a short-term medication could be added to current treatment for example (e.g. a hypnotic to aid sleep, or a benzodiazepine to help anxiety). There is also an option to increase doses of regular medicines within BNF limits and if plasma levels allow.[2,4] This could be part of a patient's relapse prevention plan.

Stopping medication

The risk of relapse remains even if patients have been in remission for a long time, therefore this should be considered if the medication is to be discontinued.[2,4] If there is a clinical need to stop or change medication, then this should be done slowly and the patient should be monitored for signs of relapse – they should be seen by a healthcare professional for a mental state examination at least 2 weeks following a dose reduction and then at least monthly for 6 months following the discontinuation.

This may vary depending on the individual, and monitoring frequency may depend on risks during relapse and previous medication reductions. However, if the patient develops mania from an antidepressant or lithium toxicity, these medications may need to be stopped suddenly.[3,4] In these cases, monitoring for mental state would be more frequent.Patients should be made aware of signs and symptoms of relapse and what to do if these occur.[13]

Medication reduction should be done slowly over weeks to months and the patient's mental state should continue to be monitored even after the medication has stopped. Early relapse to mania is a common adverse effect of discontinuation of lithium, therefore it should be done cautiously.[20]

Drug interactions

Table 4.10 outlines the main drug interactions for mood stabilisers and how to manage them.

Managing special groups

Older adults

Older adults may be more sensitive to adverse effects of medicines compared to younger people, and as they have poorer renal function they are at a higher risk of developing lithium toxicity – the half-life of lithium is increased two-fold in the elderly, therefore it is recommended to start at a lower dose and titrate at a slower rate than in younger adults with additional monitoring.[20] They are also likely to have more comorbidities and so be taking more medicines which may interact with their mood stabilisers.[7]

If valproate is prescribed to older adults they should be closely monitored for sedation and effects on their motor function.[24] Care must be used when prescribing anticholinergic medication such as procyclidine and other medicines with high cholinergic burden due to the anticholinergic effect on cognition and mobility.[7,29]

Women of childbearing potential

All women of childbearing age with bipolar should be given the opportunity to discuss contraception and family planning as not only are there risks from certain medicines during pregnancy, but pregnancy and postpartum can be stressful and there is a risk of relapse.[30]

The use of mood stabilisers, such as lithium and sodium valproate, in early pregnancy increases the risk of congenital malformations and may affect the neurodevelopment of the infant. The risk increases with the use of more than one mood stabiliser; therefore, combinations of mood stabilisers should be avoided.[4,30]

Some medicines used to treat bipolar may reduce fertility[30] – there is an increased incidence of polycystic ovary syndrome with valproate (reversible on stopping medication)[24], and some antipsychotics can increase prolactin which may impair ovulation.[4,30]

Table 4.10: *Main drug interactions for mood stabilisers and how to manage them*[19,23,24,25,27,28]

Medication	Main interaction route	Increased levels	Decreased levels	Others
Lithium	Drugs that are renally excreted	Reduced renal clearance: NSAID, ACE inhibitor, angiotensin II receptor antagonists Water retention: antidiuretics, tetracyclines	Increased lithium clearance: xanthines, sodium bicarbonate containing products, diuretics, urea, calcitonin	Additive neurotoxic effects: antipsychotics, carbamazepine, methyldopa, calcium channel blockers Drugs which prolong QTc interval: antipsychotics, methadone and some antibiotics Drugs which cause serotonin syndrome: antidepressants, tramadol and triptans Drugs which lower seizure threshold: antipsychotics, ciprofloxacin and tramadol
Sodium valproate	CYP enzymes CYP substrate and inhibitor	Enzyme inhibitors: rifampicin Highly protein bound drugs: aspirin	Levels decreased by enzyme inducers: carbamazepine, phenytoin and antimalarial drugs	Sodium valproate is an enzyme inducer and increases plasma levels of various drugs including carbamazepine and lamotrigine. May potentiate effects of psychotropics in particular olanzapine Adverse effects such as sedation may be exacerbated
Carbamazepine	CYP3A4	Inhibitors of CYP enzymes will increase levels of carbamazepine	Inducers of CYP enzymes will reduce levels	Carbamazepine is an enzyme inducer and so can reduce the plasma level of a number of medicines. e.g. warfarin, antipsychotics such as clozapine and antiepileptics such as sodium valproate Structurally similar to tricyclics, therefore cannot be given within 2 weeks of MAOI antidepressant
Lamotrigine	CYP enzymes	Sodium valproate inhibits glucuronidation of lamotrigine, therefore a reduced dosage regimen is required for lamotrigine when they are used in combination	Medicines which induce enzymes such as carbamazepine will reduce plasma levels of lamotrigine, therefore a special dosage regimen is require for lamotrigine	Lamotrigine does not significantly induce or inhibit CYP enzymes

Children and young people

Diagnosis in children and young people can be challenging as there are no specific diagnostic criteria for this age group and differential diagnosis with other childhood conditions can complicate the diagnosis.[2] The evidence for the use of medicines for children with bipolar is limited – most medicines used to treat bipolar are not licensed for use in children with the exception of lithium (licensed for those aged over 12 years)[20] and aripiprazole.[31,32]

In children prescribing of psychotropics, in general, should start at lower doses which should be guided by the BNF for Children, and they should be monitored closely for adverse effects as they are more prone to developing these.[2,31] Children are at an increased risk of switching into mania if they are prescribed an antidepressant, so these are usually avoided.[2]

Referral

Information on when to refer people with bipolar and the urgency required are detailed in *Table 4.11*.

Table 4.11: *When to refer*

When	Where	Urgency
You suspect someone is becoming unwell Signs of mania or depression	Mental health team – this can be done via the GP, or via community mental health team	Same day referral (with patient agreement) to prevent relapse
Adverse effects from medicines	Prescriber – they can offer advice (e.g. if sedating, take the medication at night) The choice and medication website available from local trust has lot of helpful advice on how to manage adverse effects[9]	Depends on severity – can advise person to discuss at their next clinical appointment unless severe
Suspected toxicity	A&E	Needs urgent blood tests and advice; advise to attend for blood test that day
Risk of harm to self or others	A&E	Immediately via ambulance or police
Patient wishes to change medicines	Prescriber	Advise person to discuss at next appointment – or you can contact prescriber and pass on their advice

Useful management advice

Box 4.2: Useful management advice

- Antidepressants should be discontinued if mania is suspected.
- Lithium is the most effective long-term treatment for bipolar and should be considered first line if not contraindicated.
- Lithium may not be the most appropriate treatment for patients in whom compliance is an issue.
- Lithium should be prescribed by brand due to its difference in bioavailability.
- Valproate should not be prescribed for women of childbearing age due to the risks of teratogenic risks associated with its use in pregnancy.[33]
  - If there is no suitable alternative and the woman of childbearing age agrees that sodium valproate is the best option, then she should be counselled on the risks and adequate contraception should also be prescribed.
- Carbamazepine interacts with many medicines – this should be considered if carbamazepine is to be prescribed.
- Remember with bipolar it is about treating the condition not just the episode – try to involve the patient with decisions about medication as this will help with compliance.

Useful resources

- www.nice.org.uk contains the NICE guidelines: Bipolar, which is the national guidance on treating patients with bipolar.
- BAP guidelines: Bipolar Journal of Psychopharmacology 2016, Vol. 30(6) 495–553. DOI: 10.1177/0269881116636545. 'The British Association for Psychopharmacology guidelines specify the scope and targets of treatment for bipolar disorder. The third version is based explicitly on the available evidence and presented, like previous Clinical Practice Guidelines, as recommendations to aid clinical decision making for practitioners: it may also serve as a source of information for patients and carers, and assist audit.'
- www.time-to-change.org.uk aims to reduce stigma associated with mental health. It provides information for patients and carers about mental health, includes fact sheets and real life stories – it hopes to bring an end to mental health discrimination.
- www.choiceandmedication.org offers patient information on medicines used in mental health, as well as handy fact sheets about mental health conditions, side effects and comparison charts for medications.
- www.rethink.org is a charity for people with mental illness and those who care for them.
- www.mind.org.uk is a mental health charity. Their website provides advice and directs patients to places where they can seek extra help.
- www.youngminds.org.uk is aimed at young people with mental health – it advises on mental health medications and conditions.

References

1. Mind and Rethink. Time to Change (2018). Mental health-bipolar. www.time-to-change.org.uk
2. Goodwin GM *et al*. Evidence based guidelines for treating bipolar disorder: revised third edition - recommendations from the British Association for Psychopharmacology. *Journal of Psychopharmacology* 2016; 30(6): 495-553.
3. Bleakley S, Henry, R. Understanding bipolar disorder. Pharmaceutical Journal 2010. www.pharmaceutical-journal.com/learning/learning-article/understanding-bipolar-disorder/11006346.article
4. National Institute for Health and Care Excellence (2014). Bipolar disorder: the assessment and management of bipolar disorder in adults, children and young people in primary and secondary care. www.nice.org.uk/guidance/cg185
5. Geeky medics (2018). Mental state examination: OSCE guide. www.geekymedics.com/mental-state-examination
6. World Health Organization (1992). The ICD-10 classification of mental and behavioural disorders. Geneva: World Health Organization.
7. National Institute for Health and Care Excellence (2015). Medicines optimisation: the safe and effective use of medicines to enable the best possible outcomes. www.nice.org.uk/guidance/ng5
8. Rethink mental illness (2018). The mental health act 1983. UK: Rethink mental illness. www.rethink.org/advice-and-information/rights-restrictions/mental-health-laws/mental-health-act-1983
9. Taylor D *et al. Maudsley prescribing guideline*, 13th edn. UK: Willey-Blackwell, 2018.
10. Choice and medication (2019). Information about medications. Mistura Enterprise Ltd. www.choiceandmedication.org
11. Rang, H *et al. Rang and Dale's pharmacology*. Edinburgh: Elsevier, Churchill Livingstone, 2016.
12. Mitchell PB *et al*. The management of bipolar disorder in general practice. *Medical Journal of Australia* 2006; 184(11): 566.
13. Perry A *et al*. A randomized controlled trial of the efficacy of teaching patients with bipolar mood disorder to identify early symptoms of relapse and obtain treatment. *BMJ* 1999; 318: 149-153.
14. Bipolar caregivers (2013). Helping with bipolar warning signs. www.bipolarcaregivers.org/supporting-the-person/helping-with-bipolar-warning-signs
15. Colom F *et al*. Clinical factors associated with treatment noncompliance in euthymic bipolar patients. *J Clin Psychiatry* 2000; 61: 549-555.

16. National patient safety agency (2009). Safer lithium therapy (archived). www.sps.nhs.uk/articles/npsa-alert-safer-lithium-therapy-2009

17. Harris E, Barraclough B. Excess mortality of mental disorder. *British Journal of Psychiatry* 1998; 173(1): 11-53.

18. Mental Health foundation (2018). Physical health and mental health. www.mentalhealth.org.uk/a-to-z/p/physical-health-and-mental-health

19. Cipriani A *et al*. Comparative efficacy and acceptability of antimanic drugs in acute mania: a multiple-treatments meta-analysis. *Lancet* 2011; 378: 1306-1315.

20. Summary of Product Characteristics for Lithium LI-Liquid 509 mg/mL (2018). www.medicines.org.uk

21. Joint Formulary Committee (2019). British National Formulary. London: British Medical Association and Royal Pharmaceutical Society of Great Britain. www.bnf.nice.org.uk

22. MHRA (2019). Drug Safety Update: Valproate use by women and girls. www.gov.uk/guidance/valproate-use-by-women-and-girls

23. Geddes JR *et al*. Lithium plus valproate combination therapy versus monotherapy for relapse prevention in bipolar I disorder (BALANCE): a randomised open-label trial. *Lancet* 2010; 375: 385-95.

24. Summary of Product Characteristics for Epilim 500 mg gastro-resistant tablets (2018). www.medicines.org.uk

25. Summary of Product Characteristics for Lamictal tablets (2018). www.medicines.org.uk

26. Summary of Product Characteristics for Tegretol 200 mg tablets (2019). www.medicines.org.uk

27. Cleare A *et al*. Evidence-based guidelines for treating depressive disorders with antidepressants: A revision of the 2008 British Association for Psychopharmacology guidelines. *J Psychopharmacol* 2016; 29: 459-525.

28. MedicinesComplete. Stockley's Interactions Checker. www.medicinescomplete.com

29. Boustani M *et al*. Impact of anticholinergics on the aging brain; a review and practical application. *Aging Health* 2008; 4:3; 311-20.

30. National Institute for Health and Care Excellence (2014). Antenatal and Postnatal Mental Health. www.nice.org.uk/guidance/cg192

31. Pediatrics Formulary Committee (2019). British National Formulary for Children. London: British Medical Association and Royal Pharmaceutical Society of Great Britain. www.bnf.nice.org.uk

32. National Institute for Health and Care Excellence (2103). Aripiprazole for treating moderate to severe manic episodes in adolescents with bipolar I disorder. NICE technology appraisal guidance 292.

33. UKTIS (2019). Best use of medicines in pregnancy. www.toxbase.org/Bumps/Medicine--pregnancy

Case studies

Case study 1

Ben, aged 55 years, attends the pharmacy to buy some analgesia – he tells you he would like some more ibuprofen as he has been using his wife's supply for the last week and now there is none left. He explains that he twisted his ankle last week playing golf, but since he started taking the ibuprofen he has been feeling nauseous and dizzy.

He asks whether this is a known side effect and tells you he has bipolar and that he takes a mood stabiliser. Ben gives you permission to check his Summary Care Record (SCR) and you can see that he is taking lithium.

Points to consider

- Are nausea and dizziness adverse effects of ibuprofen?
- Are nausea and dizziness adverse effects of lithium?
- Is there an interaction between ibuprofen and lithium? If so, what is the likely outcome?
- Which reference sources would you consult?

You explain to him that there is an interaction between lithium and ibuprofen and suspect that the effects he has been feeling may be signs of high lithium levels.

Points to consider

- What is the correct therapeutic range for lithium?
- What can contribute to high lithium levels?
- What are signs or symptoms of lithium toxicity?
- What are the consequences of high lithium levels?
- Which reference sources would you consult?

You ask to see his lithium book, but he does not have it with him and says he last had his levels checked a few months ago.

Points to consider

- How often should lithium levels be checked?
- What other monitoring is required for patients taking lithium?

You advise him not to take any more ibuprofen, but to use paracetamol instead for his pain and to use the RICE principles (rest, ice, compression and elevation). You advise him to attend his GP practice to get his lithium level checked.

Ben takes your advice and his lithium levels were found to be raised: 1.15 mmol/L (prophylactic range is 0.4-0.8 mmol/L). The GP advised him to omit his lithium for one day and stop taking ibuprofen.

Ben comes back to see you next week and you have a meeting about his lithium – you talk through his purple book and discuss signs and symptoms of toxicity and what to do if he experiences them. You also discuss other potential drug interactions, as well as diet and fluid intake which can also affect levels.

Points to consider

- Are there any additional sources of information you can direct Ben to?

Case study 2

Hannah, aged 26 years, is admitted to the emergency department. She was found in central London climbing on a monument and shouting.

You are a pharmacist working on the medical admission unit (MAU) where she has been admitted. It is suspected that she has an infection as she has a raised white blood cell count (WBC) and an elevated temperature. Her partner, Simon, has come into the hospital to see her and has brought in her medicines.

You speak to her about her medication prior to admission to complete her medicines reconciliation. She gives you permission to access her Summary Care Record (SCR) and you see she is prescribed carbamazepine 800 mg twice daily and procyclidine 5 mg twice daily; you are aware this is often used to treat adverse effects of antipsychotics, but there are no antipsychotics prescribed on her SCR. However, there is a record of adverse drug reactions:

- Olanzapine – weight gain
- Risperidone – raised prolactin
- Allergy to penicillin – rash

> **Points to consider**
>
> - Are the doses of prescribed medicines within the normal range?
> - How would you verify whether Hannah is receiving antipsychotic treatment?
> - Why would details of antipsychotic treatment not be listed in the SCR?

Hannah gives you permission to speak with her partner, Simon, so you ask him about antipsychotics and he tells you she also gets an injection from her community mental health team and you know these are often not included on SCRs. You contact the team and find out she is on zuclopenthixol decanoate 400 mg every four weeks – she is due a dose next week.

You ask her about illicit drugs and alcohol use, and she tells you she does not use these. However, when you ask about OTC medicines, she explains that her mood was low recently, so she took a herbal medicine for depression and this made her feel a lot better.

> **Points to consider**
>
> - What OTC medicines interact with carbamazepine?
> - What herbal products interact with carbamazepine?
> - What is the mechanism of the interaction?
> - What are the consequences of any interactions?
> - Which reference sources would you consult?

She reports that since then she has had a lot of energy and is now able to do a lot more. You notice she is wearing bright clothes and she is speaking rapidly. Simon tells you that she has not slept properly for the last two nights.

> **Points to consider**
>
> - Given Hannah's symptoms, what is the likely explanation?

You suspect she may be relapsing in her mental state. You ask Simon about the herbal product and he shows you the box as he has brought it in with him. You also ask the psychiatric liaison team to see her as you feel her mood is elated.

On checking the patient's own medication you note the herbal medication is St John's wort. You know this interacts with carbamazepine and can lower plasma levels, and as it is thought to act as an antidepressant, it has the risk of switching her mood from low to high.

Points to consider

- What reference source would you use to check the normal therapeutic levels for carbamazepine?
- What references can you use to look up usage, adverse effects and interactions of herbal medicines?

You ask the ward to take carbamazepine levels and they come back as low, 1 mg/L (after checking the BNF, you see that the range for optimum response is 4-12 mg/L).

You speak to Hannah and Simon and advise that she should not to take the St John's wort and explain why. She is started on an antibiotic for her infection – doxycycline as this is not a CYP inhibitor (unlike macrolides) and does therefore not interact with her carbamazepine.

Hannah is referred to the home treatment team who will manage her mental health at home and she is given zopiclone to help with her sleep. Prior to discharge you counsel her on the use of herbal medicines and the risk of drug interactions, and discuss adverse effects of carbamazepine and the monitoring requirements.

Case study 3

Fiona, aged 34 years, attends your prescribing clinic within the GP surgery for a prescription of her asthma inhalers. On taking her history she tells you she has been taking sodium valproate MR 1000 mg at night for four years since she had an admission to hospital for a relapse of her bipolar. She is aware of the teratogenic risks of sodium valproate and is currently on the contraceptive implant.

Points to consider

- Is the dose of sodium valproate within the normal therapeutic range?
- What reference sources would you consult to get advice about use of valproate in women of childbearing age?
- What other counselling points might you consider for someone on sodium valproate?

You discuss the main side effects of valproate and she is aware of these, she also knows to seek medical advice if she suspects she has an infection or sore throat as this could be a sign of agranulocytosis.

During the discussion, Fiona mentions she has a new partner and they have been discussing having a family in the future and that she knows that if she wants a family she should stop the sodium valproate. She asks how long after stopping valproate she can start trying for a family.

Points to consider

- How should the situation be managed?
- What reference sources would you consult to determine how to achieve Fiona's aims while ensuring she gets treatment she requires?
- What are the possible options?

You discuss with her the risks of stopping medication and risks of relapse – she is still currently seeing a psychiatrist in community and has a care co-ordinator. You explain that it may be best to discuss the issue with them as they may wish to put her on a different mood stabiliser which is safe to use in pregnancy, or they may wish to reduce the valproate slowly and monitor her more closely before they advise stopping the medication and trying for a baby.

Points to consider

- What reference sources would you consult to check whether medicines are safe to use in pregnancy?

Fiona agrees this is a good idea and will make a plan to go and see the team. You refer her to the BUMPS (best use of medication in pregnancy) website which has lots of information about use of medications in pregnancy as well as the choice and medication website specific to her trust, where she can look at different mood stabiliser options.

She comes back to see you in three months and the team have agreed to switch her to aripiprazole which she has now been on for two months. She feels well and plans to have her contraceptive implant removed next month. The team cross tapered her sodium valproate to aripiprazole and monitored her mental state more closely during this time.

You discuss adverse effects of aripiprazole with her and ask her to complete a GASS (Glasgow Antipsychotic Side effect Scale) tool. She is happy with the outcome and that she was involved in the decisions about her medication and felt empowered to be able to discuss this with her mental health team.

CHAPTER 5

Coronary heart disease

Helen Williams

Overview

Coronary heart disease (CHD) is a general term for a spectrum of diseases of the heart caused by insufficient blood supply to the heart muscle e.g. atherosclerotic coronary artery disease (CAD), angina and acute coronary syndromes (ACS) which comprise unstable angina, non-ST elevation and ST-elevation myocardial infarction. CHD can also be referred to as ischaemic heart disease (IHD), and is one of the group of related conditions known collectively as cardiovascular disease (CVD), which also includes cerebrovascular disease (stroke and transient ischaemic attack) and peripheral arterial disease.

CHD occurs when the demand for blood and oxygen by the heart muscle exceeds the supply. With increased demand, for example under emotional stress or physical exertion, an insufficient supply of oxygenated blood to the heart muscle manifests as chest pain or discomfort, known as angina.

A reduced flow of blood to the heart muscle is most often caused by the build-up of cholesterol-rich plaques which narrows the blood vessels – this is known as atherosclerosis. Other causes of reduced flow of blood to the heart muscle include blood clots (thrombus) or constriction of the coronary arteries. If the artery becomes partially or fully occluded, it can lead to a myocardial infarction (MI), which is a medical emergency and is usually characterised by crushing chest pain radiating to the left arm and/or neck/jaw, breathlessness, a cold sweat, nausea and dizziness.

CHD is one of the UK's leading causes of death and the most common cause of premature death (deaths below the age of 75 years). It is responsible for around 64,000 deaths in the UK each year which equates to an average of 180 people each day, or one death around every 8 minutes. One in seven men and one in 12 women die from CHD.

In the UK more than 100,000 hospital admissions each year are due to MI; that's 280 admissions each day, or one admission for an MI every 5 minutes. In the 1960s more than 7 out of 10 heart attacks in the UK were fatal, however, today, at least 7 out of 10 people survive. It is estimated that around 1.4 million people alive in the UK today have survived a heart attack – around 1 million men and 380,000 women.[1]

CHD and other forms of CVD do not suddenly occur at the point a patient experiences a heart attack or a stroke or other symptoms – it develops asymptomatically over the decades beforehand. How quickly CVD develops depends on the modifiable and non-modifiable risk factors present for an individual, as well as the other comorbidities. See *Box 5.1* and *Box 5.2*.

Box 5.1: Practice point: risk factors for CHD

Risk factors that increase a person's risk of developing cardiovascular disease can be categorised as:
- Non-modifiable – these include older age, being male, family history of CVD, ethnic background (for example, people of South Asian origin have an increased risk of CVD compared with people of European origin), as well as socioeconomic status.
- Modifiable – these include smoking, high levels of non-high density lipoprotein (non-HDL) cholesterol, lack of physical activity, poor diet, excess alcohol intake and being overweight or obese.

> **Box 5.2: Practice point: comorbidities that increase risk of developing CHD[2]**
>
> - Hypertension
> - Diabetes mellitus
> - Chronic kidney disease
> - Dyslipidaemia
> - Rheumatoid arthritis
> - Influenza
> - Serious mental health problems
> - Periodontitis

In people without established CVD, a cardiovascular (CV) risk assessment should be undertaken using a validated risk assessment tool. Details of CV risk assessment can be found in **Chapter 12**. If CV risk assessment indicates that a patient is at significant risk of developing CVD, lifestyle modification, as well as drug therapies, such as statins and antihypertensive therapies, may be indicated, even before the patient has experienced any symptoms, to reduce the risk of experiencing a CV event. This is known as primary prevention and is aimed at delaying the onset of symptomatic CVD.

The remainder of this chapter will focus on the diagnosis and management of patients with established CHD.

Once a patient has become symptomatic with CHD, the prognosis is good if the disease is detected in the early stages. With aggressive lifestyle modification and appropriate medical therapy, patients can expect a reduction in anginal symptoms. Optimal medical therapy includes drugs to prevent a CV event – known as secondary prevention – plus anti-anginal therapies to prevent or reduce the frequency and severity of episodes of anginal pain. With optimal medical therapy, 58% of patients can expect to be free of angina within one year.[3]

Ischaemic heart disease is a dynamic process. Even with aggressive medical management and lifestyle changes, some patients may experience recurrence or worsening of anginal symptoms due to progression of atherosclerotic disease. Up-titration of anti-anginal medications may resolve these symptoms. Patients on optimal doses of two anti-anginal therapies who are still experiencing episodes of chest pain should be referred for consideration for revascularisation to improve symptom control – a third anti-anginal agent may be prescribed while the patient is waiting for cardiology review.[4]

> **Box 5.3: Practice point: coronary revascularisation**
>
> Coronary revascularisation is used to mechanically restore the supply of blood to the heart muscle.
> - Percutaneous coronary intervention (PCI) uses balloon angioplasty with or without insertion of a stent to widen the lumen of the coronary arteries and improve blood flow.
> - Coronary artery bypass grafting (CABG) is a surgical procedure in which the arterial blood flow is diverted through grafts which bypass the narrowed areas of the blood vessels. In the acute setting, such as myocardial infarction, early revascularisation with PCI reduces mortality and morbidity. In people with stable ischaemic heart disease, such as angina, revascularisation reduces symptoms and improves quality of life, but does not affect prognosis.

Diagnosis

The diagnosis of CHD begins with a thorough history, including an assessment of the frequency, type and severity of chest pain and any related symptoms. Patients with stable symptoms indicative of angina should be referred for a series of cardiac investigations to confirm or exclude the diagnosis.[5] Those with more acute symptoms, suggestive of acute coronary syndrome should be triaged accordingly, with transfer to the emergency department for urgent care.[5] Acute coronary syndromes include ST-elevation myocardial infarction (STEMI), non-ST elevation MI (NSTEMI) and unstable angina. Indicators of possible acute coronary syndromes include:

- known coronary artery disease
- clammy, unwell patient
- exertional chest pain
- heavy, tight, pressure type chest pain
- pain radiating to left arm, right shoulder or both arms
- association with nausea or vomiting
- known history of coronary artery disease
- family history of premature coronary artery disease
- male sex
- new electrocardiogram (ECG) changes: ST elevation, pathological Q waves, left bundle branch block (LBBB), ST depression, T wave inversion
- positive troponin.[6]

Acute ischaemic events will be accompanied by an increase in the blood levels of troponin, an enzyme indicating myocardial damage, as well as characteristic changes in the ECG. For example, a classic ST-elevation myocardial infarction will present with raised troponin and ST elevation on the ECG.

Pharmacy input

In order to delay the progression of CHD and reduce the risk of CV events, all pharmacists should support people to adopt a healthy lifestyle; for example, by offering advice on diet and physical activity, as well as providing smoking cessation services and weight management programmes.

Pharmacists should be aware of the potential for patients to present with stable or unstable symptoms of ischaemic heart disease and should ensure they are appropriately referred for further assessment and management.

Once diagnosed, the mainstay of therapy are medications designed to reduce the risk of future CV events. Pharmacists in acute care, general practice and the community setting should be able to support patients to adhere to their secondary prevention medications, with prescribers supporting drug and dose optimisation.

Pharmacy review

All patients with a diagnosis of CHD will need at least an annual review by primary care, and practice-based pharmacists are well placed to undertake this role, although other pharmacists may be able to do so depending on their skills and experience. Assessment should explore any symptoms of CHD that the patient may be experiencing. Ask about chest pain:

- Frequency
- Type
- Severity

Note whether these have changed since the last review, identify any specific precipitants of chest pain (such as exertion, cold weather or emotional stress) and ask how the pain responds to rest and/or to sublingual GTN. Enquire about other non-specific symptoms of ischaemic heart disease such as dizziness, fatigue, nausea, shortness of breath and sweating.

Patients whose symptoms have progressed may need:

- an increased dose of their existing anti-anginal therapy

- addition of another anti-anginal drug
- referral for a cardiology review with a view to revascularisation by percutaneous coronary intervention (PCI) or coronary artery bypass grafting (CABG).

Check the person's blood pressure (BP) while sitting and standing if they complain of dizziness or light headedness to identify a postural drop (>20 mmHg systolic BP drop on standing)[6] which may be exacerbated by anti-anginal therapy. Consider anti-anginals with little effect on BP, such as nitrates, nicorandil or ivabradine, if BP is low or there is a postural drop.

Perform blood tests including renal function, HbA1c, lipid levels and liver function tests.

Discuss lifestyle issues (diet, physical activity, body weight, smoking, alcohol intake) and encourage the patient to identify areas that they may wish to address. Refer them or signpost to local services, for example, smoking cessation or weight management, for support where appropriate.

Medicines, including secondary prevention strategies and anti-anginal therapies, should be reviewed.

Box 5.4: Practice point: angina

If a patient is experiencing angina symptoms at the time of any clinical assessment, an ECG should be performed and the presence of any red flags identified which could indicate the need for hospital admission:[7]
- Heart rate >130 beats per minute (bpm)
- Respiratory rate >30 breaths per min
- Systolic BP <90 mmHg
- O_2 saturations <92%
- Reduced consciousness
- High temperature

Medication

Managing CHD, including secondary prevention

Following a diagnosis of CHD, patients will firstly need to be optimised on secondary prevention therapies to reduce their risk of future CV events and should be prescribed anti-anginal therapies to control episodes of chest pain. In addition, medication review should identify those drugs which should be stopped or have a dose reduction at specified time points during treatment.

Stable angina

For a patient with stable angina, secondary prevention consists of:
- an antiplatelet agent, usually aspirin 75 mg daily
- low dose rivaroxaban (2.5 mg twice daily) plus aspirin indefinitely is recommended by NICE and the SMC as an option for preventing atherothrombotic events in adults with CHD at high risk of ischaemic events. Adults at high risk of ischaemic events suitable for rivaroxaban are defined as those;
  — aged 65 or over, or
  — with atherosclerosis in at least two vascular territories (such as coronary, cerebrovascular, or peripheral arteries), or
  — with two or more of the following risk factors: current smoking, diabetes, chronic kidney disease, heart failure or previous non-lacunar ischaemic stroke[8,9]
- a high dose high-intensity statin, such as atorvastatin 80 mg daily.[10]
  To prevent episodes of chest pain:
- Beta blockers, such as bisoprolol, are usually used first line to protect against episodes of tachycardia

which may precipitate chest pain.[4] The dose of beta blocker should be increased as required to control chest pain, aiming for a target heart rate of between 50 and 60 beats per minute.

- A second anti-anginal, for example, a dihydropyridine calcium channel blocker (CCB) (e.g. amlodipine), should be prescribed if the patient remains symptomatic following dose optimisation.[4]
- If beta blockers are unsuitable first line, then a rate-controlling CCB, such as verapamil or diltiazem, may be considered instead.[4]
- Other anti-anginal therapies that may be considered include nitrates, nicorandil, ivabradine and ranolazine if first-line options are contraindicated or not tolerated.[4]
- All people with a diagnosis of CHD should be given sublingual glyceryl trinitrate (GTN) for use in the event of an acute episode of chest pain. Those using GTN more frequently than twice a week should have their oral anti-anginal therapy escalated.
- If a patient with stable angina is on maximum tolerated doses of two anti-anginal medications and remains symptomatic, they should be referred to cardiology for consideration for revascularisation by PCI or CABG.[4]

Acute coronary syndromes

Patients who have experienced an acute coronary event, such as a myocardial infarction, will need additional secondary prevention strategies:

- Dual antiplatelet therapy – low dose aspirin 75 mg daily, plus
  - Clopidogrel 300 mg loading dose then 75 mg daily, or
  - Prasugrel 60 mg loading dose then 10 mg daily (reduce dose to 5 mg if age >75 years or weight <60 kg), or
  - Ticagrelor 180 mg loading dose then 90 mg twice daily[11]

At the end of one year of dual antiplatelet therapy, people at high risk of further CV events, defined as those with diabetes mellitus requiring medication, chronic renal dysfunction, age ≥65 years, evidence of multivessel CAD or a second prior MI, should be considered for ticagrelor 60 mg twice daily for up to a further 3 years.[12,13] All others should revert to aspirin monotherapy indefinitely with consideration of low dose rivaroxaban if they meet the criteria outlined in the section above.[8,9]

- High-dose high-intensity statin – such as atorvastatin 80 mg daily, continued indefinitely[10]
- An ACE-inhibitor – such as ramipril, continued indefinitely[11]
- A beta blocker – such as bisoprolol, for at least 12 months but indefinitely in people with evidence of heart failure with reduced ejection fraction.[11] As length of hospital stay post-MI is now very short (often only 48 hours), ACEI and beta blocker therapy will need dose optimising post-discharge in primary care. ACEI doses should be titrated, if tolerated to achieve the doses used in the clinical trials, for example, ramipril 10 mg, lisinopril 10 mg or perindopril 8 mg. The dose of beta blockers should be increased to achieve a resting heart rate between 50-60 bpm aiming for the maximum tolerated dose within the licensed dose range. Dose titration should take into account blood pressure, heart rate and renal function, as appropriate.
- Aldosterone antagonist – such as eplerenone, should be used in people with symptoms of heart failure and evidence of left ventricular dysfunction post-MI (LVEF <40%). Potassium should be checked at initiation and at regular intervals to ensure that K^+ ≤5 mmol/L.[11]
- Anti-anginal therapies should be prescribed. If required to manage episodes of chest pain and sublingual GTN should be provided to reduce the frequency and severity of any future episodes of acute anginal pain. Once optimised, medication should be reviewed at least annually to:
- assess effectiveness – ask about episodes of chest pain
- identify any adverse effects
- address adherence to treatment alongside any concerns the patient may have
- take bloods to assess renal function, HbA1c, lipid levels and liver function tests.

Antiplatelet therapy

Aspirin at low dose (75 mg daily) has been shown to reduce the risk of death and major cardiovascular events in people with CHD. People taking aspirin, even at low dose, are at an increased risk of gastrointestinal (GI) bleeds, and those with other risk factors for GI bleeding should be considered for gastroprotection with a proton pump inhibitor or H_2 antagonist – they should also be encouraged to take the dose of aspirin with or after food.

Aspirin is no longer used for primary prevention of CVD because any benefits in terms of CV event reduction are offset by the increase in GI bleeding. Other adverse effects of aspirin include nausea, indigestion, bruising and increased bleeding times. A small proportion of the population has aspirin hypersensitivity resulting in asthma, angioedema, urticaria or rhinitis, which will require discontinuation. Clopidogrel monotherapy (75 mg daily) may be considered as an alternative where aspirin is contraindicated or not tolerated.[14]

Dual antiplatelet therapy reduces the risk of major cardiovascular events in people following an acute coronary syndrome or insertion of an intra-coronary stent, but at the expense of an increased risk of bleeding. Dual antiplatelet therapy is usually prescribed for one-year post ACS event or cardiac intervention, but ticagrelor can be continued for a further 3 years in combination with aspirin at a lower dose in patients at high risk of further events.[12,13] At the end of the period of dual antiplatelet therapy, patients should be continued on aspirin monotherapy indefinitely. Rivaroxaban low dose may also be considered in addition to aspirin for patients with CHD who meet the high-risk criteria outlined previously.[8,9]

One of the biggest issues with dual antiplatelet therapy is adherence and persistence – early discontinuation of antiplatelet therapy is the leading cause of stent thrombosis which carries a high mortality rate (up to 45%).[15]

All dual antiplatelet therapy regimens are associated with increased bruising and bleeding. Patients should be encouraged to report bleeding where it occurs and efforts made to address this where possible. For example, people who experience frequent nose bleeds should be considered for cauterisation of the nose. Excessive bleeding may necessitate a change in the dual antiplatelet regimen, for example moving from prasugrel or ticagrelor to clopidogrel, which is a lower intensity antiplatelet agent and therefore associated with lower bleeding rates. Seek advice from cardiology before making changes to the prescribed dual antiplatelet regimen.

A proportion of the population is resistant to clopidogrel due to a reduced ability to metabolise clopidogrel to the active drug, and therefore show little, if any, response to treatment in terms of the degree of platelet inhibition – if clopidogrel resistance is proven (often following a further CV event), then an alternative antiplatelet agent should be prescribed. In general, clopidogrel is well tolerated, but some patients experience rashes which can initially be treated with antihistamines, but may necessitate a switch to a different agent if the rash cannot be tolerated.

Prasugrel in combination with aspirin is licensed for the prevention of atherothrombotic events in adults with acute coronary syndrome only where the patient is undergoing primary or delayed percutaneous coronary intervention. It is contraindicated in patients with prior stroke or TIA, and in the clinical study showed no net clinical benefit in people over the age of 75 years or <60 kg bodyweight, which complicates its use in the setting of an acute coronary syndromes (ACS).[16] As a more potent antiplatelet agent than clopidogrel, prasugrel is associated with more bleeding.

Ticagrelor in combination with aspirin is licensed for the prevention of atherothrombotic events in adult patients with ACS and for those with a history of MI and a high risk of developing an atherothrombotic event. It is taken twice daily and is shorter acting than both clopidogrel and prasugrel, so adherence to the prescribed regimen is essential. On initiation, ticagrelor can cause transient dyspnoea in a small proportion of patients which usually resolves within a few days – but patients may need reassurance where it occurs, as breathlessness is also a symptom of ACS. As with prasugrel, ticagrelor is a more potent antiplatelet agent than clopidogrel, and is therefore associated with more bleeding. Neither prasugrel nor ticagrelor are licensed for monotherapy.

Statins

High dose high-intensity statins, such as atorvastatin 80 mg, are recommended in all patients with a diagnosis of CHD, while a lower dose of a high-intensity statin is used in primary prevention (e.g. atorvastatin 20 mg daily).[10] The aim should be to lower non-HDL cholesterol (calculated by subtracting the HDL level from the total cholesterol level) by 40% or more, partly as a marker of adherence to treatment.

Myalgia is the most common adverse effect of statins and can significantly impact on adherence to treatment. In people with muscle pain, statin-induced myositis (inflammatory muscle damage characterised by severe muscle pain and weakness) should be excluded by checking the creatine kinase level, and then consideration given to reducing the dose or switching to an alternative statin.

A statin intolerance pathway has recently been published by the Accelerated Access Collaborative in England which helps clinicians manage suspected statin-induced muscle pain.[17] Other adverse effects of statins include GI disturbance, headache, dizziness and insomnia. Rashes and alopecia have been less commonly reported. These adverse effects may be dose-related or specific to the agent prescribed – lower doses of the same statin or an alternative statin should be considered.

Additional lipid-lowering therapies can also be considered, for example, ezetimibe, which is licensed as an adjunct to statin therapy or as monotherapy in patients who cannot tolerate, or who have contraindications to statins. It has a CV risk reduction indication for patients with CHD and history of ACS when added to ongoing statin therapy or initiated concomitantly with a statin, and can also be used in familial hypercholesterolaemia.[18]

If LDL cholesterol remains elevated, patients should be considered for referral to a lipid specialist for consideration of a PCSK9 inhibitor – evolocumab or alirocumab. These agents are recommended by NICE for people with CHD at high risk of CV events if LDL >4 mmol/L and those at very high risk of events with LDL >3.5 mmol/L. High risk of CVD is defined as a history of any of the following: ACS, coronary or other arterial revascularisation procedures, CHD, ischaemic stroke or peripheral arterial disease. Very high risk of CVD is defined as recurrent cardiovascular events or cardiovascular events in more than one vascular bed.[19,20]

ACE inhibitors

ACE inhibitors (ACEIs) are used in all patients following an ACS, due to a significant reduction in mortality and morbidity, but are not routinely recommended in those with stable angina or for primary prevention. Doses of ACEI should be increased to achieve those used in the clinical trial setting or to the maximum tolerated dose. Dose titration can be limited by symptomatic low blood pressure, declining renal function, hyperkalaemia and a persistent dry cough – in the latter, consider an angiotensin receptor blocker (ARB), such as valsartan, as an alternative.

All people prescribed an ACEI or ARB should have a blood test to check renal function, potassium and sodium levels at baseline, 2-4 weeks after initiation or any dose change, and annually throughout treatment. Blood pressure should also be checked before and within 2-4 weeks of initiation and each increase in dose, although asymptomatic systolic BP as low as 90 mmHg should not preclude dose titration.

Beta blockers

Beta blockers have been shown to reduce mortality, sudden cardiac death and hospitalisations for at least 12 months post-ACS. Longer-term effects beyond 12 months are not well established except in those with heart failure due to reduced ejection fraction. Beta blocker doses should be increased to achieve those used in the clinical trial setting or to the maximum tolerated dose. Patients prescribed beta blockers should have their BP and heart rate checked within 2-4 weeks of initiation and any dose change. Potential risks and benefits should be discussed at 12 months, and if the beta blocker is to be stopped, then the dose should be reduced gradually and not stopped suddenly due to risk of rebound tachycardia and ischaemia precipitation.

Dose titration can be limited by symptomatic hypotension, bradycardia, declining reversible airways disease, tiredness or fatigue and erectile dysfunction. Other adverse effects include cold extremities (hands and feet), nausea, sleep disturbance or nightmares – these can be minimised by using a cardioselective agent such as bisoprolol. Beta blockers are also used in CHD to prevent episodes of anginal chest pain.

Calcium channel blockers

Calcium channel blockers (CCBs) are used to prevent episodes of angina chest pain and reduce the severity of episodes that do occur. They have not been shown to improve prognosis. Rate-controlling agents, such as diltiazem or verapamil, are used where beta blockers are contraindicated or not tolerated, whilst dihydropyridine agents, such as amlodipine, can be added into beta blocker therapy as a second agent. Verapamil, and diltiazem to a lesser extent, can cause constipation, limiting tolerability. Aside from that, CCBs are generally well tolerated but can be associated with headaches and flushing in the first few days of treatment and can also cause ankle swelling and gum hypertrophy. Patients prescribed CCBs should have their BP and heart rate checked within 2-4 weeks of initiation and any dose change.

GTN

Sublingual GTN, supplied as tablets with a short shelf life, or more commonly as a spray, is used to treat episodes of acute chest pain. If angina pain develops, patients should be advised to sit down and:

- Spray one or two sprays of GTN under the tongue, without breathing in the spray. The mouth should be closed immediately after using the spray. Pain should ease within a minute or so. If the first dose does not work, the spray should be used again after five minutes. If the pain continues for 15 minutes despite using the spray twice then urgent medical advice should be sought (999).
- Place one tablet under the tongue and allow it to dissolve. Pain should ease within a minute or so. If the first tablet does not work, take another tablet after five minutes. If the pain continues for 15 minutes despite taking three tablets then urgent medical advice should be sought (999).

Sublingual GTN can also be used prior to an episode of physical activity to prevent pain developing. Adverse effects of GTN include a throbbing headache, hypotension, flushing and nausea.

Drug interactions

For important drug interactions and how to manage them, see *Table 5.1*.

Table 5.1: *Drug interactions*

Drug class	Interacting drug	Interaction	Management
Calcium channel blockers	Dantrolene	Risk of lethal ventricular fibrillation	Concomitant use contraindicated
Rate-controlling calcium channel blockers	Amiodarone, digoxin, beta blockers, other antiarrhythmics	Increased risk of bradycardia	Caution when combined – use under close supervision and monitor ECG on initiation
	Other antihypertensive drugs	Enhanced antihypertensive effect may occur	Monitor blood pressure after inhalation and dose increases
	Verapamil with carbamazepine or phenytoin	Verapamil increases plasma concentrations	Monitor plasma levels
	Verapamil with digoxin	Plasma concentrations of digoxin increased	Check digoxin level reduce dose if required
	Verapamil with atorvastatin, lovastatin or simvastatin	Plasma concentrations of statins may be increased	Consider a reduction in the statin dose and titrate dose against serum cholesterol concentrations
	Diltiazem with lithium	Increased risk lithium-induced neurotoxicity with diltiazem	Caution with concomitant use – check lithium levels

Table 5.1: *Drug interactions (continued)*

Drug class	Interacting drug	Interaction	Management
Rate-controlling calcium channel blockers (cont.)	Diltiazem or verapamil with ciclosporin	Increase in circulating ciclosporin level with diltiazem and verapamil	Reduce ciclosporin dose, monitor renal function, check circulating ciclosporin levels and adjust dose during combined therapy and after discontinuation of diltiazem
Dihydropyridine CCBs	Amlodipine with simvastatin	Co-administration of multiple doses of 10 mg of amlodipine with 80 mg simvastatin resulted in a 77% increase in exposure to simvastatin compared to simvastatin alone	Limit the dose of simvastatin to 20 mg daily in people on amlodipine
Antiplatelets (e.g. clopidogrel, prasuragrel, ticagrelor)	Drugs affecting clotting including anticoagulants, NSAIDs, SSRIs	Increased risk of bleeding	Avoid concomitant use where possible
	Omeprazole and esomeprazole	Platelet inhibiting effects of clopidogrel reduced (maintenance dose)	As a precaution, concomitant use of omeprazole or esomeprazole with clopidogrel should be discouraged
	Co-administration of ticagrelor with strong CYP3A4 inhibitors (e.g. ketoconazole, clarithromycin, nefazodone, ritonavir and atazanavir)	May lead to a substantial increase in exposure to ticagrelor	Concomitant use is contraindicated
	Ticagrelor with potent CYP3A inducers (e.g. rifampicin, phenytoin, carbamazepine, phenobarbitone)	May decrease exposure and efficacy of ticagrelor	Concomitant use is discouraged
	Ticagrelor and amiodarone	Increased exposure to ticagrelor	Use with caution or avoid
	Ticagrelor and digoxin	Increased digoxin levels	Monitor digoxin levels and adjust dose accordingly
	Ticagrelor and simvastatin	Rhabdomyolysis risk	Limit simvastatin dose to max 40 mg daily
Statins	Potent CYP3A4 inhibitors (e.g. including itraconazole, ketoconazole, erythromycin, clarithromycin, telithromycin and HIV protease inhibitors)	Increased exposure to statins	All are contraindicated with simvastatin Avoid if possible: consider temporary suspension of atorvastatin if interacting drug is taken for short period Itraconazole: do not exceed 40 mg atorvastatin daily Clarithromycin: do not excess 20 mg atorvastatin daily HIV protease inhibitors: monitor lipid levels to ensure lowest necessary dose of atorvastatin is used
	Ciclosporin	Increased exposure to statins	Do not exceed 10 mg simvastatin daily. Do not exceed 10 mg atorvastatin daily. Rosuvastatin is contraindicated
	Danazol	Increased risk of rhabdomyolysis	Do not exceed 10 mg simvastatin daily
	Verapamil, amiodarone	Increased exposure to statins	Do not exceed 20 mg simvastatin daily. Monitor lipid levels to ensure lowest necessary dose of atorvastatin is used
	Diltiazem	Increased exposure to statins	Do not exceed 40 mg simvastatin daily. Monitor lipid levels to ensure lowest necessary dose of atorvastatin is used
	Warfarin/coumarin	INR may be affected	Monitor INR before starting treatment and regularly during treatment, especially with dose changes
	Fibrates	Increased risk of myopathy when used with fibrates Gemfibrozil increased systemic exposure to simvastatin, atorvastatin and rosuvastatin	Do not exceed 10 mg simvastatin daily (except with fenofibrate)
	Ezetimibe	Additive risk of myopathy cannot be ruled out	Advise people to report any unexplained muscle pain, tenderness or weakness

For interactions for beta blockers, ACEIs, ARBs, and aldosterone antagonists, see **Chapter 11**. For interactions for rivaroxaban, see **Chapter 3**.

Advice for patients

People diagnosed with CHD will need information and advice about the condition and the treatments. *Box 5.5* outlines the important counselling points to consider.

Box 5.5: Practice point: counselling points

It is important to ensure patients are aware of the following issues:
- CHD is a chronic condition which increases their risk of future CV events, such as stroke, myocardial infarction and kidney disease.
- CV risk is driven largely by modifiable risk factors which can be addressed through lifestyle modification and medication.
  - Lifestyle modification can include smoking cessation, weight loss, improved diet and physical activity and alcohol moderation.
- Prevention medications, including antiplatelet therapies, statins and, following an acute coronary syndrome (ACS), ACEI and beta blockers, reduce the risk of experiencing future cardiovascular events related to CHD – and must be taken as prescribed to confer their protective effects.
  - Doses of some agents may need to be increased over several weeks to ensure maximal protection from future CV events.
- In patients who have had an ACS, dual antiplatelet therapy (aspirin plus another antiplatelet agent) is usually prescribed for at least one year.
  - Patients should not stop taking dual antiplatelet therapy earlier than recommended.
- Anti-anginal therapies, including beta blockers and CCBs, prevent chest pain and reduce the severity of episodes of chest pain.
- Sublingual GTN should be used to treat episodes of acute chest pain when they occur.
  - Urgent medical advice should be sought if chest pain does not resolve after treatment with sublingual GTN.
- Patients experiencing adverse effects due to their medications, such as muscle pain while on a statin or a rash on clopidogrel, should not stop these medicines but should seek advice from a clinician to allow their drug therapy to be adjusted to reduce or eliminate the adverse effects.
- Patients with a diagnosis of CHD should be reviewed at least annually, but they should seek advice earlier if their symptom control deteriorates.

Useful resources

- CPPE Elearning package. Ischaemic heart disease. www.cppe.ac.uk/gateway/ihd
- NICE (2020). Acute coronary syndromes. www.nice.org.uk/guidance/ng185
- NICE (2016). Stable angina management. www.nice.org.uk/guidance/cg126
- NICE (2013). Myocardial infarction: cardiac rehabilitation and prevention of further cardiovascular disease. www.nice.org.uk/guidance/cg172
- RPS (2019). Pharmacy: Helping to prevent and support people with cardiovascular disease. www.rpharms.com/recognition/all-our-campaigns/policy-a-z/cardiovascular-disease
- SIGN (2016). Acute coronary syndrome. www.sign.ac.uk/assets/sign148.pdf
- SIGN (2018). Management of stable angina. www.sign.ac.uk/media/1088/sign151.pdf

References

1. British Heart Foundation (BHF). BHF statistics factsheet. London: BHF; 2020. www.bhf.org.uk/what-we-do/our-research/heart-statistics

2. National Institute for Health and Care Excellence (NICE) Clinical Knowledge Summaries. CVD risk assessment and management. London: NICE; 2019. www.cks.nice.org.uk/topics/cvd-risk-assessment-management/

3. Boden WE *et al*. COURAGE Trial Research Group. Optimal medical therapy with or without PCI for stable coronary disease. *N Engl J Med* 2007; 356(15): 1503-16.

4. NICE. Stable angina management [CG126]. London: NICE; 2016. www.nice.org.uk/guidance/cg126

5. NICE. Recent-onset chest pain of suspected cardiac origin: assessment and diagnosis [CG95]. London: NICE; 2016. www.nice.org.uk/guidance/cg95

6. NICE. Hypertension in adults: diagnosis and management [CG136]. London: NICE; 2019. www.nice.org.uk/guidance/ng136

7. Murphy J. What are the red flags for chest pain? *B J Family Med* 2019 [online]. www.bjfm.co.uk/blog/what-are-the-red-flags-for-chest-pain

8. NICE. Rivaroxaban for preventing atherothrombotic events in people with coronary or peripheral artery disease [TA607]. London: NICE; 2019. www.nice.org.uk/guidance/ta607

9. Summary of Product Characteristics for Xarelto 2.5 mg film-coated tablets. www.medicines.org.uk/emc/product/3410/smpc#gref

10. NHS England (NHSE). Summary of national guidance for lipid management for primary and secondary prevention of CVD. London: NHSE; 2020. www.england.nhs.uk/aac/wp-content/uploads/sites/50/2020/04/lipid-management-pathway-guidance.pdf

11. NICE. Myocardial infarction: cardiac rehabilitation and prevention of further cardiovascular disease [CG172]. London: NICE; 2013. www.nice.org.uk/guidance/cg172

12. NICE. Ticagrelor for preventing atherothrombotic events after myocardial infarction [TA420]. London: NICE; 2016. www.nice.org.uk/guidance/ta420/chapter/1-Recommendations

13. Summary of Product Characteristics for Brilique 60 mg film coated tablets. www.medicines.org.uk/emc/product/7606/smpc#gref

14. NICE. Clopidogrel and modified-release dipyridamole for the prevention of occlusive vascular events [TA210]. London: NICE; 2010. www.nice.org.uk/Guidance/TA210

15. Morton K *et al*. *The Interventional Cardiac Catheterization Handbook*, 4th edn. London: Elsevier, 2018.

16. Wiviott SD *et al*. Prasugrel versus clopidogrel in patients with acute coronary syndromes. *N Engl J Med* 2007; 357: 2001-2015.

17. NHS England (NHSE). Statin intolerance Pathway. London: NHSE; 2020. www.england.nhs.uk/aac/wp-content/uploads/sites/50/2020/08/statin-intolerance-pathway-16072020.pdf

18. Summary of Product Characteristics for Ezetrol 10 mg tablets. www.medicines.org.uk/emc/medicine/12091/SPC/Ezetrol+10mg+Tablets/#gref

19. NICE. Evolocumab for treating primary hypercholesterolaemia and mixed dyslipidaemia [TA394]. London: NICE; 2016. www.nice.org.uk/guidance/ta394

20. NICE. Alirocumab for treating primary hypercholesterolaemia and mixed dyslipidaemia [TA393]. London: NICE; 2016. www.nice.org.uk/guidance/ta393

Case studies

Case study 1

Daniel is a white British male, 56 years old, who has recently been discharged from hospital following a non-ST elevation myocardial infarction treated by primary percutaneous coronary intervention with insertion of a drug-eluting stent to the left anterior descending artery.

On discharge he is prescribed:

- Aspirin 75 mg daily
- Ticagrelor 90 mg twice daily
- Ramipril 2.5 mg daily
- Bisoprolol 2.5 mg daily
- Atorvastatin 80 mg daily
- Omeprazole 20 mg daily
- GTN spray 1-2 puffs PRN

His discharge summary notes a left ventricular ejection fraction (LVEF) of 60%. Prior to the MI, Daniel was a smoker and overweight with a BMI of 31. Admission bloods indicate total cholesterol of 5.8 mmol/L and HDL cholesterol of 0.9 mmol/L. His renal function was normal in hospital with a serum creatinine of 82 micromol/L and eGFR of 85 mL/min.

Two weeks post-discharge he attends the GP practice for a review and issue of his new medications. He seems a little anxious about the change in his health and circumstances – he tells you he is currently signed off work as an HGV driver and he is scared to do too much in case he has another heart attack.

He is due to start cardiac rehabilitation in about a week but wonders if this will be any use to him.

On examination, his BP is 156/96 mmHg with a heart rate of 78 bpm. You order bloods to check his renal function and HbA1c.

Points to consider

- What are the priorities for this consultation?

Daniel has experienced a major cardiovascular (CV) event so you know it's important to check his understanding of his condition and reassure him that he will be able to get back to a 'normal' life. You also explain that he should make some changes to his lifestyle and take medications to protect himself from further CV events – for a previously apparently healthy man, a heart attack can have a significant psychological impact, even precipitating clinical depression, so it is important to explore the mental as well as the physical impact.

You encourage him to attend cardiac rehabilitation as it has been shown to improve long-term outcomes following a MI, it will build his confidence in becoming more physically active and educate him on the lifestyle changes he should make to reduce his future CV risk.

Points to consider

- What lifestyle factors need to be identified and addressed?

Smoking, diet and physical activity are all issues that may need to be addressed, and you also assess his alcohol intake – whilst smoking cessation would have the most impact on CV risk, Daniel will need to set his priorities and goals in terms of lifestyle change, with referral or signposting to appropriate support services.

In the short-term, cardiac rehabilitation will provide education, support and encouragement to make the necessary lifestyle changes, including a safe environment in which to begin to increase his physical activity.

Points to consider

- What do you need to consider about his medication?

You want to ensure that Daniel's secondary prevention medication is optimised and that he is involved in a discussion about his treatment.

Daniel has been discharged on five medicines for secondary prevention of CVD, including:

- Dual antiplatelet therapy which is to continue for one year – you make a note on the computer system that the ticagrelor should be stopped at the end of the year as Daniel does not currently fulfil the criteria for lower dose ticagrelor therapy. You discuss the importance of adherence to the dual antiplatelet therapy for the full year as this is critical to preventing a blood clot forming in his drug-eluting stent. He should not allow anyone to stop his dual antiplatelet therapy, even temporarily, for example for dental treatment, without consulting the cardiologist first.
- High dose high-intensity statin which should continue lifelong – you explore Daniel's attitude to statins as there have been many negative articles in the media which have been shown to impact on patient behaviour. Statins improve mortality and risk of recurrent events post-MI and are generally well-tolerated. You reassure Daniel that should he experience side effects, such as muscle pain, you will help to address them. You arrange to check his cholesterol levels 3 months after initiation, alongside a check of his liver function, which should be repeated at one year.
  - You should consider adding in ezetimibe if the non-HDL cholesterol has not been reduced by 40% or more from baseline and/or non-HDL-C remains greater than 2.5 mmol/L on atorvastatin 80 mg; assuming you are confident that the patient is adhering to treatment.
- An ACE inhibitor, ramipril, which should be continued indefinitely – this requires dose titration aiming for 10 mg daily.
  - However, you may wish to await the results of the renal function check before increasing the dose of ACEI. If the renal function is stable, the ACEI dose can be increased to 5 mg daily, and then further increased to 10 mg daily after 2-4 weeks if the systolic BP remains >90 mmHg and renal function remains stable.
- A beta blocker, bisoprolol, which should be continued for at least one year post-MI – this also needs dose titration to achieve the evidence-based dose of 10 mg daily.
  - In view of Daniel's BP and heart rate, the bisoprolol dose can be doubled to 5 mg daily. You counsel him that he may feel more tired and lethargic in the few days after the dose increase. The dose can be further increased to 10 mg daily after four weeks, assuming the systolic BP remains above 90 mmHg and the heart rate remains above 60 bpm.

Points to consider

- How would you confirm a diagnosis of hypertension?
- How would you optimise antihypertensive therapy?

Daniel should already have been referred for an ABPM to confirm hypertension and should be treated to achieve a BP target of less than 140/90 mmHg. He is currently having ACEI and beta blocker therapy optimised which may also reduce his BP to target, but if it remains above target once both have been optimised, you may need to consider a calcium channel blocker (CCB), such as amlodipine and/or a thiazide diuretic, such as indapamide.

Points to consider

- What other assessment should be carried out?
- What additional information and advice should you give him?

You ask Daniel if he is experiencing any symptoms of angina. You also confirm he knows what his GTN spray is for, and he knows how and when to use it.

You discuss the importance of adherence, explore his attitudes and address any concerns.

Points to consider

• What follow-up is required?

You follow up Daniel every few weeks whilst his medication is being optimised and then review him annually.

Case study 2

You are undertaking an annual review of patients on the CHD register and have called in Rosie, aged 72 years, an ex-school teacher who has had angina for more than 10 years, as well as a history of hypertension, asthma and depression.

She is currently prescribed:

• Aspirin 75 mg daily
• Simvastatin 20 mg daily
• Amlodipine 5 mg daily
• Ramipril 5 mg daily
• Indapamide 2.5 mg daily
• Symbicort 200/6 two puffs twice daily
• Terbutaline PRN

You notice she has not collected her aspirin or statin for many months. Her blood pressure is 122/68 mmHg and heart rate is 98 bpm. During the consultation, she tells you she has been having weekly episodes of chest pain on exertion, which resolve on resting. Her blood test results indicate good renal function, but her total cholesterol is 5.4 mmol/L and HDL cholesterol is 1.1 mmol/L.

Points to consider

• What are the priorities for this consultation?

Rosie is complaining of episodes of chest pain, so you undertake a full assessment of the frequency, type, duration and severity of these episodes. You also assess for any other angina-related symptoms and exclude any red flags which would warrant urgent referral.

Rosie should have sublingual GTN, so you ensure that she has a supply and confirm that she knows how to use this if she experiences angina.

Points to consider

• What other aspects of Rosie's treatment may need to be addressed?

Rosie is only taking amlodipine as an anti-anginal, although it was probably originally prescribed for hypertension. Ideally, she should be on a rate-controlling anti-anginal agent, and in view of her history of asthma, it may be best to avoid a beta blocker.

Changing the amlodipine to a rate-controlling CCB will help to lower her heart rate and may reduce the frequency of episodes of angina. If she remains symptomatic after optimising the dose of the CCB, a second agent, for example, a nitrate may be added. Her blood pressure and heart rate should be monitored after each change in therapy.

Points to consider

• What other issues should you discuss?

You chat to Rosie about adherence and she admits that she does not take her aspirin or simvastatin because she was getting some side effects (nausea after the dose with aspirin and muscle pain with the statin), and when she stopped taking them temporarily she did not notice any ill effects, so she has not been taking them for some months now.

Points to consider

- How would you address these issues?

You explain that aspirin-related nausea can be reduced by taking the dose on a full stomach, but as this is already causing poor adherence, you consider switching Rosie to clopidogrel 75 mg daily as an alternative.

Switching to an alternative statin with a lower rate of muscle adverse effects and at a low dose is an option – for example, atorvastatin 20 mg daily, with a view to increasing the dose if tolerated.

If muscle pain occurs with atorvastatin, a water-soluble agent, such as rosuvastatin, is an alternative.

Points to consider

- What are the options if Rosie refuses to take a statin?

You discuss the benefits of the statin as well as aspirin and emphasise that these two drugs are not intended to help with her angina symptoms, but that they will reduce her risk of having a heart attack or stroke in future, and hence long-term adherence is important. You also reassure her that if she does experience more side effects, you are happy to see her to review the medicines again. If Rosie still refuses to take the statin, you should consider ezetimibe 10 mg daily instead.

You ensure that her LFTs are checked three months after switching statin and at 12 months and arrange a cholesterol check to confirm adherence to the new treatment.

CHAPTER 6

Chronic obstructive pulmonary disease

Toby Capstick and Helen Meynell

Overview

Chronic obstructive pulmonary disease (COPD) is a common, preventable and treatable disease that is characterised by persistent respiratory symptoms and airflow limitation that is due to airway and/or alveolar abnormalities usually caused by significant exposure to noxious particles or gases.[1] Generally the airflow limitation does not vary from day to day, resulting in persistent breathlessness, sputum production and/or cough.

Exacerbations of COPD are an acute worsening of respiratory symptoms that is beyond normal day-to-day variations, specifically a significantly increased level of breathlessness, cough and/or sputum production (volume/colour).

Airflow obstruction results from a mixture of small airways disease (such as obstructive bronchiolitis) and destruction of lung parenchyma (emphysema) as a consequence of chronic inflammation. These processes cause narrowing of the small airways and loss of alveolar attachments to the small airways, with a consequential reduction in elastic recoil of the lung, making the airways prone to collapse during expiration and a reduction in gas transfer.

There are two main pathological components of COPD that are often described: emphysema and chronic bronchitis. Emphysema describes the destruction of lung parenchyma and gas exchanging surfaces, whilst chronic bronchitis describes the presence of cough and sputum production for at least three months in each of two consecutive years.

The most common cause of COPD is tobacco smoke, but it can also develop as a result of exposure to other particles and gases, including outdoor, occupational and indoor air pollution. Occupational causes may result from mining, steelworks or similar occupations where there may be exposure to inorganic dust, chemical agents and fumes. In the developing world, indoor pollution is an important cause of COPD, such as from open fires or cooking with poorly functioning stoves, especially where ventilation is limited. People with alpha-1 antitrypsin deficiency are predisposed to early onset of emphysema and accounts for 1-2% of all COPD cases.

It's estimated that 1.2 million people in the UK have been diagnosed with COPD,[2] although it's thought that a further 2 million people remain undiagnosed. Annually, there are 140,000 UK hospital admissions and 25,000-30,000 deaths.

Box 6.1: Practice point: COPD

- COPD is a common and preventable condition that affects 1.2 million people in the UK.
- COPD is an irreversible obstruction of the airways.
- Risk factors for COPD include tobacco smoke and smoke from other causes and air pollution, occupational exposure to dusts, vapours, fumes, gases and other chemicals and genetic factors.
- Patients experience persistent shortness of breath that is progressive with time and worse on exercise, and chronic cough, with or without sputum production.
- Spirometry that demonstrates airflow limitation is required to support the diagnosis.

Diagnosis

A diagnosis of COPD may be suspected due to chronic symptoms of breathlessness, cough and sputum production, a history of lower respiratory symptoms and a history of exposure to causative agents. The diagnosis is made by post-bronchodilator spirometry that demonstrates persistent airflow obstruction confirmed by a ratio of forced expiratory volume in one second (FEV_1) to forced vital capacity (FVC) less than 0.7.

Box 6.2: Practice point: spirometry

- The forced vital capacity (FVC) measures the volume of lung breathed out during a forced expiratory effort after breathing in as far as possible.
- The forced expiratory volume in one second (FEV_1) measures the volume of air exhaled during the first one second of a forced expiratory effort.
- The FEV_1/FVC ratio represents the proportion of a person's vital capacity that they are able to exhale during a forced expiratory effort.
  - If a person has healthy lungs and no airway obstruction, they should be able to breathe out more than 70% of their vital capacity within the first one second of a forced expiratory effort.

Pharmacy input

Pharmacists in all sectors of practice have the opportunity to provide education and support for patients with COPD. Possible roles include:

- referral when patients present at community pharmacy with potential symptoms of COPD
- regular assessment of inhaler technique for new or ongoing inhaled therapies
- adherence monitoring through monitoring of repeat prescriptions of maintenance therapies
- highlighting worsening symptom control through overuse of reliever inhalers
- educating patients on the aims of the different treatments used for COPD.

Community pharmacists, in particular, can help to identify patients at high risk of COPD, for example, people with a significant smoking history (or history of chronic exposure to other sources such as fumes and chemicals) exhibiting characteristic symptoms of chronic and progressive breathlessness that might be affecting their ability to perform their usual activities, and cough with repeated requests for cough medicines.

Studies have demonstrated that community pharmacists can also effectively undertake case finding of COPD using a handheld micro-spirometer, with the potential to provide cost savings to the NHS and improve quality of life.[3]

GP practice-based pharmacists may also set up COPD clinics to perform annual COPD reviews or medication reviews. Pharmacists with training and expertise in this area are able to assess COPD health status and symptom control, monitor adherence through prescription collection data and optimise treatments in line with local and national guidelines. It is important that there are clear policies to refer patients when necessary to other members of the multidisciplinary team, such as community respiratory nurses, physiotherapists, occupational therapists, social services, dieticians, and palliative care services.

Hospital pharmacists may interact with people with COPD during hospital admissions and outpatient clinics. During hospital admissions, the pharmacist and pharmacy technicians should always assess patients' inhaler technique and check their adherence to their current medications as this can be a cause of COPD exacerbations. Throughout hospital admissions, the pharmacist is responsible for ensuring that the patient is receiving the appropriate treatment and providing education on new treatments that are prescribed. At discharge, a final check of inhaler technique and the patient's understanding of their medication will help to ensure that they continue to use their treatment correctly at home. Where necessary, patients can be referred to their local community pharmacist to further support patients after discharge.

Pharmacy review

Whilst it is recognised that there are the 'missing millions' who have COPD but have not been diagnosed, there is also another issue in that a number of large primary care audits have identified that 20-25% of people on GP Practice Quality and Outcomes Framework COPD registers do not have evidence of airflow obstruction on spirometry.[4,5,6] Consequently, pharmacists managing the care of people with COPD should be familiar with the interpretation of spirometry to be assured of the correct diagnosis, particularly where there is a poor response to treatment.

Assessment of patients with a confirmed diagnosis of COPD focuses on determining the severity of airflow limitation, the severity of symptoms and future risk of exacerbations, which aid decision making on treatment plans.

Box 6.3: Practice point: information and advice

- Pharmacists in all sectors have opportunities to provide education for people with COPD and may be able to identify those at risk of COPD.
- Pharmacists roles include:
  - referral when patients present at community pharmacy with potential symptoms of COPD
  - education on COPD and the role of different medicines used for COPD, how they work and when they should be used
  - regular assessment of inhaler technique for new or ongoing inhaled therapies
  - adherence monitoring, through monitoring of repeat prescriptions of maintenance therapies
  - highlighting worsening control through increased use of reliever inhalers.

Severity of COPD

The severity of airflow limitation is determined using spirometry to measure post-bronchodilator FEV_1 and is graded from mild to very severe (see *Table 6.1*). It is important to realise that the severity of airflow limitation is only weakly correlated with symptoms and health-related quality of life, and at each stage of severity, patients may have anything between well-preserved and very poor health status. Consequently, measures of the severity of symptoms are essential components when assessing overall health status in COPD during consultations in all sectors of practice.

Table 6.1: *Grading of the severity of airflow in COPD in people with FEV/FEV_1 <0.70*

GOLD[1] grade	NICE[7]	Severity	Post-bronchodilator FEV_1
GOLD 1	Stage 1	Mild	≥80% predicted
GOLD 2	Stage 2	Moderate	50-80% predicted
GOLD 3	Stage 3	Severe	30-49% predicted
GOLD 4	Stage 4	Very severe	<30% predicted

GOLD: Global Initiative for Chronic Obstructive Lung Disease; NICE: National Institute for Heath and Care Excellence.

The severity of COPD symptoms can be assessed in two ways: the British Medical Research Council (MRC) dyspnoea scale (see *Table 6.2*), which measures the severity of breathlessness and relates well to health status and predicts future mortality risk. A score of 3-5 identifies people with COPD with 'more breathlessness', and 1-2 indicates 'less breathlessness'. It can be used by asking patients 'Which statement most closely applies to you?'. This tool is familiar to most healthcare professionals and widely used across the UK, but since it focuses on only one symptom of COPD, it does not give a holistic assessment of the impact of COPD on patients.

Table 6.2: *British Medical Research Council (MRC) dyspnoea scale*

MRC score	Degree of breathlessness related to activity
1	Not troubled by breathlessness except on strenuous exercise
2	Short of breath when hurrying or walking up a slight hill
3	Walks slower than contemporaries on the level because of breathlessness, or has to stop for breath when walking at own pace
4	Stops for breath after walking about 100 metres or after a few minutes on the level
5	Too breathless to leave the house, or breathless when dressing or undressing

An alternative tool that is commonly used in practice and clinical trials is the COPD Assessment Test (CAT™, http://catestonline.org/),[8] which is a validated 8-item patient-completed questionnaire designed to measure the impact of COPD on a person's life, and how this changes over time (see *Figure 6.1*). It is quick and simple for patients to complete either before or during a consultation. Results correlate closely with health-related quality of life questionnaires such as the St George's Respiratory Questionnaire (SGRQ).[9] It is available to download from the website in over 50 languages.

Although it is not a diagnostic tool, the results of the CAT questionnaire allow patients and healthcare professionals to understand the impact of COPD, and identify where COPD has the greatest effect on each patient's health and daily life. The score is used by healthcare professionals to guide the management of patients and can assist discussions and decisions about managing COPD. The questionnaire may be repeated every two to three months to detect changes and trends in the CAT score.

The CAT questionnaire has a scoring range of 0-40. A change of 2 or more in the score over a two to three month period indicates a clinically significant change in health status. A score of:

- less than 10 indicates a low impact of COPD on a person's life
- 10-20 indicates a medium and significant impact of COPD on a person's life, including breathlessness, wheeze, cough and/or sputum production on most days
- 21-40 indicates a high to very high impact of COPD on a person's life, such that their COPD stops them doing most things that they want to do.

COPD exacerbations

Avoiding COPD exacerbations is an important aspect of disease management as these are associated with increased lung function decline, deterioration in health status and increased risk of death. As a result, it is important to determine each patient's future risk of exacerbations at each COPD review to ensure they are prescribed the appropriate medication to prevent them.

COPD exacerbations vary in severity from mild (requiring treatment with short-acting bronchodilators only), to moderate (requiring treatment with short-acting bronchodilators plus oral corticosteroids with or without antibiotics), to severe (requiring A&E attendance or hospitalisation). Whilst most exacerbations are triggered by viral infections, other causes include bacterial infection, pollution and ambient temperature, and patients should be advised to avoid known precipitating factors.

The best predictor of future risk of exacerbation is having previous exacerbations – people are at highest risk if they have a history of at least two in the past 12 months or one hospitalisation. Whilst declining airflow limitation is also associated with an increased risk of exacerbations, as well as hospitalisation and death, the FEV_1 itself is not a good predictor of exacerbation risk.

Figure 6.1: *CAT score*[8]

How is your COPD? Take the COPD Assessment Test™ (CAT)

This questionnaire will help you and your healthcare professional to measure the impact that COPD (Chronic Obstructive Pulmonary Disease) is having on your wellbeing and daily life. Your answers and test score can be used by you and your healthcare professional to help improve the management of your COPD and gain the greatest benefit from the treatment.

If you wish to complete the questionnaire by hand on paper, **please click here** and then print the questionnaire.

For each item below, place a mark (X) in the box that best describes your current situation. Please ensure that you only select one response for each question.

Example: I am very happy (0) (1) (X) (3) (4) (5) I am very sad

SCORE

I never cough	0 1 2 3 4 5	I cough all the time	
I have no phlegm (mucus) on my chest at all	0 1 2 3 4 5	My chest is full of phlegm (mucus)	
My chest does not feel tight at all	0 1 2 3 4 5	My chest feels very tight	
When I walk up a hill or a flight of stairs I am not out of breath	0 1 2 3 4 5	When I walk up a hill or a flight of stairs I am completely out of breath	
I am not limited to doing any activities at home	0 1 2 3 4 5	I am completely limited to doing all activities at home	
I am confident leaving my home despite my lung condition	0 1 2 3 4 5	I am not confident leaving my home at all because of my lung condition	
I sleep soundly	0 1 2 3 4 5	I do not sleep soundly because of my lung condition	
I have lots of energy	0 1 2 3 4 5	I have no energy at all	

TOTAL SCORE

Available at: https://www.catestonline.org. The IP in the COPD Assessment Test CAT is owned by GlaxoSmithkline and it is reproduced with the company's permission.

The Global Initiative for Chronic Obstructive Lung Disease (GOLD)[1] advises that assessments of symptoms and exacerbation history should be combined at the point of diagnosis to categorise COPD patients into one of four clinical phenotypes (GOLD categories A, B, C, and D), as this will guide initial treatment.

- Category A: low symptoms, non-frequent moderate or severe exacerbations
- Category B: high symptoms, non-frequent moderate or severe exacerbations
- Category C: low symptoms, frequent moderate or severe exacerbations
- Category D: high symptoms, frequent moderate or severe exacerbations

In primary care, it is often also useful to perform oximetry and exercise tolerance testing. Pulse oximetry should be used for anyone with signs suggestive of respiratory failure or right-sided heart failure to assess the need for supplemental oxygen. Patients with oxygen saturation less than 92% on room air should be referred for an oxygen assessment. Exercise tolerance is commonly assessed using either a shuttle walk test or a 6-minute walking test to determine how far or how long a patient can walk, the effectiveness of pulmonary rehabilitation, or as a predictor of prognosis since this will decline in the year before death.

A final key assessment for patients with COPD is to assess and optimise any coexisting comorbidities such as cardiovascular disease, osteoporosis, depression, anxiety, and lung cancer.

Information and advice

Patients diagnosed with COPD are likely to require treatment with at least one inhaler and potentially oral medicines as well. Despite this, many patients have a poor understanding of what COPD is and what their medicines do.

Patient education is a key intervention to ensure that they understand their diagnosis and how to self care, and taking the time to discuss the basics is appreciated by many patients as part of routine COPD consultations and medicines reviews.

Pharmacists can tailor the content of consultations by gauging each patient's current level of knowledge by asking then what they understand about their diagnosis and treatment, and whether they know when and why to take their medicines. The British Lung Foundation has produced useful consultation guides for pharmacists to support the delivery of patient-centred care (www.blf.org.uk/health-care-professionals/supporting-pharmacists), which although were designed for the Medicines Use Review service, they are a useful resource to guide consultations in all sectors. Examples of useful questions to ask patients include:

- How much do you know about your respiratory diagnosis and its treatment?
- Do you know what each of the medicines are for?
- How are you getting on with taking your medicines?
- Do you know how your medicines work?

Basic information on what COPD is and how this affects their airways in terms of inflammation and narrowed, obstructed airways with increased sputum production, may help patients understand the condition and how this manifests in symptoms of breathlessness, cough and sputum production. This can aid understanding the role of different medicines in controlling these symptoms: relievers open up the airways, preventers control the disease and prevent flare-ups, some medicines help cough up sputum.

A discussion about adherence is useful to identify any potential medication-related reasons for poor symptom control or frequent exacerbations, which can be supported through monitoring of repeat prescription collection. Community and GP practice-based pharmacists are well positioned to monitor this due to their access to prescription and dispensing data, as well as having regular contact with patients. Where poor adherence is identified, the reasons for this should be explored in a non-confrontational manner to identify and address both unintentional and intentional causes of poor adherence. These are discussed in more detail in **Chapter 2**.

Patients with COPD often have multiple comorbidities treated with a large number of medicines, and so the complexity of their medication regimen can make it difficult to adhere to their prescribed therapies.

Simplifying inhaled regimens through use of combination inhalers (such as dual long-acting bronchodilators, or triple therapy - ICS/LABA/LAMA) can be appreciated by many patients to reduce the number of inhalers they have to use each day.

It is also important to discuss the signs and symptoms of a flare-up (exacerbation) of COPD so that patients understand how to recognise it early, know to increase the frequency of their SABA inhaler, and when to contact their GP for a course of oral corticosteroids or antibiotics.

Some patients may be given a rescue pack of oral corticosteroids and sometimes an antibiotic as well on prescription, and in some regions these may be made available as part of a patient group direction. It is important that patients are given clear instruction on when each rescue medication should be started, and when it is not appropriate to start them.

Advise them that their reliever (SABA) inhaler is sufficient to manage episodes of breathlessness, but if this is much worse than normal and persists despite using their inhaler, then they should start a course of oral corticosteroids. Antibiotics should only be started if they are coughing up more sputum than normal, or if it has changed colour, as this increases the probability that they are suffering from a bacterial chest infection. Patients should be advised that if they have started a rescue pack, then they should contact their GP or healthcare professional within two days to arrange a review and monitor recovery.

Whilst the prompt and appropriate use of oral corticosteroids and antibiotics for a COPD exacerbation can minimise the risks of hospitalisation, overuse can be harmful due to the risks of long-term adverse effects and antibiotic resistance. Consequently, patients who are prescribed rescue packs should be monitored for excessive use suggesting either poor control of COPD or lack of knowledge about when it is appropriate to commence treatment. GP practice-based pharmacists will be able to identify patients on their COPD registers with high levels of antibiotic and oral corticosteroid use. This could prompt a case review to ensure that patients are followed up appropriately following each exacerbation, or to review whether their medicines need optimising and whether they are self-managing their COPD correctly.

This can be supported with patient information leaflets, such as those produced by the British Lung Foundation (www.blf.org.uk). Patients can be supported with managing their COPD by providing them with a self-management plan, which provides written information on COPD, an action plan to self-manage exacerbations and to complete a daily symptom and mood diary to monitor their condition. Plans are available from the British Lung Foundation or may be produced locally.

Lifestyle advice

Patients should also be advised on the importance of non-pharmacological management of COPD, including keeping active, how to control breathlessness, eating well to maintain a healthy weight and to take care of their emotional wellbeing.

Patients should be asked about how often they feel breathless to the extent that it stops them from doing the things that they want to do, and advised that regular exercise may help with breathing and overall health status by maintaining physical fitness and strengthening muscles to improve exercise tolerance and quality of life. Patients should be advised to exercise at their own pace, but not to overstrain themselves. Exercise should be taken for 30 minutes on 5 days a week, at a pace that causes mild breathlessness. This may include walking or gardening, joining an exercise class, or activities such as yoga, dancing or tai chi.

Pulmonary rehabilitation (PR) is a multidisciplinary programme comprising a 6 to 8-week course of twice-weekly group exercise classes, with combined educational sessions designed to optimise each patient's physical and social performance and autonomy, and improve quality of life, exercise tolerance and breathlessness. Patients who meet the criteria and should be referred to PR services are those who feel functionally disabled by COPD and are breathless walking at their own pace on the level (MRC grade ≥3), or who have had recent hospitalisation for an exacerbation of COPD.

Breathing techniques can help people cope with breathlessness, and can be taught by physiotherapists and other trained healthcare professionals. Simple advice is also available from the British Lung Foundation.

A healthy balanced diet is essential for people with COPD to maintain a healthy weight and lead an active life. Patients should be asked during COPD consultations about how their diet is, and whether they have noticed any changes in their weight; either weight gain or loss. People who are overweight should be encouraged to lose weight as the excess weight will require more effort to breathe and move around. However, some people with COPD may lose too much weight because they may become too breathless whilst eating or preparing food, and these patients should be encouraged to eat smaller, more frequent meals. Maintaining a good level of hydration can help with sputum clearance, and so patients should be advised to drink at least 6 to 8 cups a day of water, juice, tea, coffee or milk.

Anxiety and depression are common, normal reactions to living with COPD, and these should be identified by asking whether their symptoms increase their anxiety or cause them to worry, particularly if they find it hard to control. Patients with anxiety or depression should be provided with support through medication, counselling, and social support. Further information is available in **Chapter 1**.

Interventions

It is important that all healthcare professionals understand the most cost-effective interventions in COPD management. Non-pharmacological interventions such as flu vaccination, smoking cessation and pulmonary rehabilitation are more cost-effective than inhaled medication and should be offered to all patients.[10]

All COPD patients should be asked about their vaccination status, since ensuring patients are up-to-date with their immunisations can reduce hospital admissions due to pneumonia and influenza and reduce their mortality risk. People with COPD should be strongly advised to have a flu vaccination each year, and a single pneumococcal vaccination as an adult, which will protect for life.

Stopping smoking is the single most important intervention that can be made in COPD, regardless of disease severity. Stopping smoking is one of the most cost-effective interventions that can be made in COPD, will slow disease progression, and will have health benefits for other conditions. One of the most effective ways of ensuring that patients access local stop smoking services is to give very brief advice:[11] 'Ask, Advise and Act' since this will give them the best chance to successfully stop smoking. Pharmacists may wish to undertake online training on smoking cessation advice from the National Centre for Smoking Cessation Training (www.ncsct.co.uk).

- ASK and record smoking status and whether they live with a smoker.
- ADVISE patient of health benefits of quitting and inform them that the best way to quit is with a combination of trained support and medication.
- ACT on patient's response and refer smokers who want to quit to their local NHS stop smoking service.

Depending on local arrangements you may be able to support the patient with some of these interventions, however, if you are unable to, you should be aware where patients can access them and signpost or refer as appropriate.

Medication

The majority of medications used to treat COPD symptoms and reduce the risk of exacerbations are inhaled, so ensuring good inhaler technique is essential. See *Table 6.3* for information about the variety of inhalers available.

The choice of inhaler device to prescribe is dependent on patient preference, cost, local formulary and patient's ability to use that device. In particular, many elderly or frail patients may struggle to generate sufficient inspiratory effort to use a dry powder inhaler or may need to use a spacer with their MDI devices due to difficulties with coordination.

It is important to identify whether patients can inhale at the correct speed to use their inhaler device: either quickly and deeply using a dry powder inhaler, or slowly and steadily to use an aerosol inhaler.[12] Inhaler technique videos for patients and healthcare professionals are available on the Asthma UK website (www.asthma.org.uk/advice/inhaler-videos).

Table 6.3: *Inhalers for treating COPD*

Drug class	Example	Brand	
Individual drug			
Short-acting beta$_2$ agonist (SABA)	Salbutamol	• Airomir • Airsalb • Salamol	• Salbulin • Ventolin
	Terbutaline	• Bricanyl	
Long-acting muscarinic antagonist (LAMA)	Aclidinium	• Eklira	
	Glycopyrronium	• Seebri	
	Tiotropium	• Braltus • Spiriva	
	Umeclidinium	• Incruse	
Long-acting beta$_2$ agonist (LABA)	Formoterol	• Atimos • Modulite	• Foradil • Oxis
	Indacaterol	• Onbrez	
	Olodaterol	• Striverdi	
	Salmeterol	• Neovent • Serevent	• Soltel • Vertine
	Vilanterol	• n/a	
Combination drugs			
LAMA/LABA	Umeclidinium/vilanterol	• Anoro	
	Aclidinium/formoterol	• Duaklir	
	Tiotropium/olodaterol	• Spiolto	
	Glycopyrronium/indacaterol	• Ultibro	
Inhaled corticosteroid (ICS)/LABA	Fluticasone propionate/salmeterol	• AirFluSal • Fusacomb	• Seretide • Stalpex
	Budesonide/formoterol	• DuoResp • Fobumix • Symbicort	
	Beclometasone/formoterol	• Fostair	
	Fluticasone furoate/vilanterol	• Relvar	
ICS/LABA/LAMA	Fluticasone furoate/vilanterol/umeclidinium	• Trelegy	
	Beclometasone/formoterol/glycopyrronium	• Trimbow	

Short-acting beta$_2$ agonist (SABA)

All patients should be prescribed a SABA inhaler to be used when needed for fast-acting relief of breathlessness and wheezing. They have a fast onset within 5 minutes but are short-acting with a duration of response of 4-6 hours.

Adverse effects tend to occur with frequent use or larger doses given as a nebuliser and include tremor, palpitations and headache. If these are experienced regularly or become problematic, a review of patient's medication should be undertaken to optimise their treatment regimen in an attempt to reduce their need for using the SABA inhaler as frequently.

Long-acting muscarinic antagonists (LAMA)

These are more effective than short-acting relievers, producing larger improvements in lung function, breathlessness and quality of life, and reductions in hospitalisations. They are recommended for patients with more significant COPD symptoms (CAT score ≥10; MRC ≥3) and are used once a day (except aclidinium, which is used twice a day). Tiotropium and glycopyrronium are both renally cleared; tiotropium should be used with caution in patients with moderate to severe renal impairment (creatinine clearance ≤50 mL/min), and glycopyrronium should be used with caution in patients with severe renal impairment.

Dry mouth is the most common adverse effect, which can be managed by rinsing the mouth after use, or in severe or persistent cases it may require a switch to an alternative within this class.

LAMA inhalers are usually not recommended to be given at the same time as short-acting muscarinic antagonists (e.g. ipratropium) due to concerns about additive adverse effects without additive clinical benefits.

Long-acting beta$_2$ agonist (LABA)

These are more effective than short-acting relievers, producing larger improvements in lung function, breathlessness and quality of life, and reductions in hospitalisations. They are recommended for patients with more significant COPD symptoms (CAT score ≥10; MRC ≥3), and are used once a day (indacaterol, olodaterol, vilanterol (not available as monotherapy)) or twice a day (formoterol, salmeterol).

Adverse effects include tremor, palpitations, headache and muscle cramps, which may occur more commonly where there is also high use of SABA. Where these occur and are distressing or troublesome, a review of the patient's treatment should be undertaken to optimise their regular medication in an attempt to reduce the need for SABA use. In other cases, a change in inhaler device or ensuring correct inhaler technique may reduce systemic adverse effects.

LAMA/LABA

Combining two classes of long-acting bronchodilator produces greater increases in lung function, breathlessness, quality of life and exercise tolerance than using only one long-acting bronchodilator. Dual long-acting bronchodilators have also been shown to have greater improvements in lung function, quality of life and greater reductions in exacerbation rates with a lower risk of pneumonia than combination inhaled corticosteroid and long-acting beta$_2$ agonist inhalers.[13]

Whilst there are no studies available to determine the effect of using combination LABA/LAMA inhalers on adherence or patient preference in comparison to using separate inhalers, the cost of these is lower. There are currently no convincing data to suggest the superiority of any one LABA/LAMA inhaler over another, and as each of the four currently available licensed preparations have the same NHS list price, the choice of which to prescribe is likely to depend on patient preference and their ability to use each device.

Adverse effects are likely to be similar to those observed with each single agent, i.e. dry mouth, tremor, palpitations, headache, muscle cramps. If these are severe or troublesome, they may be managed by checking and optimising inhaler technique, changing inhaler device, switching to an alternative drug within the class, or optimising the treatment regimen.

Corticosteroid (ICS)/LABA

In vitro data have shown that ICS only has a limited effect on inflammation in COPD, and are not licensed as monotherapy in COPD. In severe COPD in patients at high risk of exacerbations (at least two moderate or one severe exacerbation in the past 12 months), ICS in combination with LABA is more effective than either drug alone in improving lung function, health status and preventing exacerbations.[14] However, recent studies have shown that ICS may have a beneficial effect in patients with higher blood eosinophil counts (>300 cells per microlitre),[15,16] but are less effective in patients with low blood eosinophil counts (100 cells per microlitre).[16] Eosinophils are associated with inflammation in the airways and consequently, patients with higher blood eosinophil counts are thought to be more likely to respond to inhaled corticosteroids.

Local adverse effects from ICS include oral thrush and dysphonia (hoarse voice), which can be managed by rinsing the mouth with water after use, using a spacer with MDI, or switching to an alternative drug/device. Other adverse effects include skin thinning and bruising, osteoporosis and pneumonia. Patients at high risk of pneumonia include current smokers, aged over 55 years, low body mass index less than 25 kg/m^2, more severe airflow limitation and low blood eosinophil counts.

Pharmacists should also bear in mind that patients with emphysema or a low BMI are at higher risk of osteoporosis in addition to using ICS, and so consideration should be made for high-risk patients to request a DEXA scan and prescribe bone protection, especially in patients requiring frequent courses of oral corticosteroids. Consequently, caution should be applied when prescribing ICS in COPD, and they should only be used in patients expected to respond to treatment where the advantages of treatment outweigh the risks of adverse effects. They should be prescribed in the lowest effective licensed dose, and inhaler technique checked and optimised to reduce the risk of systemic adverse effects. Patients prescribed a high dose ICS/LABA should be issued with a high dose inhaled steroid warning card.

ICS/LABA/LAMA

Combining an inhaled corticosteroid with two classes of long-acting bronchodilator produces greater increases in lung function, breathlessness and quality of life, and significant reductions in exacerbation rate than using either dual long-acting bronchodilator,[17,18] or an ICS/LABA.[18,19]

Mucolytics

Mucolytics such as carbocisteine (Mucodyne) and acetylcysteine (NACSYS) may reduce sputum viscosity and reduce COPD exacerbations in patients receiving inhaled corticosteroids.[20] NICE recommends them for COPD patients with a chronic cough associated with sputum production, and continue them where there is symptomatic improvement.[7]

Adverse effects are not common, but occasionally patients may experience dyspepsia, abdominal pain, nausea, vomiting, and diarrhoea. Where these are severe and persistent, mucolytic therapy should be stopped.

Phosphodiesterase-4 (PDE4) inhibitors

Roflumilast (Daxas) inhibits PDE4, causing an increase in intracellular concentrations of cyclic adenosine monophosphate in inflammatory cells which causes a reduction of inflammatory mediators and cytokines. It is available in tablet form and is recommended as an option for severe COPD with chronic bronchitis, only if there is severe airflow obstruction (FEV$_1$ <50% of predicted) and frequent exacerbations (at least 2 in the previous 12 months), despite triple inhaled therapy with LAMA + LABA + ICS,[21] where it may achieve a small reduction in the rate of moderate and severe COPD exacerbations.[22]

The starting dose is 250 micrograms daily for 28 days, titrated to 500 micrograms daily.

Adverse effects include diarrhoea, nausea, sleeplessness, psychiatric disorders, weight loss (mandating weight monitoring throughout treatment), and it should be avoided in patients with immunosuppression, cancers, congestive heart failure (NYHA grade 3/4) and mild hepatic impairment. Patients experiencing severe adverse effects, or any unexplained weight loss or psychiatric symptoms, should have their treatment discontinued.

Methylxanthines

Methylxanthines, theophylline (Uniphyllin, Nuelin SA) and aminophylline (Phyllocontin) are thought to act as non-selective phosphodiesterase inhibitors with bronchodilator activity and produce additive improvements in lung function when used in combination with long-acting beta$_2$ agonists.

Dose-related toxicity is a particular issue with theophylline and aminophylline as they have a narrow therapeutic window. At therapeutic doses, common adverse effects include nausea, indigestion and headache, which generally resolve with time; whilst at toxic doses, serious adverse effects include atrial and ventricular arrhythmias (which can be fatal) and seizures.

Drug-drug interactions are common as theophylline is metabolised by cytochrome P450, and include drugs such as macrolide and fluoroquinolone antibiotics, necessitating theophylline dose reductions. Consequently, therapeutic drug monitoring is recommended to ensure a therapeutic dose is prescribed, whilst avoiding toxic serum levels.[1,7]

Antibiotics

Long-term azithromycin may reduce COPD exacerbations in patients experiencing frequent exacerbations through an anti-inflammatory effect. NICE recommends a trial of treatment in non-smokers if their pharmacological therapy has been optimised and they have been referred for pulmonary rehabilitation, but continue to experience either frequent (more than four) exacerbations with sputum production, prolonged exacerbations with sputum production, or exacerbations resulting in hospitalisation.[7]

The recommended dose varies from 250 mg three times a week in some guidelines,[7] to 500 mg three times a week, or 250 mg once a day in others.[1] In practice, a pragmatic approach is to start at the lowest dose, which can then be increased according to clinical response and adverse events.

Adverse effects include bacterial resistance, prolongation of the QTc interval and tinnitus. Consequently, monitoring of ECG and hearing is recommended, and treatment should only be commenced where coexisting mycobacterial infection has been excluded due to the risk of developing resistance.

Oral corticosteroids

Oral corticosteroids, such as prednisolone, have no role in the long-term management of COPD due to the risk of significant systemic adverse effects and limited evidence of benefit in stable disease.

Medication changes

Patients on treatment should be reviewed regularly to assess their symptoms and risk of future exacerbations. In patients who have worsening breathlessness and/or frequent exacerbations, their adherence to their current prescription and inhaler technique should be assessed prior to increasing their pharmacological treatment.

GOLD and NICE agree that occasional mild symptoms require PRN SABA alone, supported by non-pharmacological interventions. For patients who continue to experience high levels of symptoms, but infrequent exacerbations on SABA alone, GOLD recommends the addition of a single long-acting bronchodilator therapy (either a LABA or LAMA), and then to step up to dual long-acting LABA/LAMA bronchodilator therapy as a second-line option in patients who remain symptomatic or with poor health status despite treatment with monotherapy.[1]

In contrast, NICE advises that patients who continue to be limited by symptoms or have exacerbations despite treatment with SABA alone, and who do not have any features of asthma or steroid responsiveness, should be optimised to LABA/LAMA dual long-acting bronchodilator therapy from the outset, as this is more cost-effective than single long-acting bronchodilator therapy.[7]

The approach that NICE recommends may be a more pragmatic and appropriate approach for many COPD patients because many continue to experience significant symptoms on single long-acting bronchodilator therapy, irrespective of whether they had mild to moderate or severe to very severe airflow limitation.[23] Optimising the treatment of symptomatic patients with moderate severity COPD with dual long-acting bronchodilator therapy produces significant improvements in lung function and breathlessness.[24]

Persistent breathlessness on dual inhaled therapies

For patients who experience persistent breathlessness or exercise limitation despite an adequate trial (at least 6-8 weeks) of ICS/LABA treatment, both GOLD and NICE recommend the addition of a LAMA (i.e. triple inhaled therapy with ICS/LABA/LAMA).[1,7] Alternatively, the ICS/LABA could be switched to a LABA/LAMA if there is no indication for ICS, such as in patients with no history of exacerbations, lack of response, and/or adverse effects necessitating withdrawal of treatment (e.g. pneumonia).

In patients using a LABA/LAMA dual long-acting bronchodilator who continue to have day-to-day symptoms that adversely affect their quality of life despite an adequate trial (at least 6-8 weeks) of treatment, NICE also recommend a trial of adding an ICS in patients (i.e. triple inhaled therapy with ICS/LABA/LAMA).[7]

Exacerbations

For patients experiencing frequent exacerbations on SABA alone, particularly where blood eosinophil count is low (<300 cells per microlitre), it may also be prudent to commence dual long-acting bronchodilators (LABA/LAMA) as there are data demonstrating superiority in exacerbation prevention compared to ICS/LABA, with a reduction in pneumonia risk.[25]

However, in patients with a history of asthma or features suggesting steroid responsiveness (e.g. a higher blood eosinophil count (≥300 cells per microlitre), substantial variation in FEV_1 or peak expiratory flow), stepping up to an ICS/LABA may be a preferable approach.[1,7]

In patients who continue to experience exacerbations despite LABA/LAMA or ICS/LABA treatment, stepping up to triple inhaled therapy (ICS + LABA + LAMA) is recommended.[1,7] The addition of an ICS to dual long-acting bronchodilator (LABA/LAMA therapy) is particularly recommended where the eosinophil count is greater than 300 cells per microlitre. However, if the eosinophil count is low (<100 cells per microlitre), the evidence that ics will have a beneficial effect is limited. consequently, addition of azithromycin or roflumilast may be preferable[1] (although this is outside of NICE guidelines).[7]

See *Figure 6.2* which outlines a pharmacological treatment pathway for people with COPD.

For inhaled triple therapy (ICS/LABA/LAMA), there are no studies assessing the effectiveness of using combination ICS/LABA/LAMA inhalers on adherence or patient preference in comparison to using separate inhalers. However, the cost of combination inhalers is lower than using separate inhalers, allowing the possibility of financial savings whilst simplifying treatment for patients.

The TRIBUTE[18] and IMPACT[19] studies provide good evidence for the benefits of using a three-drug ICS/LABA/LAMA inhaler compared to an ICS/LABA, or even a LABA/LAMA inhaler. There are concerns with the study design and patient recruitment for both studies such as recruitment of mainly low-exacerbating patients in TRIBUTE, and rapid de-escalation of ICS at the start of the study rather than at the start of the run-in period in IMPACT. This reduces confidence that triple inhalers should be used routinely in place of two-drug FDC inhalers, and certainly from IMPACT, concerns about pneumonia with ICS continue. It may well be prudent to prescribe Trelegy Ellipta and Trimbow MDI for COPD patients who continue to experience frequent exacerbations despite good adherence and good inhaler technique with two-drug FDC inhalers containing either LABA/LAMA or ICS/LABA, which is advised by NICE[6] and GOLD.[1]

Figure 6.2: *NICE COPD inhaler algorithm 2019[7]*

Chronic obstructive pulmonary disease in over 16s: non-pharmacological management and use of inhaled therapies

Confirmed diagnosis of COPD

Fundamentals of COPD care:
- Offer treatment and support to **stop smoking**
- Offer **pneumococcal** and **influenza vaccinations**
- Offer **pulmonary rehabilitation** if indicated
- Co-develop a personalised **self-management plan**
- Optimise treatment for **comorbidities**

These treatments and plans should be revisited at every review

Start inhaled therapies only if:
- all the above interventions have been offered (if appropriate), and
- inhaled therapies are needed to relieve breathlessness and exercise limitation, and
- people have been trained to use inhalers and can demonstrate satisfactory technique

Review medication and assess inhaler technique and adherence regularly for all inhaled therapies

Offer SABA or SAMA to use as needed

If the person is limited by symptoms or has exacerbations despite treatment:

No asthmatic features or features suggesting steroid responsiveness[a]

Asthmatic features or features suggesting steroid responsiveness[a]

Offer LABA + LAMA

Consider LABA + ICS[b]

Person has day-to-day symptoms that adversely impact quality of life

Person has 1 severe or 2 moderate exacerbations within a year

Person has day-to-day symptoms that adversely impact quality of life, or has 1 severe or 2 moderate exacerbations within a year

Consider 3-month trial of LABA + LAMA + ICS[b,c]

Consider LABA + LAMA + ICS[b,c]

Offer LABA + LAMA + ICS[b,c]

If no improvement, revert to LABA + LAMA

Explore further treatment options if still limited by breathlessness or subject to frequent exacerbations (see guideline for more details)

[a] Asthmatic features/features suggesting steroid responsiveness in this context include any previous secure diagnosis of asthma or atopy, a higher blood eosinophil count, substantial variation in FEV1 over time (at least 400 ml) or substantial diurnal variation in peak expiratory flow (at least 20%).

[b] Be aware of an increased risk of side effects (including pneumonia) in people who take ICS.

[c] Document in clinical records the reason for continuing ICS treatment.

This is a summary of the recommendations on non-pharmacological management of chronic obstructive pulmonary disease and use of inhaled therapies in people over 16. The guideline also covers diagnosis and other areas of management. See www.nice.org.uk/guidance/NG115

See the NICE website for information on how we use offer and consider to show strength of recommendations.

© NICE 2019. All rights reserved. Subject to Notice of rights. Last updated May 2019.

NICE National Institute for Health and Care Excellence

Reproduced with permission from NICE.

Patients who continue to experience frequent exacerbations should be referred to a specialist COPD service. In such cases, the diagnosis should be reviewed and confirmed, the treatment of any comorbidities optimised, and their adherence to treatment and inhaler technique checked and optimised. If this does not resolve the problem, then the addition of azithromycin or roflumilast should be considered in eligible patients.[1,7]

Stopping inhaled corticosteroids

There is an emerging consensus in the respiratory community that ICSs are largely over-prescribed in COPD, and that they should be avoided in the majority of patients unless they are frequent exacerbators, very symptomatic, and potentially if they have an elevated blood eosinophil count. Furthermore, there are concerns about an increased risk of pneumonia in COPD patients treated with ICS[26] and those of older age, lower body mass index, more severe airflow limitation, more frequent COPD exacerbation rates and low eosinophil counts.

LABA/LAMA combination inhalers have been shown to be effective at preventing exacerbations compared to ICS/LABA inhalers with a lower risk of pneumonia, and so withdrawal of ICS in patients at risk of pneumonia where there is likely to be no clinical benefit is likely to be beneficial.

Two studies (WISDOM[27] and SUNSET[28]) have shown that ICS withdrawal in patients taking triple inhaled therapy (ICS + LABA + LAMA) in patients with moderate to very severe COPD, with or without a history of exacerbations, was well tolerated and did not result in an increase in exacerbation rates in the overall population. Conversely, a potentially high-risk group of patients with an eosinophil count ≥300 cells per microlitre was identified on subgroup analyses, as these had a higher risk of subsequent exacerbations after ICS withdrawal. This suggests that patients with high eosinophil counts are more likely to benefit from ICS/LABA/LAMA than LABA/LAMA.

De-escalation of therapy should be performed with caution due to the lack of long-term follow-up data, and patients should be monitored closely to ensure that a return of worsening symptoms or exacerbations does not occur.

Box 6.4: Practice point: COPD treatment

- There are currently two guidelines commonly used in the UK to guide COPD treatment: NICE (2018) and GOLD, which are updated annually.
- The most cost-effective treatments for COPD are smoking cessation, annual flu vaccination and pulmonary rehabilitation.
- Patients should start treatment at the level most appropriate to the initial level of COPD symptoms and exacerbation history, which for most patients will be a combination of one or more bronchodilators.
- Before initiating a new drug in patients it is important to check their adherence and inhaler technique.
- Inhaled corticosteroids (ICS) should be reserved for patients who experience frequent exacerbations despite optimised treatment with dual long-acting bronchodilators.
- Patients should be referred to specialist COPD services if they are not controlled on triple inhaled therapies.
- Mucolytics may be beneficial in patients with a chronic productive cough.
- Roflumilast and azithromycin may have a role in selected patient groups, and are usually restricted to specialist use only.

Monitoring

Long-term follow-up of COPD patients is recommended as the condition will progress over time even with the best available management. Pharmacists based in GP practice and hospital outpatient clinics are well placed to take on this responsibility with support from other members of the multidisciplinary team.

Routine investigations include spirometry and assessment of exercise capacity and oxygenation. Annual spirometry is recommended to measure annual decline in FEV_1 and identify patients with rapidly declining lung function. Exercise endurance can be measured using the 6-minute walking or shuttle test, and patients referred for pulmonary rehabilitation if they meet local eligibility criteria. Oxygen saturation at rest should also be measured to identify the need for supplemental oxygen.

During COPD consultations, and at least annually, pharmacists or other healthcare professionals should measure health status and symptoms of COPD using the CAT score and MRC dyspnoea scale, as these will allow assessment of changes in health status and response to treatments. Community pharmacists in some regions provide dedicated inhaler technique training services, and measuring health status before and several weeks after providing the service can provide invaluable information on the performance of this service.[29,30]

Patients should be asked about the frequency, severity and causes of exacerbations, including the presence or absence of increased sputum volume and purulence during exacerbations, and how they have been managed. The frequency of use of rescue packs, oral corticosteroids and antibiotics should be determined to assess whether they have been used appropriately, or whether maintenance therapy needs escalating.

COPD treatment should be reviewed and optimised on an annual basis, and if patients have deteriorated. This should include an assessment of adherence, inhaler technique, and appropriateness of treatment (including response and adverse effects) to determine whether any therapies need escalating or de-escalating. Blood eosinophils may be a useful measure to determine the need for ICS. Uptake of the annual flu vaccine should also be checked as this is an important intervention for the prevention of avoidable exacerbations.

Patients should also be asked about their smoking history at each annual review, and current smokers offered advice and support to stop smoking, as a key intervention in COPD.

Follow-up and referral

Most people with COPD should have a routine review of their condition and treatment on an annual basis, although those with very severe COPD should be reviewed every six months.[7] More frequent reviews may be required where there is a clinical need, such as in patients experiencing an increased number of exacerbations or hospitalisations, or worsening chronic symptoms.

When changes are made to a patient's treatment regimen, a follow-up appointment should be offered to assess the impact of any changes made and can be measured with tools such as the CAT score. In some situations, a telephone consultation may be the most efficient mechanism to do this, although face-to-face follow-up consultations can often be more useful, particularly where inhaler technique needs to be assessed.

It is important that pharmacists are aware of the multidisciplinary team and local services available to help support people with COPD in the community. Routine referral pathways in COPD include community respiratory nurses, physiotherapists, occupational therapists, social services, dieticians, palliative care, as well as community pharmacists.

Community respiratory nurses can provide additional care of the patient in their home and support those requiring home oxygen or ventilation, and to provide psychological and emotional support for the patients and their families. Respiratory physiotherapists help patients with breathing techniques to help reduce the work of breathing associated with respiratory disease and to improve peripheral and respiratory muscle fitness and function. Community pharmacy services are available to support patients with taking their medicines and to teach and reinforce good inhaler technique.

Patients should be referred to a specialist where there is any uncertainty in the diagnosis, in the presence of severe COPD or where there has been a rapid decline in FEV_1 at the onset of cor pulmonale.

Patients should be referred urgently to a doctor if there is presence of any red flag symptoms consistent with any urgent medical conditions, including: where the cough changes in nature or lasts for more than three weeks, in the presence of haemoptysis, unexplained weight loss, chest pain, cyanosis, worsening oedema, severe fatigue, inability to speak sentences, night sweats or finger clubbing.

Useful resources

- GOLD. Global strategy for diagnosis, management, and prevention of COPD. 2020. www.goldcopd.org
- NICE. Chronic obstructive pulmonary disease in over 16s: diagnosis and management. NICE guideline [NG115] 2018. www.nice.org.uk/guidance/ng115
- NICE. Chronic obstructive pulmonary disease (acute exacerbation): antimicrobial prescribing. NICE guideline [NG114] 2018. www.nice.org.uk/guidance/ng114
- Clinical Knowledge Summary. www.cks.nice.org.uk/chronic-obstructive-pulmonary-disease
- British Lung Foundation. Supporting Pharmacists. www.blf.org.uk/health-care-professionals/supporting-pharmacists
- National Centre for Smoking Cessation Training. www.ncsct.co.uk
- Asthma UK. Inhaler technique videos. www.asthma.org.uk/advice/inhaler-videos
- RightBreathe. www.rightbreathe.com

References

1. GOLD (Global Initiative for Chronic Obstructive Lung Disease). Global strategy for diagnosis, management, and prevention of COPD. 2020. www.goldcopd.org

2. British Lung Foundation. The battle for breath – the impact of lung disease in the UK. 2016. www.blf.org.uk/policy/the-battle-for-breath-2016

3. Wright D *et al*. Chronic obstructive pulmonary disease case finding by community pharmacists: a potential cost-effective public health intervention. *International Journal of Pharmacy Practice* 2015; 23: 83-85.

4. Jones RCM *et al*. Accuracy of diagnostic registers and management of chronic obstructive pulmonary disease: the Devon primary care audit. *Respiratory Research* 2008; 9: 62.

5. Enright P *et al*. Can nurses successfully diagnose and manage patients with COPD? *Primary Care Respiratory Journal* 2014; 23: 12-13.

6. Fisk M *et al*. Inaccurate diagnosis of COPD: the Welsh National COPD Audit. *Br J Gen Pract* 2019; 69: e1-e7.

7. National Institute for Heath and Care Excellence (2018). Chronic obstructive pulmonary disease in over 16s: diagnosis and management. NICE guideline [NG115]. London: NICE. www.nice.org.uk/guidance/ng115

8. Jones PW *et al*. Development and first validation of the COPD Assessment Test. *Eur Respir J* 2009; 34: 648-654.

9. Jones PW. St. George's Respiratory Questionnaire: MCID. COPD. 2005; 2: 75-9.

10. NHS Networks. LRN's COPD Value Pyramid. 2014. www.networks.nhs.uk/nhs-networks/london-lungs/latest-edition-of-thorax-publication

11. National Institute for Heath and Care Excellence (2018). Stop smoking interventions and services. NICE guideline [NG92]. London: NICE. www.nice.org.uk/guidance/ng92

12. Usmani O *et al*. Choosing an appropriate inhaler device for the treatment of adults with asthma or COPD. *Guidelines* [online] 2017. www.guidelines.co.uk/respiratory/inhaler-choice-guideline/252870.article

13. Horita N *et al*. Long-acting muscarinic antagonist (LAMA) plus long-acting beta-agonist (LABA) versus LABA plus inhaled corticosteroid (ICS) for stable chronic obstructive pulmonary disease (COPD) (Review). *Cochrane Database of Systematic Reviews* 2017, Issue 2.

14. Calverley P *et al*. Salmeterol and Fluticasone Propionate and Survival in Chronic Obstructive Pulmonary Disease. *N Engl J Med* 2007; 356: 775-789.

15. Pascoe S *et al*. Blood eosinophil counts, exacerbations, and response to the addition of inhaled fluticasone furoate to vilanterol in patients with chronic obstructive pulmonary disease: a secondary analysis of data from two parallel randomised controlled trials. *Lancet Respir Med* 2015; 3: 435-42

16. Bafadhel M *et al*. Predictors of exacerbation risk and response to budesonide in patients with chronic obstructive pulmonary disease: a post-hoc analysis of three randomised trials. *Lancet Respir Med* 2018; 6: 117-26.

17. Papi A *et al*. Extrafine inhaled triple therapy versus dual bronchodilator therapy in chronic obstructive pulmonary disease (TRIBUTE):a double-blind, parallel group, randomised controlled trial. *Lancet* 2018; 391(10125): 1076-1084.

18. Lipson DA *et al*. Once-daily Single-Inhaler Triple versus Dual Therapy in Patients with COPD. *New Eng J Med* 2018; 378: 1671-1680.

19. Singh D *et al.* Single inhaler triple therapy versus inhaled corticosteroid plus long-acting β2-agonist therapy for chronic obstructive pulmonary disease (TRILOGY): a double-blind, parallel group, randomised controlled trial. *Lancet* 2016; 388(10048): 963-973.

20. Wedzicha JA *et al.* Prevention of COPD exacerbations: a European Respiratory Society/American Thoracic Society guideline. *Eur Respir J* 2017; 50: 1602265.

21. National Institute for Heath and Care Excellence (2017). Roflumilast for treating chronic obstructive pulmonary disease. Technology appraisal guidance [TA461]. London: NICE. www.nice.org.uk/guidance/TA461

22. Martinez FJ *et al.* Effect of roflumilast on exacerbations in patients with severe chronic obstructive pulmonary disease uncontrolled by combination therapy (REACT): a multicentre randomised controlled trial. *Lancet* 2015; 385: 857-66.

23. Dransfield MT *et al.* Disease severity and symptoms among patients receiving monotherapy for COPD. *Prim Care Respir J* 2011; 20: 46-53.

24. Vogelmeier CF *et al.* CRYSTAL study investigators Efficacy and safety of direct switch to indacaterol/glycopyrronium in patients with moderate COPD: the CRYSTAL open-label randomised trial. *Respir Res* 2017; 18(1): 140.

25. Wedzicha JA *et al.* Indacaterol-glycopyrronium versus salmeterol-fluticasone for COPD. *New Engl J Med* 2016; 374: 2222-2234.

26. Kew KM, Seniukovich A. Inhaled steroids and risk of pneumonia for chronic obstructive pulmonary disease. *Cochrane Database of Systematic Reviews* 2014, Issue 3.

27. Watz H *et al.* Blood eosinophil count and exacerbations in severe chronic obstructive pulmonary disease after withdrawal of inhaled corticosteroids: a post-hoc analysis of the WISDOM trial. *Lancet Resp Med* 2016; 4(5): 390-398.

28. Chapman KR *et al.* Long-term triple therapy de-escalation to indacaterol/glycopyrronium in patients with chronic obstructive pulmonary disease (SUNSET): a randomized, double- blind, triple-dummy clinical trial. *Am J Respir Crit Care Med* 2018; 198: 329-339.

29. Community Pharmacy West Yorkshire. Enabling Patient Health Improvements through COPD (EPIC) Medicines Optimisation within Community Pharmacy: a prospective cohort study. www.cpwy.org/doc/1433.pdf

30. The Cambridge Consortium. Evaluation of inhaler technique improvement project. 2012. Cambridge, UK: Cambridge Inst. for Research Education and Management (CiREM).

Case studies

Case study 1

Robert, aged 57 years, attends his local community pharmacy with a prescription for salbutamol 100 micrograms MDI 2 puffs four times a day when required, and you realise from your PMR that this is the fifth prescription for this in the past three months. You ask him how he's getting on with his inhaler, and he tells you that it doesn't seem to be helping much even though he's using it every day, so you ask him into your consultation room for a chat about his treatment.

He tells you that he'd been getting breathless for some time and had noticed that he was struggling to walk to the pub. His GP diagnosed him with COPD earlier in the year after doing some breathing tests and gave him a blue inhaler which he's used at least four times a day.

Points to consider

- What are the causes of poor response to salbutamol?
- How can you assess the severity of his symptoms?
- Does he understand when to use his salbutamol?
- Is he using his inhaler correctly?

Robert tells you that he feels a bit on his own, and is not really sure what his diagnosis means or what his medicines are for, so you discuss these with him. He tells you he smokes 20 cigarettes a day and you complete a COPD Assessment Test and record a score of 15/40 indicating a medium impact of COPD on health. His MRC score is 3.

You explain that he should only have to use his salbutamol inhaler on an as required basis (not regularly) and he clearly requires something stronger to reduce his need for salbutamol. Assessing his inhaler technique, you find that he is only able to inhale quickly and deeply.

Points to consider

- What class(es) of drug therapy should Robert be prescribed next?
- What type of inhaler device might be suitable for Robert?
- What other interventions would you make for people with COPD?

With Robert's permission, you speak to his GP to discuss your consultation and assessment of his symptoms. You agree that he needs to step up his treatment to Anoro 55/22 Ellipta 1 puff once a day and Easyhaler salbutamol 100 micrograms 2 puffs when required. Later that day, Robert returns with a prescription for his new inhalers and you assess his inhaler technique with both devices as good. He understands when and why to use both inhalers.

Points to consider

- What patient support groups could you recommend to Robert?
- When and how should his response to treatment be reassessed?

Case study 2

Lisa, aged 67 years, is brought into the emergency department with an oxygen saturation of 92% on 28% oxygen via venturi facemask, her respiratory rate is 35 breaths per minute, blood pressure 85/60 mmHg and weight 52 kg.

Her blood tests show a urea of 8 micromoles/L, creatinine 75 mmol/L, haemoglobin 140g/L, white cell count 15×10^9/L, eosinophils 0.01×10^9/L, CRP 170 mg/L and chest X-ray shows bibasal consolidation. A diagnosis of severe multilobar community-acquired pneumonia is made on the background of COPD; the third admission for pneumonia in the past 12 months. She is prescribed:

- Ceftazidime 1 g three times a day
- Prednisolone 30 mg once a day
- Salbutamol 2.5 mg nebules four times a day
- Ipratropium 500 microgram nebules four times a day

Points to consider

- Does the antibiotic regimen comply with local antibiotic formularies?
- How long are intravenous antibiotics required for?
- Are any other acute medicines required?
- What monitoring is required?

The first doses of her medicines are administered urgently in the emergency department prior to her transfer to the respiratory high dependency unit. You speak to her about her medication history and get permission to access her medical records to complete the medicines reconciliation. You confirm her drug history, which she has been prescribed for 18 months:

- Seretide 500 Accuhaler 1 puff twice a day
- Spiriva 18 micrograms once a day
- Salbutamol 100 micrograms 2 puffs when required
- Uniphyllin 400 mg twice a day
- Carbocisteine 750 mg twice a day
- No known drug allergies

Points to consider

- Could her medication be contributing to her acute illness?
- What are the consequences of using inhaler devices that require different inspiratory manoeuvres?
- Should Spiriva be prescribed with ipratropium nebules?

24 hours after admission, Lisa is responding to treatment and you check her inhaler technique and find that she has a weak inspiratory effort. On discussion with the medical team, you propose that the inhaled corticosteroid should be stopped. You agree to switch her Seretide and Spiriva to Spiolto 2.5/2.5 micrograms Respimat 2 puffs once a day, and she has good technique with this device.

Points to consider

- Can the inhaled corticosteroid be stopped suddenly, or should it be reduced slowly?
- What advice should be given to avoid adverse effects from Spiolto?
- How many times can a new refill canister be used in a reusable Respimat?

A few days later Lisa is stepped down to oral co-amoxiclav and clarithromycin to complete the course of treatment.

Points to consider

- How would you manage any drug interaction with her regular medication?
- What support could you arrange for her after discharge?

CHAPTER 7

Chronic pain

Deborah Steven, Suzanne Saunders and Karen Somerville

Overview

The International Association for the Study of Pain (IASP) defines pain as 'An unpleasant sensory and emotional experience associated with actual or potential tissue damage, or described in terms of such damage'.[1] Pain can be described by its severity, temporal characteristic, type, location or underlying pathophysiology.

Chronic pain may be considered as pain lasting longer than 3-6 months or 'pain that extends beyond the expected period of healing'. The terms chronic or persistent pain are interchangeable. This chapter will focus on chronic pain although some information will apply to acute and cancer pain.

Chronic pain is a multidimensional phenomenon that can affect everyday function and quality of life. It occurs as a result of complex mechanisms that are not fully understood;[1] it may or may not be associated with an underlying cause (see *Table 7.1*). It can often be the pain pathway itself at fault, involving mechanisms such as central sensitisation; it is not merely an extension of acute pain over time.[2]

Table 7.1: *Conditions associated with pain*

Underlying condition	Clinical features
Chronic low back pain	Pain, muscle tension or stiffness localised below the costal margin and above the inferior gluteal folds, with or without sciatica.
Osteoarthritis (OA)	The most common chronic joint condition. It occurs when the protective cartilage on the ends of bones breaks down and the bones within the joint rub together, causing pain, swelling and problems moving the joint. OA occurs most often in older people, although it can occur in adults of any age.
Rheumatoid arthritis (RA)	An autoimmune disorder that causes pain, swelling and stiffness in the joints; other systemic features can be present. The most commonly affected joints are the small joints of the hands and feet, however, any joint may be affected, typically on both sides of the body.
Peripheral neuropathy	Occurs when there is damage to peripheral nerves. Diabetic neuropathy is a common cause. Symptoms are usually constant, but can be intermittent and include numbness, tingling, burning, shooting or stabbing pain. There may also be loss of balance or muscle weakness.
Fibromyalgia or fibromyalgia syndrome (FMS)	A persistent and often debilitating syndrome which is more common in women. It is characterised by widespread muscle pain and stiffness, non-restorative sleep and fatigue. Other somatic complaints such as irritable bowel or cognitive impairment may be present.
Functional neurological disorder (FND)	No structural abnormality is identified – it is also called 'medically unexplained' neurological symptoms. Presence of neurological symptoms such as weakness, difficulty walking or controlling and moving limbs, sensory symptoms and blackouts. Symptoms may fluctuate or be there most of the time causing a lot of distress.
Complex regional pain syndrome (CRPS)	CRPS is a poorly understood condition in which there is persistent, severe and debilitating pain, often confined to one limb, usually after an injury. CRPS is believed to be caused by damage to, or malfunction of, the peripheral and central nervous systems.

It is estimated that between a third to a half of the UK population have chronic pain, classed as moderate to severe intensity in up to 14.3% of them.[3] People with chronic pain consult their GP around five times more frequently than those without, and it accounts for 22% of primary care consultations, which results in a significant impact on healthcare resource.[4]

Risk factors for the development of chronic can be:[5]

- physical – female gender, genetics, older age, obesity or previous injury
- psychological – history of depression, anxiety or childhood trauma
- social – lower socioeconomic groups, lack of social support and occupational risk factors.

Chronic pain is unlikely to resolve, but with appropriate pain management strategies there is potential for improvement. Many patients find their own ways to manage, whilst others require advice and support from primary care clinicians and some benefit from more specialist input. Treatment aims for chronic pain can differ from acute or cancer pain, and medication alone is unlikely to achieve complete pain relief. The application of the biopsychosocial model (see *Figure 7.1*) of illness to chronic pain[6] has become the accepted paradigm and all dimensions should be considered in assessment and treatment to provide the best outcomes for patients.

Figure 7.1: *Biopsychosocial model with examples of factors affecting pain experience*

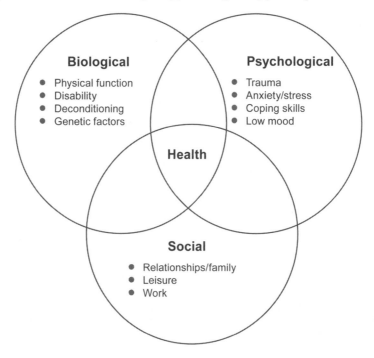

Diagnosis

When pain persists past the normal healing time of 3-6 months, understandably patients want to know what is going on and seek a specific diagnosis.

If chronic pain is associated with a pathological diagnosis, such as osteoarthritis or rheumatoid arthritis, this can be reassuring for patients and support the interventions offered. Similar tests are used to rule out disease and severe pathology, but this can be confusing and distressing for patients as they wonder why the tests do not find a medical cause for their pain that can be 'fixed'. Direct measurement of pain presents a challenge and investigations such as X-ray or MRI are not an accurate measure or account of an individual's pain.

If 'chronic/persistent pain' is considered as the diagnosis then the assessment and management are similar, irrespective of the underlying cause. At the same time, it is important that if you identify specific indicators of a yet undiagnosed condition, you refer appropriately for assessment (e.g. mirror image joint pain with inflammation in rheumatoid arthritis).

Pharmacy input

All pharmacists, irrelevant of setting can use their core skills in managing people with chronic pain by providing ongoing assessment and review to ensure medication is optimised, effective and safe. Some suggested interventions that may be suitable depending on your knowledge and skill levels are outlined in *Table 7.2*.

Advice on non-pharmacological strategies should also be given, with signposting to other services, supporting the biopsychosocial approach to pain management.

Table 7.2: *Pharmacist interventions in managing chronic pain*

Core interventions	● Ensure medicines use is effective and safe.
	  − Identify uncontrolled or poorly managed pain and suggest strategies to improve management.
	  − Provide advice on driving restrictions, tolerance, dependency, or addiction issues.
	  − Ensure patient is aware of maximum dosage, which medicines should be regularly used, and which should be used when required basis.
	  − Support patients to step down medication if their pain is well controlled, is causing adverse effects, or is ineffective.
	  − Assess GI risk of NSAIDs and whether a PPI is required for gastroprotection.
	  − Manage common adverse effects, such as constipation with opioids.
	● Advise on non-pharmacological treatment options.
	● Signpost to local service and third sector agencies.
	● Implement local or national prescribing initiatives.
	● Liaise between different sectors regarding interface issues.

Community pharmacist	● Ensure regular contact with chronic pain patients.
	● Conduct ad hoc reviews or identify specific patient groups for review.
	  − Identify and offer support to patients who are self-managing chronic pain with over-the-counter (OTC) medicines. Opportunity to provide advice on NSAIDs or codeine. Participation in safety initiatives (e.g. NSAID safer care bundle www.ihub.scot/media/6476/20190627-nhs-his-sc-toolkit-guidance-booklet-240x190mm.pdf).
	  − Patients taking NSAIDs may be eligible for medicine review services provided by community pharmacy.

Pharmacist working in GP practice	● Develop and/or implement a practice policy on high risk medication for chronic pain. ● Provide information on prescribing data and trends. ● Reconcile medicines including when patients are discharged from hospital. ● Conduct ad hoc reviews or identify specific patient groups for review.
Pharmacist working in secondary care clinic or ward	● Take an accurate medication history, including OTC medicines and illicit drugs. ● Identify if the presenting complaint could be attributed to medication (e.g. serotonin syndrome). ● Ensure discharge/clinic information is clear (e.g. short-term acute or post-op pain relief).
Independent prescriber – chronic pain	● Optimise current medication. ● Change medicines within therapeutic group when required. ● Assess/monitor renal function and adjust doses where appropriate.
Specialist chronic pain independent prescriber	● Manage patient expectations. ● Manage complex medication regimens and discuss more complex prescribing issues or decisions (e.g. risk of QT prolongation with TCAs + SSRIs). ● Use non-formulary medication where appropriate. ● Liaise with consultants regarding complex patients and medication regimens. ● Work within multidisciplinary team to provide holistic pain management to patients. ● Develop and review formulary guidance and prescribing resources

Informal or ad hoc reviews can be undertaken in any pharmacy setting, initiated with simple statements such as: 'I see you are on pain medicines at the moment, how is your pain?', or 'Do you feel your medicines are helping you?'. This may allow a brief intervention or lead to a more formal planned review.

Pharmacy review

When undertaking a review in people with chronic pain, assessment of the benefits of their pain medication is fundamental, but this should be part of a wider holistic assessment of their pain experience, including an overview of their activity, sleep, mood and understanding of their condition.

There are a variety of tools to support the assessment of pain (see *Table 7.3*), such as body descriptor charts, pain diaries or questionnaires which can be completed by the patient in advance and prompt discussion during the assessment.

Table 7.3: *Pain assessment tools*

Pain assessment tools	Comment	Benefits	Limitations
Body descriptor chart (see *Figure 7.2*)	Can be completed by patient or clinician with patient support to indicate areas affected	May help identify patterns such as mirror joint pain in rheumatoid arthritis or fibromyalgia (pain in all 4 quadrants)	Indicates site but not intensity or type of pain
Numerical rating scale (NRS) – an 11-point numerical scale	Self-reported; the scale is from 0 (no pain at all) to 10 (worst pain imaginable)	Quick – useful in acute pain to determine level of intervention needed	Only valid at that point in time unless contextualised as: 'Over the last 2 weeks, how would you rate your pain?'
Verbal rating scale (VRS) Variety available, score attributed to descriptor.	Self-reported as: No pain = 0 Mild = 1 Moderate = 2 Severe = 3 Excruciating = 4	Quick – useful in acute pain to determine level of intervention needed	Same as NRS
Faces scale (see *Figure 7.3*)	Illustrative, can be linked to NRS/VRS	Useful to overcome language barriers	Same as NRS
Pain diary	Completed by patient; may note pain severity, activities and medication taken at different times of the day and may include comment on mood	Can be useful to identify issues with over/under-activity or issues with timing of doses	Time consuming for patient to complete
FLACC (Face, Legs, Activity, Cry, Consolability scale)	Observational tool to support carers/clinicians identify levels of pain in children or others unable to communicate their pain	Validated and easy to use	Physical impairments (e.g. muscle tone) may lead to underestimation from facial expressions
PAINAD (Pain Assessment IN Advanced Dementia)	Observational tool to support carers/clinicians identify levels of pain in cognitively impaired	Validated tool which allows pain assessment in patients unable to communicate	Consideration should be given to alternative cause of 'pain behaviour'; Is patient too cold?
POMI – Prescription Opioid Misuse Index (see *Box 7.4*)	A 6-point questionnaire with strong predictive ability for opioid use disorder	Allows identification of inappropriate opioid use	Only validated for opioids
GAD-7 (generalised anxiety disorder – 7 questions)	Self-reported measure for screening levels of anxiety	Helps identify whether patient needs further support or clinical review for anxiety	Only focuses on generalised anxiety, not validated for other disorders (e.g. post-traumatic stress disorder).
PHQ-9 (patient health questionnaire – 9 questions)	Self-reported measure for screening for levels of depression	Helps identify whether patient needs further support or clinical review for depression	Validated in primary care; not a diagnostic tool for use in an acute psychiatric episode

*All tools are easily accessible online.

As pain is multifactorial, ideally, assessment should be too, not only focussing on diagnosis and medication but also including discussing any underlying concerns that the patient may have. Assessment can include as much or as little of *Table 7.4* as time, experience, competence and accessibility to patient records allow. When supporting patients with chronic pain, recognition and assessment of how the pain is impacting on many aspects of their life, not just the physical sensation or intensity, will help those patients that have not yet recognised the application of the biopsychosocial model to do so and show that you are interested in them as a whole person.

Table 7.4: *Assessment of pain*

Assessment	Questions to consider	Rationale
Pain • Location • Severity/intensity • Description • Temporal • Red flags • Diagnoses (if known) • Physical examination (if skilled in this area)	• Where is the pain? • How bad is the pain on a 0-10 scale? (NRS) • Can you describe it? • What makes your pain worse? • What helps your pain? • Is it worse at certain times of the day?	• The description can help identify the type of pain (mechanical/inflammatory/neuropathic) and guide the choice of analgesic. • Does the patient describe something that merits further investigation or onward referral? And how urgently? (for red flags – see *Box 7.2*). • Physical examination may identify red, swollen joints or physical limitations (e.g. Heberden nodes on hands).
Patient concerns and understanding • Establish whether they have a diagnosis • Clarify their understanding and expectations	• What do you think is causing your pain? • What do you understand by your diagnosis? • Do you have any concerns about your diagnosis?	• Patients may wonder why they have not had specific tests. • Sometimes patients are afraid of what has been missed (i.e. do they have cancer?). • Not addressing these issues may hinder progression in self-management.
Medication • Current pain medication. Confirm doses & timings of dose (pain diary can help) • Previous pain medication • Non-pain medication • Adverse effects • OTC medicines, vitamins/supplements/alternative substances they use for pain • Assess against comorbidities and risk factors (e.g. renal/hepatic/anticholinergic burden/weight/frailty/ hypertension/cardiovascular or GI risk) • Patient concerns • Assessment of potential dependence/addiction	• What are you currently taking to manage your pain? • Do you feel it is helping your pain? • Is it causing you any side effects? • What concerns do you have about your pain medication? • What have you used before? Why did you stop? • Is there anything you use that you buy or borrow, legal or illegal that helps your pain? • Consider use of POMI questionnaire (see *Box 7.4*).	• Build a picture of medication use and their expectations from it. • Explain the different types of medication for different types of pain. • Simple explanation of things like duration of action may help patients accept tablet load for example. • Identify opportunities to optimise either dosing or timings or stop ineffective or potential harm-causing medicines. • Manage adverse effects if pain relief is beneficial. • It is important to have a comprehensive picture including other POM medicines borrowed from friends or relatives, or regular use of alternative substances such as cannabis or alcohol or CBD oils to manage pain. Building rapport with your patient will develop a level of trust and allow the best advice about their medicines to be given. Patient may not recognise opioid use disorder and resent the implication.
Self-management • Use of heat or cold • Use of TENS • Activity (e.g. Tai chi/yoga) • Relaxation • Pacing of activity	• What do you do to manage your pain? • Do you benefit from use of heat or cold? (e.g. baths/showers/hot water bottles/wheat packs/cool packs) • When you are distracted doing an activity you like, is your pain better?	• This helps establish whether the patient is focused on medication alone as the solution to their pain, or whether they are taking steps towards self managing the pain.
Background • Home circumstances • Partners or dependents • Working/retired/unemployed	• What type of house do you live in? Does it have stairs? • How does your partner help with your condition? • Do you have any caring responsibilities for others? • Are you off work due to ill health?	• Can help identify if patient is struggling with physical environment of home or emotional aspects of over/under supportive partner. • Caring for others may be preventing aspects of self care as they 'push on through'. • Are there financial implications adding to stress?

Table 7.4: *Assessment of pain (continued)*

Assessment	Questions to consider	Rationale
Observational • Visible wellbeing or pain behaviours such as grimacing • Walking/gait – use of a walking aid (crutches/stick) • Use of wheelchair • Physical positioning in chair	These features are observed.	• May help identify functional limitation, or if they would benefit from a walking aid. • Would they benefit from cushions/lumbar rolls? • Possible referral to podiatry for GAIT assessment.
Function and quality of life	• How active are you? • Is it stopping you from doing anything? (e.g. work/hobby/socialising/activities of daily living such as cleaning or shopping)	• Patients want to feel involved and have as 'normal' a life as possible. If they are unable to do tasks of daily living or work they may develop feelings of worthlessness and experience loss of identity.
Mood • Ask about mood • Consider use of GAD-7 and PHQ-9	• How do you feel your mood has been over the last few weeks? • Any significant changes?	• Chronic pain can have a negative impact on mood, even leading to suicidal thoughts or thoughts of self-harm. • Assess if patients needs additional support, safety net by giving advice and options and signpost accordingly.
Sleep • Assess duration and quality	• How is your sleep pattern? • Are you able to get to sleep ok? • Are you woken overnight by your pain? • Do you feel refreshed on waking in the morning? • Do you have daytime naps?	• Persistent poor sleep will have a negative effect on physical and emotional wellbeing. • Is sleep being hampered by poor pain control over 24-hour period or other factors including dietary (caffeine), lack of activity (not physically tired) or inability to get into a comfortable sleeping position?

The more facets the assessment has, the more opportunities there are to suggest non-pharmacological strategies that may improve quality of life and function, in addition to ensuring any medicines used are safe and effective. However, shorter, briefer interventions are also beneficial.

Box 7.1: Practice point: brief interventions

- While comprehensive assessments can improve quality of life, don't be put off undertaking brief interventions.
- Small changes can make big differences.
  - A patient takes paracetamol 500 mg, two in the morning and night, they feel the benefit, but it then wears off. Explaining paracetamol dosing is short-acting and that it can be used four times daily may improve overall pain relief for longer over the 24-hour period.

Pain is closely aligned to comorbidities of anxiety and depression (see **Chapter 1**) and they can have a detrimental effect on each other. Low mood, social isolation, lack of motivation and poor sleep pattern can be associated with chronic pain, or similarly an underlying untreated depressive condition. It is therefore important to consider mood as part of your assessment when you can.

When assessing pain, be alert to red flags (see *Box 7.2*). Red flag symptoms require onward referral for further assessment, and in the case of cauda equina symptoms (see *Box 7.3*) may require immediate presentation at accident and emergency.

Box 7.2: Practice point: musculoskeletal red flags

Be aware of red flag symptoms, including:
- bladder or bowel incontinence
- difficulty swallowing
- drop attacks
- dysphasia
- family history or previous history of cancer
- night sweats
- saddle anaesthesia
- thoracic pain
- unable to lie supine
- unexplained weight loss
- unremitting night pain.

Box 7.3: Cauda equina warning symptoms:[7]

Advise people to seek medical help immediately if they experience any combination of the following symptoms:
- loss of feeling/pins and needles between inner thighs or genitals
- numbness in or around back passage or buttocks
- altered feeling when using toilet paper to wipe themselves
- increasing difficulty when trying to urinate
- increasing difficulty when trying to stop or control flow of urine
- loss of sensation when urinating
- leaking urine or recent need to use pads
- not knowing when bladder is either full or empty
- inability to stop a bowel movement or leaking
- loss of sensation when passing a bowel motion
- change in ability to achieve an erection or ejaculate
- loss of sensation in genitals during sexual intercourse.

As pharmacy professionals, our focus is on ensuring any medicines used are initiated correctly, safely used and effective. However, your interaction will be enhanced and have greater benefit if you can place it in the context of the wider umbrella of pain self-management, encouraging and supporting the use of other interventions, such as:

- pacing activity – finding the optimum balance between activity and rest, breaking tasks down into bitesize achievable chunks
- participating in exercise
- good sleep hygiene
- other non-medicinal pain management strategies.

Reliance on medicines alone to resolve chronic pain will result in high failure rates and disappointment and frustration, which in turn, may increase pain levels.

Patient's managing chronic pain can become less active and therefore less able to participate in exercise, work or activities of daily living such as shopping, washing hair and looking after children. They can become socially isolated, withdrawing from hobbies and other social situations and become less motivated or have low mood, preventing them from doing the things they love. Anything you can do to encourage them to be active and engaged in themselves, their families, friends and activities and manage their pain more effectively can have a positive impact on improving their health and wellbeing.

Pain management should be patient-centred, consider what is important to the patient and focus on improving pain (where possible), quality of life and function.

In some cases review is about managing expectations, particularly in relation to the benefits of medication and physical activity. It is important to be active but not in a way that flares up their pain.

While other chronic conditions such as hypertension or diabetes have an objective measurement of control (e.g. blood pressure or HbA1c), in contrast pain is subjective and based on the patient's account. Pain is 'what the patient says it is' and the most useful measures for chronic pain come from the patient.

You can ask questions such as 'Is this a good day or a bad day?', or 'Over the last week have you had more good days than bad?' and values can be ascribed, such as the numerical rating scale (see *Table 7.3*), but this is only useful as a measure for that specific patient at that point in time. This gives a reference point to compare a patient's progress or whether an intervention is helping. Other improvements in physical functioning, mental health, quality of life or meeting personal goals are measures of progress too. The British Pain Society published a report on outcome measures appropriate for pain management which may help you identify tools that work for you.[8] Below are examples of a body descriptor chart and a variation of a 'faces scale'.

Figure 7.2: *Body descriptor chart*

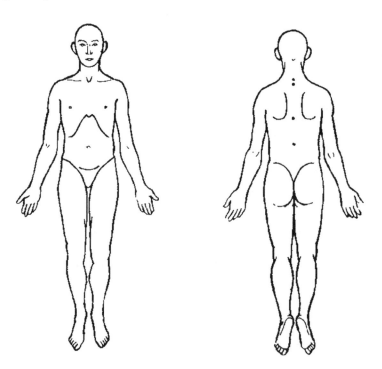

Figure 7.3: *Fife Pharmacy face pain scale*

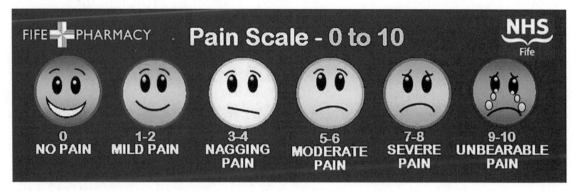

Medicines

Medicines should be safe, effective and include flexibility to empower patients to alter medication as their pain changes and to help manage 'flare-up'. You can help manage expectations that complete pain relief is rarely achieved in chronic pain and that a 30-50% reduction in pain levels or improved function is considered a good outcome – it could be the difference between the patient being able to participate in an activity or not. If you suspect issues of dependence or addiction you can utilise the POMI questionnaire[9] and offer appropriate support or utilise other services if an issue is identified.

Box 7.4: POMI – Prescription Opioid Misuse Index[9]

This tool can be used during a consultation or issued to the patient to complete pre- or post-consultation.
1. Do you ever use MORE of your medication, that is, take a higher dosage, than is prescribed for you?
2. Do you ever use your medication MORE OFTEN, that is, shorten the time between dosages, than is prescribed for you?
3. Do you ever need early refills for your pain medication?
4. Do you ever feel high or get a buzz after using your pain medication?
5. Do you ever take your pain medication because you are upset, using the medication to relieve or cope with problems other than pain?
6. Have you ever gone to multiple physicians including emergency room doctors, seeking more of your pain medication?
Answering 'Yes' to more than one question classifies an individual as an opioid misuser, with high sensitivity and specificity.

Most analgesics work well but only in a small number of people[10] and only a trial of a medicine will allow this to be determined. It is reasonable to trial a range of pain medications, but it is important to review treatment within 1-2 months of initiation, where only the most effective medications with the fewest adverse effects are continued.

Any risk factors need to be assessed when initiating or reviewing treatment (e.g. anticholinergic burden, renal and liver function, high-risk medicine combinations, risk of medication abuse).

Developed and validated for the treatment of cancer pain, the WHO pain ladder has little quality evidence to support its use for managing chronic pain. However, some may still find it useful to use the concept of the WHO pain ladder for explaining pain medication strategy to patients, emphasising that it is a ladder and that you step pain medication down the ladder as well as stepping up. *Figure 7.4* shows that it also encompasses standard pain medication.

Figure 7.4: *Variation of WHO ladder*

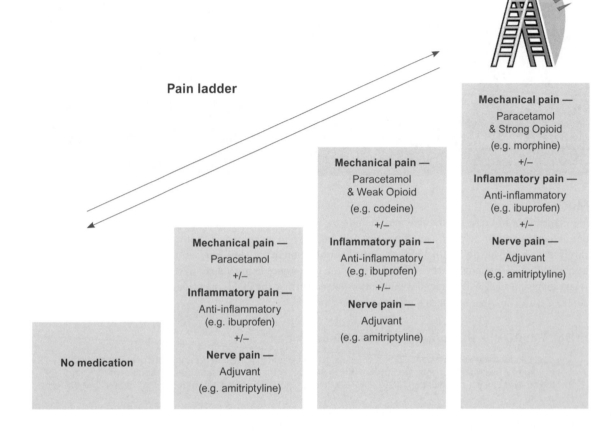

When discussing the initiation of new pain medicines or carrying out a review, consider the following steps:

- Weigh up potential treatment options based on information gathered during the assessment.
- Use the WHO ladder structure to describe how pain medicines can help manage pain and that multiple pain medications may be needed.
- Discuss and explore patients' expectations and goals, as well as explaining the risks and benefits of the current medicines or any new medications being considered.
- Explain the criteria for stopping or continuing medication (e.g. benefit to pain and function, adverse effects).
- Start with low doses and go slowly, stepping up the dose to assess any benefit or adverse effects.
- If possible, consider starting only one medicine at a time and likewise if reducing medication, reduce only one medication at a time and assess response.
- Review regularly to determine effectiveness, tolerability and compliance.
- Reinforce the message that medicine is part of overall therapy in conjunction with other self-management strategies.

Box 7.5: Practice point: key messages for patients

- Medicines are just a small part of managing pain.
- Appropriate use of pain management medications can help control pain sufficiently to allow increased activity and effective self-management, which in turn may allow a reduction in analgesic use over time.
- With an increased knowledge and understanding, patients can make the most of their medicines.
- Patients should have some flexibility to alter their medication according to their pain, as pain levels can fluctuate.
- Patients should have a plan to assess ongoing benefit and then reduce and safely stop medication at appropriate times.

The pain experienced and response to medicines will be different for every patient. It is important for patients to understand this as often they will compare their experience with that of family, friends and acquaintances.

Choice of pain medicine depends on the type of pain and severity. It can be helpful to group medicines into categories suitable for different types of pain. Broadly speaking, pain can be categorised as mechanical, inflammatory or neuropathic (although more than one type can coexist). See *Table 7.5* for the clinical features of these types of pain and suitable treatment options.

Table 7.5: *Types of pain and treatment options*

Type of pain	Clinical features	Treatment options
Mechanical/nociceptive	Involves bones and muscles Described as aching, gnawing, grinding, sharp	Paracetamol Nefopam Opioids (e.g. codeine, morphine)
Inflammatory/nociceptive	Easier to see if in a joint such as a knee as it will be red, swollen, warm	NSAIDs (e.g. ibuprofen, naproxen, diclofenac)
Neuropathic	Direct involvement of a nerve or nerves and/or central sensitisation where the patient's whole nervous system is on high alert and thus being more sensitive to pain Described as pricking, tingling, pins and needles, burning, painful cold, electric shocks	Antidepressants (e.g. amitriptyline, imipramine, duloxetine) Gabapentinoids (e.g. gabapentin, pregabalin)

Paracetamol

Paracetamol is considered one of the safer medicines used for supporting pain management, although recently it's safety has been questioned as adverse effects such as gastrointestinal bleeds and decreased renal function have been identified.[11]

It is usually worth considering a trial of regular paracetamol three or four times daily for a period of 2-4 weeks and then assessing efficacy. If the patient has no perceived benefit and/or is experiencing intolerable adverse effects then discontinue. Standard dosing for a healthy adult of average weight is 500-1000 mg every 4-6 hours (4 g in 24 hours). For patients with low body weight (>33 kg <50 kg), the maximum daily dose is 60 mg/kg and no more than 3 g in 24 hours.

If the patient has risk factors for hepatoxicity (e.g. excess alcohol consumption, concomitant medications that induce liver enzymes) or there is likely to be reduced glutathione levels (e.g. eating disorders, cystic fibrosis or HIV), the maximum daily dose should also be reduced to 3 g in 24 hours. In frail elderly people aged over 75 years, it is worthwhile checking local guidance as some geriatricians may prefer the dose to be limited. Paracetamol adverse effects are rare, however cases of hypersensitivity including skin rash have occurred. Symptoms of paracetamol toxicity include pallor, anorexia, nausea, vomiting and abdominal pain. If significant quantities are ingested over a short period of time then signs of hepatic failure may present as liver tenderness and jaundice. The risk of developing toxicity depends on the total dose that has been taken in 24 hours. Annual liver function tests should be considered for people taking a regular maximum dose over a long period of time.

Nefopam

Nefopam is a non-opioid medication thought to be centrally acting but its mode of action is unclear. It should be avoided in patients with a history of epilepsy due to the risk of convulsions.

There is limited evidence on effectiveness in treating acute or long-term pain, however, it may be considered for persistent unresponsive pain or if other pain medicines are contraindicated. Prescribers should carefully consider whether the potential benefits outweigh the risks of adverse effects. The usual dose is 30-60 mg three times a day.

Nefopam is commonly associated with adverse drug reactions including nausea, dizziness, lightheadedness, nervousness, confusion or tremor. Less common adverse effects include dry mouth, difficulty urinating, hallucinations and numbness or tingling in hands and feet. It is toxic in overdose.

The severity of adverse effects should be weighed up against any benefit and a dose reduction considered to see if pain relief can be maintained but adverse effects reduced. If risks outweigh the benefit, then it should be discontinued. It is important to advise patients that nefopam might also colour urine pink.

Opioids

Opioids have been increasingly prescribed to treat chronic non-malignant pain, however, it is recognised that many patients prescribed opioids are dependent on them with no benefit for their pain, but there is a detrimental impact on their daily life due to adverse effects.

The goal should be to reduce pain sufficiently to facilitate engagement with rehabilitation and the restoration of useful function. The medicine can then be reduced and discontinued.

Opioids are often referred to as weak or strong, however, they can all be potent and individuals respond very differently to them. There should be a clear rationale before initiation, as well as a clear plan for assessment and review with reduction and discontinuation if the desired outcomes are not achieved.

Before initiation, undertake a comprehensive discussion with the patient. The Royal College of Anaesthetists resource Opioid Aware[12] is useful to help support understanding and discussion (See *Box 7.6*).

Box 7.6: Opioid aware information[12]

Opioids are not recommended for people:
- who have had no improvement with opioids in the past
- with sleep apnoea.

There is no clinical evidence for long-term effectiveness of opioids in the following conditions:
- headache
- non-specific low back pain
- fibromyalgia
- unexplained persistent pain.

Potential high risk/dependent patients who require closer monitoring when taking opioids include people with:
- mental health disorders
- depression and anxiety related to pain
- current or past history of substance misuse
- a family history of substance misuse.

Patients are at increased risk of adverse effects and dependence where multiple opioids are prescribed concomitantly (e.g. co-codamol and tramadol). It is important to consider the total daily morphine equivalence (see *Table 7.6*) as the risk of harm increases substantially at doses above an oral morphine equivalent of 120 mg/day.[12] Increasing above this is unlikely to yield further benefit, but exposes patients to increased harm. Opioids should be prescribed at the lowest dose for the shortest period of time.

The Scottish Intercollegiate Guidelines Network (SIGN)[13] recommends patients receiving opioid doses over 50 mg/day morphine equivalent should be reviewed regularly (at least annually) to detect emerging harms and consider ongoing effectiveness. Pain specialist advice or review should be sought before escalating doses over 90 mg/day morphine equivalent.

Table 7.6: *Opioid equivalence*

Transdermal opioids: approximate equivalence with oral morphine								
Oral morphine equivalent (mg/24 hours)	30 to 60	60 to 90	90 to 120	120 to 180	180 to 240	240 to 300	300 to 360	360
Transdermal fentanyl (mcg/hour)	12	25	37	50	62	75	87	100

Note: published conversion ratios vary and these figures are a guide. Morphine equivalences for transdermal opioid preparations have been approximated to allow comparison with available preparations or oral morphine. Patient response may be variable. Please check the most recent BNF for current conversion guide.

Oral morphine to other oral analgesics		
Conversion	Conversion ratio	Comments
Morphine to oxycodone	2:1	Oral morphine 10 mg ~ oral oxycodone 5 mg
Morphine to tramadol	1:5-1:10	Oral morphine 10 mg ~ oral tramadol 50-100 mg
Morphine to codeine	1:10	Oral morphine 10 mg ~ oral codeine 100 mg

Note: published conversion ratios vary and these figures are a guide. Patient response may be variable.

Initial adverse effects of nausea and drowsiness can wear off after a few days. All opioids can impair cognitive function – advise all patients of this and to avoid driving or operating machinery if affected. A common adverse effect that is continuous is constipation and this needs to be managed – guidelines suggest a combination of stimulant laxative and stool softener.

Opioid-induced itch occurs in around 1% of people – it is thought to be caused by a central mechanism rather than by histamine release, therefore in some cases, antihistamines are ineffective. Trial of a sedating antihistamine such as chlorpheniramine may help, but if this is not effective after a few days it should be stopped. Emollients should be used liberally if the patient has dry skin.

As well as the potential to develop tolerance and dependence, there is also the risk of possible long-term adverse effects. Opioids can have effects on the endocrine system influencing the hypothalamic-pituitary-adrenal (HPA) axis leading to hypogonadism and low bone mass. Opioids can also affect the immune system, leading to immunosuppression, and there is the possibility of opioid-induced hyperalgesia, where the patient may present with increased diffuse pain.

It is important to review patients' prescribed opioids regularly and recognise the need to withdraw opioid regimes where there is no therapeutic benefit.

Non-steroidal anti-inflammatories (NSAIDs)

There are differences in anti-inflammatory activity and adverse effects between NSAIDs, and there can be considerable variation in individual response and tolerance to these drugs. About 60% of patients will respond to any NSAID, and those who do not respond to one may well respond to another.

Pain relief starts soon after taking the first dose and full analgesic effect should normally be obtained within a week, whereas the anti-inflammatory effect may not be achieved for up to 3 weeks. If appropriate responses are not obtained within these timeframes, another NSAID should be tried.[14] The lowest effective dose should be used for the shortest duration necessary to control symptoms.

NSAIDs are associated with cardiovascular, renal and gastrointestinal risk factors. Ibuprofen in doses up to 1.2 g daily or naproxen 0.5-1 g daily are not associated with significant thrombotic or cardiovascular risks. Extra caution is required with NSAIDs in frail patients where there is an increased risk of acute kidney injury with dehydrating illness.

Careful consideration is therefore required before starting NSAIDs in people taking cardiovascular, GI, renal, and other concomitant medicines (e.g. SSRI, ACEI). The highest risk is associated with high doses for prolonged use.

Box 7.7: Sick Day Rules advice[15]

- 'Sick Day Rules' advice should be given to patients using NSAIDs regularly.
- It helps to raise awareness of potential harms, including acute kidney injury (AKI), if patients continue to take NSAIDs whilst suffering from a dehydrating illness.
- If the patient is unwell with vomiting, diarrhoea or fever type illness, advise them to stop NSAID until 24-48 hours after eating and drinking normally.

Some patients find that NSAIDs are the only pain management medication that improves their quality of life and wish to continue. A clinical decision should be taken and if continuing, the risk should be documented and reviewed again at regular intervals and renal function should be monitored annually.

Topical NSAIDs have a potentially lower risk of adverse effects and have been shown to be effective for local inflammation. They are recommended by NICE for pain relief in addition to core treatments for people with knee or hand osteoarthritis. Consider topical NSAIDs and/or paracetamol ahead of oral NSAIDs, COX-2 inhibitors or opioids[16] for management of chronic pain, particularly when smaller joints are involved.

Antidepressants

Tricyclic antidepressants (TCAs) are the class most commonly used (e.g. amitriptyline, imipramine and nortriptyline) and are generally the first-line treatment option in most guidelines. They should be initiated at a low dose and gradually titrated in small weekly or fortnightly increments to a maximum of 50-75 mg (or the highest tolerated dose).

It is important to advise patients not to expect immediate benefit, as many patients expect them to work like conventional pain medicines and have an effect on their pain within a few hours. Therapy should be trialled for 4-8 weeks before assessing benefit.

The most common adverse effects are morning hangover/drowsiness. Advise people to take the dose 10-12 hours before they normally get up in the morning to reduce or eliminate this problem. Dry mouth can also be troublesome for some patients, advise these people to carry water or sugar-free gum/sweets with them for use when required.

Amitriptyline has been associated with QTc interval prolongation or torsade de pointes (mainly in overdose). Sometimes low dose tricyclics are initiated for pain reasons in patients already prescribed an SSRI for low mood, however, these also have the potential to prolong QTc. It is prudent to consider that concurrent use might increase the risk and should be avoided. If this is not possible, it is advocated that baseline ECG should be undertaken before co-administration and rechecked at steady state.

It is important to review patients prescribed tricyclic antidepressants regularly and recognise the need to withdraw the regime if there is no therapeutic benefit.

Duloxetine, a selective serotonin and norepinephrine reuptake inhibitor (SNRI) is used to treat pain, but is only licensed for use in diabetic peripheral neuropathy (DPN). The usual starting dose is 30-60 mg daily. The maximum dose is 120 mg a day.

Common adverse effects include nausea, headache, dry mouth, sleepiness and dizziness. Less common adverse effects include loss of appetite, flushes, raised blood pressure, sleeping problems and feeling anxious or sweating. Some adverse effects can be reduced by slowly building up the dose, while others may pass after the first few doses.

Regularly review therapy and withdraw treatment if there is no therapeutic benefit.

Gabapentinoids

There are growing concerns about the rise in the prescribing of gabapentinoids (pregabalin, gabapentin) and the potential for dependency, misuse and implication in drug-related deaths. Follow local and national guidance for initiation of these medications.

Gabapentin and pregabalin have similar efficacy and adverse effect profiles, though patients may respond better or tolerate one better than the other. The dose is increased gradually to help avoid adverse effects and most patients are advised to increase by 300 mg per week up to 600 mg three times daily with a gap of 6-8 hours between doses. It can take up to 6-8 weeks to get the full benefit from gabapentin. In renal impairment, the dosage should be adjusted accordingly.

The most common adverse effects are drowsiness, dizziness, muscle fatigue, tremor and weight gain. Again, as with other pain management medicines, the severity of adverse effects should be weighed up against any benefit for the individual's pain. If risks outweigh benefit then the medication should be discontinued.

Gabapentinoids should not be stopped abruptly – they should be reduced gradually over a minimum of one week, often longer, depending on the dose and duration of treatment.

There is a risk of severe respiratory depression in the elderly, people taking concomitant CNS depressants, or with any of the following conditions: compromised respiratory function or respiratory disease, neurological disease, or renal impairment.[17]

Review regularly and withdraw if there is no therapeutic benefit. Annual monitoring of renal function is required – check local guidance for details.

Other treatments

Capsaicin cream is licensed for symptomatic relief of osteoarthritic pain or neuropathic type pain. The 0.025% is licensed for osteoarthritis of the knee and the 0.075% is licensed for postherpetic neuralgia (PHN) or DPN. There is also a high strength 8% patch available for specialist administration.[18]

In practice, it is used outside its licence to help manage localised neuropathic pain. Advise patients to use a pea-sized amount of the cream and apply to the affected area three or four times daily. It can take 4–8 weeks of regular application for the patient to achieve any benefit and if no benefit is achieved should be discontinued.

Some patients experience intense burning which they cannot tolerate and have to discontinue use. Irritation of the mucous membranes, eyes and respiratory tract (such as nasal and throat irritation) on application of capsaicin cream is rare and can result in symptoms such as coughing, sneezing and watering eyes.

Lidocaine is available in 5% plasters licensed for treatment of PHN. It is recommended if there are contraindications to first-line systemic treatments, or if they are unsuitable or ineffective. It is most often used for off-label, but there is limited evidence to support its use and it is a fairly expensive treatment.

If all other treatments are exhausted and lidocaine plasters are trialled, it should be applied to the affected area once daily for up to 12 hours in a 24-hour period, with a 12-hour plaster-free period between each application. Localised reactions at administration site are the most common adverse effect. A 2-week trial period is sufficient to determine the effectiveness and then regular assessment to assess ongoing benefit.

Topical rubefacients may contain nicotinate compounds, salicylate compounds, essential oils and camphor. They dilate blood vessels and the resulting increased blood flow to the area gives a soothing feeling of warmth; they can cause irritation and reddening of the skin. They seem to be well tolerated in the short-term, but the evidence base means uncertainty remains about the effects of salicylate-containing rubefacients for chronic pain.[19]

Currently, clinical studies on cannabinoids for the management of pain conclude that there is no positive evidence to support routine use in pain management, including neuropathic pain, chronic non-malignant pain and cancer pain. Check the British Pain Society website for the latest statement on cannabis. Other useful resources for more recent advice and evidence is the Royal Pharmaceutical Society (RPS) and Food Standard Agency (FSA) websites.

Table 7.7: *Important drug interactions*[20]

Medication combination	Risk	Action
Opioid +/- gabapentinoid +/- benzodiazepine.	Respiratory depression, sedation and increased risk of death.	Avoid where possible. If concurrent use is necessary, advise patient to be aware of symptoms and seek medical advice.
Tricyclic antidepressants and SSRIs.	Increased risk of QTc prolongation.	Avoid where possible. If concurrent use is necessary, consider ECG monitoring on initiation and dose change.
Tramadol, tricyclic antidepressants and duloxetine. Consider other co-prescribed medicines which may also cause serotonin syndrome.	Increased risk of serotonin syndrome which can be life threatening. Symptoms can include: • confusion • agitation • muscle twitching • sweating • shivering • diarrhoea.	Stop medication where safe and appropriate and advise patient to seek medical advice unless symptoms require immediate medical attention, then appropriate action should be taken.

Note: this is not an exhaustive list of drug interactions. For additional information, see Stockley's online[20]

Self-management

Some non-pharmacological self-management strategies to suggest to patients include:

- Relaxation – pain can lead to muscle tension. Learning to relax can help reduce physical tension. This helps by lowering the amount of adrenaline in the body. Relaxation can also aid sleep.
- Distraction – shifting attention away from pain can help. Participating in enjoyable activities releases endorphins which can help individuals feel better both physically and emotionally.
- Planning the day – planning enjoyable activities into the day (taking care to pace and take short breaks as necessary) gives a sense of satisfaction.
- Planning for set-back or 'flare-up' – being prepared can give a sense of control over pain.

While evidence from research is limited, many patients benefit from the use of heat and cold in various formats (e.g. gels/rubs, hot water bottles, wheat bags, gel packs that can be used hot or cold). These interventions are low cost and safe and are supported by NICE in its osteoarthritis guideline, as is the use of transcutaneous electrical nerve stimulation (TENS).[21]

The role of acupuncture, osteopathy and chiropractors has been debated with limited evidence though some patients find them beneficial. They are not routinely offered on the NHS and some patients may find them cost-prohibitive.

Supports, walking aids (sticks/rollators/crutches) and cushions such as lumbar rolls can all give benefit at an appropriate time, but may not be needed all the time.

Physical activity

Patients with chronic pain may avoid physical activity as they are worried that it might exacerbate pain or cause physical damage, which means they are less active, which over time reduces physical fitness and wellbeing. Undertaking activity in a paced, gradual way, building up capacity over time, will increase fitness and muscle strength. Consider referral or signposting to other agencies or healthcare professionals such as physiotherapists for advice.

Another key issue is the 'boom/bust' cycle. On a 'good' pain day the patient tries to do all the jobs they've been putting off (boom) and end up overdoing it and causing flare-up of their pain (bust) where it may then take several days to get over the impact of their pain. It is better to pace activity, doing things in small manageable chunks.

Meaningful activity

Chronic pain can cause people to withdraw from meaningful activity because they can't do it to the level they did before, or they struggle to maintain personal care or housework. Encourage people to remain involved, alter the way they do things to make it easier (e.g. get a supermarket shopping online) and keep up with friends and family. Occupational therapists are a key clinician to consider for additional support.

Mood

Underlying persistent low mood may need referral to other clinicians such as GPs or psychology. In the meantime, signposting to local NHS recommended websites that offer a variety of psychological-based interventions such as short online CBT courses, relaxation and advice, may help. Some patients may reveal a history of trauma or abuse; this is not unusual in patients managing chronic pain. Knowing about local support organisations would be helpful.

Sleep

Improving 24-hour pain control or using supportive positions and cushioning may improve sleep. In addition, there is lots of information available about 'good sleep hygiene'. Consider the role of caffeine and hydration in diet, restricting screen time near bedtime and winding down with a hot bath.

Other lifestyle issues

There may be more fundamental things that stop patients from engaging in pain self-management or which add to their anxiety and stress, for example, social care benefits, housing or financial issues. You may be able to signpost them to local agencies that can help, for example, Citizens Advice.

Being overweight can increase the pressure and strain on joints and patients should be encouraged to try and maintain a healthy weight and BMI. Offer weight management advice or refer to appropriate others, such as dieticians if additional support is required.

Special groups

Elderly

Supporting older people manage pain with medication becomes increasingly complicated as the older people get, the more likely they are to have other chronic conditions such as heart disease, diabetes, chronic lung disease or kidney disease.

Elderly people are at increased risk for gastrointestinal toxicity associated with NSAIDs, specifically peptic ulcers. They may be considered for people without heart disease or renal function issues, however, a gastro-protective should be considered (such as a proton pump inhibitor). Check national guidance for details of when this is appropriate and your local guidance for the preferred choice of medicine. All older people should be monitored regularly for GI, renal and cardiovascular adverse effects. Other medicines which have an increased risk of adverse effect in elderly people include:

- Opioids – constipation, nausea, gastrointestinal complications, respiratory depression, increased falls, and sleep disturbances.
- Tricyclic antidepressants – loss of equilibrium, which can contribute to an increase of falls and injuries, sudden decreases in blood pressure, sleep disturbances and arrhythmias.
- Anticholinergics – confusion, dizziness and falls. These have been shown to increase patient mortality. A number of ACB calculators can be found online where a score of 3+ is associated with increased cognitive impairment and mortality.

See **Chapter 17** for more information on medicines which are more problematic in elderly people.

Pregnancy and breastfeeding

The general principle when managing this group of patients is to minimise the use of all medications unless the potential benefit outweighs any risk of harm to mother, foetus or child. When considering pain medication for women who are trying to conceive, who are pregnant or breastfeeding, check the following websites for the latest information:

- Bumps (best use of medicines in pregnancy) – www.medicinesinpregnancy.org
- UK teratology information service – www.uktis.org

Also, raise awareness in all female patients of childbearing age that they may need to discuss their medicines with their pain specialist if they are considering trying to conceive.

Sodium valproate may be prescribed for pain indications. The MHRA advises that if a woman of childbearing age is to be prescribed sodium valproate, she must be enrolled in a pregnancy prevention programme (PPP).

Renal impairment

Managing chronic pain in patients with chronic kidney disease can be problematic. Information on dosage adjustment can be obtained from the SPC, BNF or renal drug handbook. Advice from pain or renal pharmacist or specialist teams may be required.

- Gabapentin and pregabalin – these are renally excreted therefore the dose should be adjusted accordingly. Patients with severe renal failure taking gabapentin or pregabalin have a higher incidence of neurological adverse effects and should be monitored regularly.
- Opioids – consider the drug choice as the adjustment required in people with renal impairment varies for individual opioids. Reduce doses if required and monitor closely for signs of toxicity.
- NSAIDs – avoid if possible or use with caution, contraindicated in people with eGFR <30.

Recommendations for renal replacement therapy (dialysis) patients may differ and it would be appropriate to liaise with their specialist team.

Follow-up and onward referral

Medication review is recommended every 6-12 months. The interval between reviews and the number of follow-up appointments required will depend on the intervention; it may also be dependent on patient engagement.

It is important to be aware of the referral pathways to other clinicians and services in your local area, including the local pain management team or specialists. Information can be found on local, regional or national pain services. Examples include:

- Fife pain management service – www.nhsfife.org/services/services-and-departments/pain-management-service
- The Scottish National Residential Pain Management Programme (SNRPMP) offers a 3-week residential pain management programme with patients referred from local pain services – www.snrpmp.scot.nhs.uk
- Bath centre for pain service. A nationally commissioned specialist centre providing pain rehabilitation for people with chronic pain of all ages – www.bathcentreforpainservices.nhs.uk

Table 7.8: *Onward referral options*

Circumstances	Referral options
New unusual symptoms	May require further assessment by GP
Ongoing or worsening symptoms	GP review is indicated where symptoms are ongoing or worsening despite maximum therapy
Mental health issues (e.g. depression, suicide risk, trauma or abuse)	Depending on issue and severity, GP practice, A&E, adult psychology services or a local third sector agency (e.g. www.mind.org.uk)
Possible serious adverse effects or toxicity (e.g. serotonin syndrome, GI bleeding or overdose)	GP practice or A&E
Musculoskeletal problems	Local musculoskeletal (MSK) physiotherapy; patients may be able to self refer
Substance misuse	Local addictions services or other third sector agencies. We are with you is a charity providing support for mental health, alcohol and drug misuse
Help with activities of daily living	Occupational therapy services – may be able to offer assessments and living aids
Work-related issues	Occupational health services Health Working Lives – Scotland (www.healthyworkinglives.scot)
Money, legal or social issues	Citizens Advice – free, confidential information and advice to assist people with money, legal, consumer and other problems

Useful resources

- Live Well with Pain (www.livewellwithpain.co.uk) – Developed by clinicians, for clinicians to help support patients towards better self-management of chronic pain.
- NHS Inform or NHS Choices (www.nhsinform.scot, www.nhs.uk) – National health information services providing accurate and relevant information to help make informed decisions about health.
- Pain Association Scotland (www.painassociation.com) – National charity delivering professionally-led pain management in the community.
- Pain Concern (www.painconcern.org.uk) – Provides support to people with pain and those who care for them.

- ReConnect2Life (www.torbayandsouthdevon.nhs.uk/services/pain-service/reconnect2life) – An interactive programme to help patients look at their pain and how it affects them.
- The British Pain Society (www.britishpainsociety.org) – Endeavours to increase both professional and public awareness of the prevalence of pain and the facilities that are available for its management.
- The Pain Toolkit (www.paintoolkit.org) – The Pain Toolkit is for people who live with persistent pain and healthcare teams who support them, handy tips and skills to support self-management of pain.
- West of Scotland Chronic Pain Education Group Website (www.paindata.org) – Multilingual audio, visual and print resources to assist patients and clinicians in the management of chronic pain.
- Faculty of Pain Medicine. Opioids Aware (www.fpm.ac.uk/opioids-aware) – A resource for patients and healthcare professionals to support the prescribing of opioid medicines for pain.
- CredibleMeds (www.crediblemeds.org) – Medicines information regarding QT prolongation risk.

References

1. International Association Study of Pain (IASP). Classification of Chronic Pain. Second edition (revised) 2012.

2. Voscopoulos C, Lem M. When does acute pain become chronic? *British Journal of Anaesthesia* 2010; 105(s1): 69-85.

3. Fayaz A *et al*. Prevalence of chronic pain in the UK: a systematic review and meta-analysis of population studies. *BMJ Open* 2016; 6: e010364.

4. Van Hecke *et al*. Chronic pain epidemiology and its clinical relevance. *British Journal of Anaesthesia* 2013; 111(1): 13-18.

5. Loeser JD (1982). Concepts of Pain. In: Stanton-Hicks M, Boas RA, eds. *Chronic Low Back Pain*. New York: Raven Press, 145-8.

6. Moore DS *et al*. The Costs and Consequences of Adequately Managed Chronic Non-Cancer Pain and Chronic Neuropathic Pain. *Pain Practice* 2014; 14(1): 79-94.

7. Greenhalgh S *et al*. Development of a toolkit for early identification of cauda equina syndrome. *Primary Healthcare Research & Development* 2017; 17: 559-567.

8. British Pain Society: Outcome measures 2019. www.britishpainsociety.org/static/uploads/resources/files/Outcome_Measures_January_2019.pdf

9. Knisely JS *et al*. Prescription Opioid Misuse Index: A brief questionnaire to assess misuse (POMI). *Journal of Substance Abuse Treatment* 2008; 359(4): 380-386.

10. Moore A *et al*. Expect analgesic failure; pursue analgesic success. *BMJ* 2013; 346: f2690.

11. Roberts E *et al*. Paracetamol: not as safe as we thought? A systematic literature review of observational studies. *Ann Rheum Dis* 2015; 0: 1-8.

12. Faculty of Pain Medicine. Opioids Aware: A resource for patients and healthcare professionals to support prescribing of opioid medicines for pain. www.fpm.ac.uk/opioids-aware

13. Scottish Intercollegiate Guidelines Network. Management of chronic pain (online). Edinburgh: SIGN; 2013. www.sign.ac.uk/assets/sign136_2019.pdf

14. Joint Formulary Committee. British National Formulary (online) London. BMJ Group and Pharmaceutical Press. www.new.medicinescomplete.com

15. Healthcare Improvement Scotland, Scottish Patient Safety Programme. Medicines Sick Day Rules Card. www.ihub.scot/improvement-programmes/scottish-patient-safety-programme-spsp/spsp-medicines-collaborative/high-risk-situations-involving-medicines/medicines-sick-day-rules-card

16. National Institute for Health and Care Excellence. Osteoarthritis: Care and Management (online). London: NICE; 2014. www.nice.org.uk/guidance/cg177

17. MHRA 2017 Drug Safety Update Gabapentin (Neurontin): risk of severe respiratory depression [online]. www.gov.uk/drug-safety-update/gabapentin-neurontin-risk-of-severe-respiratory-depression

18. Anand P, Bley K. Topical capsaicin for pain management: therapeutic potential and mechanisms of action of the new high-concentration capsaicin 8% patch. *British Journal of Anaesthesia* 2011; 107(4): 490-502.

19. Derry S *et al*. Topical rubefacients for acute and chronic musculoskeletal pain in adults. *Cochrane Database of Systematic Reviews* 2014, Issue 11.

20. Stockley's Interactions Checker [online]. www.new.medicinescomplete.com/#/interactions/stockley

21. National Institute for Health and Care Excellence (2018). Osteoarthritis Management. www.cks.nice.org.uk/osteoarthritis#!scenario

Case studies

Case study 1

Shona, aged 47 years, regularly comes into your pharmacy for her prescriptions and over-the-counter advice. She is in to pick up her prescription for 200 co-codamol 30/500 which she collects every four weeks and has been taking for over a year.

Whilst waiting for the prescription she asks your counter assistant for something for constipation. When the counter assistant identifies what medication she is taking she refers her to you for advice. You notice she is hobbling more than usual and looks in pain.

Points to consider

- Is there anything to be concerned about?
- What would you ask Shona?

As you hand out the prescription you ask about her pain and constipation. She states she has been troubled by her knee for about 18 months after a skiing accident where she twisted it badly. She thought it healed quite well and resumed running about 14 months ago but has been quite curtailed recently and unable to run on it. She stopped going out with her running club about 5 months ago. It can get quite swollen at times and when it does she uses frozen peas and a knee support. The co-codamol used to help but doesn't seem to be working quite so well anymore and also, it would seem, is causing her problems with constipation.

Points to consider

- What other questions would you ask Shona and why?
- What tools and resources could you make use of?

On a NRS scale, she rates her pain as 7-8/10 on her worst days and 3/10 on her best days.

She was previously quite fit and active and enjoyed running two or three times a week as part of a local running group. She also enjoys golf, but her knee has restricted her now too as she can't walk around the course and she has missed most of this season and is seriously considering giving up her membership. She's put on weight because of her inactivity and it's getting her down.

She has no other significant medical history.

Points to consider

- What are the issues that you need to consider?
- What are the priorities?

The issues you have identified are:
- Pain and discomfort have persisted beyond initial acute injury and are significantly impacting her function and quality of life.
- The co-codamol is no longer working.
- A previously very fit and active person, her activity levels have reduced significantly and she is gaining weight which will put additional pressure on the knee joint.
- She appears to have the opioid-induced adverse effect of constipation.
- She is becoming more socially isolated having stopped running club, considering giving up golf club membership and her mood is decreasing as she reports it is 'getting her down'.

Points to consider

- Are you concerned she may have developed tolerance due to regular fixed codeine intake?
- How would you assess her low mood?
- How can Shona's pain be managed better?

As a result of your discussion with Shona you suggest and agree on the following actions:

- Continue to use her knee support and frozen peas but will explore the use of heat and cold in various formats to see what gives her additional relief.
- Start a topical NSAID, such as ibuprofen 5% gel, for local inflammation – this is less likely to cause systemic adverse effects such as GI irritation.
- Trial combination therapy, substituting some paracetamol for co-codamol 30/500, altering the codeine component depending on pain levels, ensuring no more than a combination of two tablets at any one time and eight in 24 hours. This may help reduce tolerance and improve constipation.
- Initiate dietary measures including increased fluid/fruit/vegetables/fibre for opioid-induced constipation and if not adequate, trial adding a stimulant laxative such as bisacodyl or senna. A stool softener may be added if needed.
- Encourage continued activity but in a paced way, not pushing in to pain.
- Encourage social interaction – are there ways she could volunteer as an organiser with the running club? Can she meet golf friends for lunch or consider using a golf buggy?

You make an appointment with Shona to review how things are when she is next due to collect her prescription.

Shona reports a general improvement in stiffness and swelling of her knee, though some days are worse than others. She attempted to jog around her local loch at the weekend but 'paid for it' Monday through to Wednesday as she could hardly walk. Constipation has improved and she rarely needs to use the bisacodyl. She is using less co-codamol as her pain has improved, though she takes eight paracetamol-based tablets a day as she does find it helpful. Her pain is now generally 5/10, though was 10/10 after jogging. Some days her pain has almost gone which is why she tried jogging – she says, 'I won't be trying that again, it crippled me.' She has been volunteering as a timer at the weekly running club 5k.

The current issues are as follows:

- Improved pain but still impacting on physical ability
- Has literally tried to run before she can walk (any distance) causing an acute flare-up and been put off further exercise (boom/bust cycle)
- Her weight remains an issue

Points to consider

- How can the care plan be developed to address the current issues?

You develop the care plan as follows:

- Advise she could switch from topical NSAID to systemic NSAID during an acute flare-up and increase co-codamol use at that time, staying with 4 g per day paracetamol limit. She may require the addition of gastroprotection such as omeprazole for NSAID prophylaxis.
  - You consider use of capsaicin cream 0.025%.
- Signpost (or refer) for further assessment by a physiotherapist to determine whether additional intervention required and for advice on paced exercise and activity.
- Offer weight management advice or signpost for additional help.

Over the next six months you have a brief check-in when Shona collects her prescription. Her pain has improved and she completed her first 5k walk/jog. She has managed to lose weight through dietary measures and because she is more active.

Case study 2

You are working as a general practice clinical pharmacist and have been asked to review patients on high-dose gabapentin (more than 1800 mg/day). You have set up a fortnightly clinic and have invited patients for review.

Points to consider

- What information would be useful to have at that review?

You have arranged blood testing for U&Es in advance of the clinic for patients who do not have a recorded test within two years.

Shahid, aged 58 years, has had chronic low back pain for over 15 years which he says is getting worse. He's come to the appointment in the hope that you can offer him 'stronger painkillers' for his pain. He works with the local council refuse collection; he used to drive the lorry but stopped as he felt he was too tired to drive. He was then shifted to the bin collection which he was finding too physical. He's always managed to stay at work but has been off the last nine months following his back 'popping' one day. He's worried he may lose his job and he can't afford to do that.

Points to consider

- What questions would you ask Shahid?
  - About his pain?
  - About his treatment?

You ask him to describe his pain. He reports it as a widespread aching in his low back lumbar area but it sometimes shoots across his left buttock and can go down over his thigh and into his calf and makes him catch his breath. This happens once or twice a week and before gabapentin it happened every day. He also gets pins and needles in his foot and thigh. He's not sure his current medication is working. He also thinks it makes him feel really tired, and on questioning notes an occasional dry mouth. You can see from his pain diary that his sleep pattern is good; he manages at least 8 hours' sleep, struggles to get up in the morning and often has an afternoon nap as well. You note he takes his amitriptyline at 11 pm.

Points to consider

- Is Shahid's therapy optimised?

He was hoping for surgery to resolve his back, but the neurologist has told him there is no surgical target and to manage his pain. He is frustrated and thinks he should get a second opinion. His wife tells him he is bad-tempered and should stop sitting about all day watching the television. He used to read books but can't concentrate anymore and struggles with memory.

Shahid's details are as follows:
- He reports an NRS of 6/10 most of the time
- Medical history: back pain and COPD
- Height: 5 ft 9 inches
- Weight: 80 kg
- Previous smoker
- Electrolytes: normal
- Serum creatinine = 122 micromol/mL, eGFR >60 mL/min

- Current medication:
  - Amitriptyline 50 mg and 25 mg – takes 75 mg at 11pm
  - Gabapentin 300 mg – takes 3 three times daily 8am, 2pm, 8pm
  - Relvar Ellipta 92/22 mcg – one puff daily
- Previous pain medication:
  - Co-codamol 30/500 mg – he describes as useless
  - Diazepam 5 mg – had when the back was at worst, felt it helped and asks if he can have more for his really bad days

---

Points to consider

- What are the important issues to consider?
- Can you think of any solutions to help Shahid?

You have identified the following issues:
- Chronic low back pain with a neuropathic element which is controlled better than before, but is still present
- Biomedical focus on resolving pain with surgery or 'painkillers'.
- High-dose gabapentin (2700 mg daily) above recommended daily dose for his current renal function, creatinine clearance calculated using the Cockroft-Gault equation of 66 mL/min
- Takes amitriptyline late at night – appears to be experiencing dry mouth and morning sedation
- No medication for generalised ache or for flare-up – requesting a benzodiazepine
- Reduced cognitive function with poor concentration as possible adverse effects of medication
- Not undertaking any physical activity
- Low mood and bad-tempered – is this caused by his pain? His frustration at not being offered surgery? Or is it an independent concomitant depression?
- Possible financial worries creating additional stress
- No use of non-medicinal pain management strategies

You explain about different types of pain and medicines used to manage them and that in chronic pain, medication is not a pain killer and we need to adjust our expectations about what levels of relief may be achieved.

He has already indicated his nerve pain frequency is far less than before. You also discuss that pain medication is a small piece of the jigsaw in managing pain and that there is a need to focus on non-pharmacological strategies too.

You highlight the need to ensure any medication he is currently taking is effective and safe and that you want to help him get the right balance of benefit vs side effects or inconvenience of taking.

Points to consider

- What can be done to address the issues outlined above?

In discussion with Shahid you decide on the following:
- Gradual reduction of gabapentin by 300 mg weekly to 600 mg three times daily in line with renal function dosing and better dose spacing across a 24-hour period. Assessing the impact of change on nerve pain and cognitive function.
- Move amitriptyline dosing to earlier in the evening, suggesting 10-12 hours before wishing to rise and sip water or suck on sugar-free sweets to help with dry mouth.
- Trial regular paracetamol 2 four times daily and assess the impact on general ache.
- Explain that benzodiazepines are not recommended for long-term use and would only be considered in an acute flare-up with muscle spasm. Even then they would be used with caution as he has COPD and is on gabapentin and at increased risk of respiratory depression.
- Consider a trial of topical NSAID for flare-up.
- Advise on use of heat, cold and TENS.

- Encourage interaction with either websites (Pain Toolkit) or local pain management groups to help increase understanding of chronic pain and pain management.
- Encourage discussion with occupational health at work and interaction with Citizens Advice.
- Encourage gradual build-up of physical activity, highlighting local leisure options for those with long-term conditions.

Shahid is a bit sceptical of paracetamol and continues to think there must be something else that can help but is prepared to trial the suggestions and come back in four weeks for review.

On his return, he reports that the general ache is a bit better and that he quite likes the NSAID gel. He's not so tired in the morning, but unfortunately, his shooting pains in his leg are more frequent, occurring almost every day now. He likes using heat, finds it quite soothing and has read about TENS and wants to know more. He has an appointment booked at Citizen's Advice. He and his wife have been going out for short walks each day and on reading the websites he is beginning to understand the importance of non-medicinal strategies.

His current medication is now:

- Amitriptyline 50 mg and 25 mg – 75 mg at 7pm at night
- Gabapentin 300 mg – 2 three times daily 8am, 3pm, 11pm
- Paracetamol 500 mg – 2 four times daily
- Ibuprofen 5% gel – applied three times daily when required
- Relvar Ellipta 92/22 mcg – one puff daily

Points to consider

- What is the main problem Shahid is now experiencing?
- What suggestions do you have for improving the management of Shahid's pain?

It is clear that reducing the gabapentin to licensed dosing for renal function has worsened his nerve pain, so you develop a new care plan and consider a switch to pregabalin, starting at 75 mg at night increasing in weekly 75 mg increments to 150 mg twice daily if tolerated. You also show him how to use TENS and suggest using Tai Chi videos at home to support gentle stretching.

Two months later Shahid reports he is doing quite well, the nerve pain has settled again. He has been meeting with his occupational health team and manager and they are currently looking at redeployment to a less physical role so he is no longer fearful of having to give up work. His wife says he's less bad-tempered and they've both been going to local Tai Chi classes. He is not so tired during the day and is enjoying reading again – especially information around pain self-management!

Points to consider

- What are the next steps?

You explain to Shahid that it would be useful to assess the ongoing need for pregabalin or amitriptyline every 6 or 12 months by undertaking a gradual reduction and assessing impact. Making sure to attempt reduction of only one drug at a time.

If his pain was to become more problematic you could consider a trial of tramadol because of its dual action (opioid/serotonergic), but would need to consider risk of serotonergic syndrome with amitriptyline (you could advise on symptoms to watch for and reduce amitriptyline dose slightly) and risk of respiratory depression of using an opioid and gabapentinoid together.

CHAPTER 8

Dementia

Delia Bishara

Overview

'Dementia' is an umbrella term used to describe a range of cognitive and behavioural symptoms that can include memory loss, difficulties with thinking, problem solving or language and changes in personality. It is a progressive condition, so symptoms will gradually get worse and become severe enough to affect daily activities. People often have some of the same general symptoms, but the degree to which these affect each person will vary.[1,2]

There are many diseases that can result in dementia, and regardless of which type of dementia is diagnosed, each person will experience dementia differently. Symptoms can include:[3]

- **Memory problems** – problems retaining new information or remembering recent events, while having a good memory for past events. They might get lost in previously familiar places and may struggle with names or have difficulty recognising people or objects. Relatives might notice the person seems increasingly forgetful and misplacing things regularly.

- **Cognitive problems** – they may appear confused and disorientated and have difficulty with time and place, for example, getting up in the middle of the night to go to work, even though they're retired. Their concentration could also be affected. They may experience difficulties when shopping with choosing the items and then paying for them due to poor organisational skills and reduced ability to reason and make decisions. Some people develop a sense of restlessness and prefer to keep moving rather than sitting still; others may be reluctant to take part in activities they used to enjoy.

- **Communication difficulties** – they may repeat themselves often or have difficulty finding the right words. Their speech might become slow, muddled or repetitive. Reading and writing might also become challenging. They might experience changes in personality and behaviour, and suffer from mood swings, anxiety and depression. They can lose interest in seeing others socially, thus withdrawing gradually from family and friends. Since following and engaging in conversation can be difficult and tiring, formerly outgoing people might become quieter and more introverted, with their self-confidence also being affected.

- **Behavioural and psychological symptoms of dementia (BPSD)** – this describes the issues often seen in the later stages of dementia, including depression, apathy, agitation, disinhibition, psychosis (delusions and hallucinations), wandering, aggression, incontinence and altered eating habits. Often, these noncognitive symptoms are also described as neuropsychiatric symptoms. It is thought that these behaviours may occur in up to 90% of people with AD.[4]

Investigation and appropriate management of the underlying causes for the behavioural symptoms should be considered and this should include a review of the patient's medication. Behavioural problems can be exacerbated by some drugs with anticholinergic properties. These include tricyclic antidepressants such as amitriptyline, phenothiazine antipsychotics such as chlorpromazine, and anti-Parkinson's medication such as benztropine. In addition, problems can also occur with benzodiazepines and some analgesics such as tramadol.[5] The exclusion of physical causes or delirium is also important in patients with dementia. Constipation, untreated pain and infections including urinary tract and respiratory infections can cause or worsen behaviour.[6]

Causes of dementia include:

- **Alzheimer's disease (AD)** – this is the most common type of dementia. Around 60% of people diagnosed with dementia will have Alzheimer's disease. The exact cause is unknown, but it seems to be caused by abnormal amounts of proteins in the brain that create plaques and tangles which then interfere with, and damage, nerve cells. There may also be a reduction in the neurotransmitter, acetylcholine. This leads to information not being transmitted effectively and the symptoms of dementia.[3]

- **Vascular dementia** – this is caused by reduced blood supply to the brain due to diseased blood vessels. Death of brain cells can cause problems with memory, thinking or reasoning. Vascular dementia can result from transient ischaemic attacks (TIAs) or damage to the blood supply to the brain caused by atherosclerosis or haemorrhage. The symptoms of vascular dementia depend on which area of the brain has been affected. Whilst language, reading, writing and communication can be affected, memory problems may not initially be an issue in vascular dementia if this area of the brain has not been damaged, although they may occur later.[3]

- **Dementia with Lewy bodies (DLB) or Lewy body dementia (LBD)** – this is thought to account for 15-20% of all cases of dementia, although it is believed that this figure may be much higher due to under-diagnosis of this condition. In the early stages, it is often mistaken for Alzheimer's disease. Lewy body dementia particularly affects the person's ability to think and move and can cause hallucinations, fluctuations in alertness and sleep disturbances, which can be extremely distressing for the person and their family. The symptoms are largely similar to those of Parkinson's disease.

- **Frontotemporal dementia** – in people aged under 65 years, frontotemporal dementia is the second most commonly diagnosed dementia but it is less common in those aged over 65.[3] It is a group of conditions caused by the death of nerve cells and pathways in the frontal and temporal lobes of the brain. The damage to the brain is linked to abnormally forming proteins that interfere with communication between brain cells.

- **Other causes** – rarer types of dementia include alcohol-related dementia, young onset dementia and Huntington's disease, but there are many others. Mixed dementia is common and at least one in every 10 people diagnosed with dementia is diagnosed as having more than one type. The most common combination is AD and vascular dementia.

The most significant risk factor for dementia is age,[7] the older you are the more likely you are to develop the condition, but it is not an inevitable part of ageing. About two in 100 people aged between 65 to 69 have dementia, and this figure rises to one in five for those aged between 85 to 89. However, it is a common misconception that dementia is just a condition of older age; over 42,000 people under 65 years old have dementia in the UK (see *Box 8.1* for information on risk factors for dementia).

The number of people with dementia globally is estimated to be 50 million (5.2% of people over the age of 60) and this is projected to nearly triple by 2050. There are around 210,000 new cases of dementia in the UK each year and every three minutes, someone in the UK develops dementia. It is important to note, however, that the incidence of dementia in the UK has fallen, possibly due to the improvement in male cardiovascular health over the last several decades, which is a risk factor for dementia.[8]

Studies have shown that dementia has a poor prognosis. One-year mortality risks are three to four times higher in patients visiting a day clinic compared with the general population. Mortality risks of patients with dementia in the Netherlands admitted to hospital even exceeded those following cardiovascular diseases.[17]

In a UK study, males were found to have a worse prognosis than females after a diagnosis of dementia – the average survival time for females was 4.6 years compared to 4.1 years for males. Frailer patients died sooner than healthier ones, but being married, living at home and the degree of mental decline were not found to have an impact on survival. However, patients diagnosed before age 70 typically live for a decade or even longer.[18]

Box 8.1: Risk factors for dementia

- **Age** – this is the most well-known risk factor for dementia. Studies of prevalence and incidence have consistently shown an almost exponential increase with advancing age.[7] Most individuals with the disease are aged 65 years and older. After 65, the risk of AD doubles with every 5 years increase in age. Over the age of 80, there is a one in six chance of developing dementia.[3]
- **Gender** – females are at increased risk of AD, especially at old age.[7] Twice as many women over the age of 65 are diagnosed with Alzheimer's than men, whereas vascular dementia is diagnosed in slightly more men than women.[3]
- **Ethnicity** – people of South Asian, African or African-Caribbean heritage seem to develop dementia more often than white Europeans. The reason for these differences is not well understood, however specific risk factors associated with these ethnicities such as stroke, diabetes, hypertension and cardiovascular disease, as well as differences in diet, smoking, exercise and genes are thought to explain this.[3]
- **Genetics** – only a small proportion of individuals with dementia suffer from a hereditary form caused by an autosomal dominant mutation. Mutations in several genes have been shown to cause AD, but these genetic forms account for less than 5% of all cases and usually affect people aged under 65 years. Genetic factors seem to influence non-familial cases, as AD is governed by common DNA variants. The apolipoprotein E gene ε4 allele is thought to be a risk factor for AD. However, it is neither necessary nor sufficient to cause AD but operates as a genetic risk modifier.
- **Vascular risk factors** – hypertension, heart disease, diabetes and smoking have all been shown to be associated with AD, although the mechanisms linking these with AD remain unclear.[7] In addition, some studies have found that mid-life obesity is also a risk factor for AD,[9] although evidence is conflicting, as this association may change with age since being overweight or obese in later life has been associated with reduced risk of dementia.[10]
- **Diet and alcohol** – there is limited and conflicting information on the effects of various food, nutrients and vitamins on reducing dementia risk. A few cohort studies on a Mediterranean diet have suggested an association with reduced risk.[10] Small or moderate alcohol consumption by older people may decrease the risk of cognitive decline and dementia, however, the evidence is not strong enough to suggest that those who do not drink should start to do so.[10]
- **Education** – among the potentially modifiable risk factors, the most consistent evidence surrounds education and specifically the number of years of formal education. It appears that people with more years of formal education or greater literacy have a lower risk for dementia.[10]
- **Traumatic brain injury** – there is an increased risk of developing certain forms of dementia in people who have suffered moderate or severe traumatic brain injury and people who have experienced repeated head injuries (such as boxers or footballers) may be at an even higher risk.[10]
- **Depression** – a history of depression increases the risk for dementia.[11,12] The effect of treatment for depression on subsequent cognitive function is not well understood.[10]
- **Sleep** – several studies have linked sleep disturbance to increased risk for cognitive decline. One study further suggested that treatment for breathing disorders occurring during sleep may reduce the risk of cognitive decline. Again, it is not yet known whether the sleep disturbance is a cause or a related precursor to dementia.[10]
- **Anticholinergic medication** – there is growing evidence linking the long-term use of anticholinergic medication in older people with increased risk of cognitive decline, dementia and mortality.[13] Some studies have found a robust association between some classes of anticholinergic drugs and future dementia incidence.[14,15] There is a nationwide drive to review and reduce the anticholinergic burden of drugs in older people as a precaution. The Anticholinergic Effect on Cognition (AEC)[16] scale can be used to establish which medications have an anticholinergic effect on cognition; the online tool can be accessed at www.medichec.com.

Diagnosis

There is no single test for dementia. A diagnosis is based on a combination of things:[1]

- A comprehensive medical history
- A physical examination and investigations (e.g. blood tests) to exclude other possible causes for the symptoms

- Cognitive testing (e.g. memory, thinking) – simpler tests will be carried out by a nurse or doctor, more specialist tests by a psychologist
- A brain scan if this is required to confirm the diagnosis (e.g. MRI or CT scan)

Treatment

There is still no cure for dementia and no available treatment has shown to either modify or reverse the progression of the disease. Therapeutic interventions are targeted at managing symptoms or improving cognitive function for a limited amount of time.

Despite this having been questioned over the years, the cholinergic hypothesis remains the basis for medication used in dementia. Three cholinesterase inhibitors (donepezil, rivastigmine and galantamine) are currently licensed in the UK and elsewhere for the treatment of mild to moderate AD, although these are also now often used in severe cases of AD as well. In addition, rivastigmine is licensed in the treatment of dementia associated with Parkinson's disease.

Memantine is licensed in the UK for the treatment of moderate to severe AD. It is thought to exert its therapeutic effects by acting as non-competitive N-methyl-D-aspartate (NMDA) receptor antagonist that binds preferentially to open NMDA receptor-operated calcium channels. This is thought to mitigate the effects of sustained and pathologically elevated levels of glutamate that may lead to neuronal dysfunction.[19]

Whilst these medicines are not yet licensed for other forms of dementia (other than AD), NICE guidance recommends the following:

- For dementia with Lewy bodies:[2]
  - Offer donepezil or rivastigmine to people with mild to moderate dementia with Lewy bodies
  - Only consider galantamine for people with mild to moderate dementia with Lewy bodies if donepezil and rivastigmine are not tolerated
  - Consider donepezil or rivastigmine for people with severe dementia with Lewy bodies
  - Consider memantine for people with dementia with Lewy bodies if acetylcholinesterase inhibitors (AChEIs) are not tolerated or are contraindicated
- For Parkinson's disease dementia, the NICE Parkinson's disease guideline states:
  - Offer a cholinesterase inhibitor for people with mild or moderate Parkinson's disease dementia
  - Consider a cholinesterase inhibitor for people with severe Parkinson's disease dementia
  - Consider memantine for people with Parkinson's disease dementia, only if cholinesterase inhibitors are not tolerated or are contraindicated

Pharmacy input

There are several areas in which pharmacists can provide value in the prevention and management of dementia. This will vary depending on skills, experience and knowledge:

- Review medication and optimise therapy – review of unnecessary or inappropriate medication.
  - Community and hospital pharmacists of all levels and skills should be able to do this.
- Ensure there are no drug interactions involving the combination of an anticholinergic drug and an AChEI, resulting in the lack of efficacy of the AChEI.
  - This should be checked by all pharmacists at any level, although in reality, specialist old age pharmacists or mental health pharmacists for older people are more aware of this drug interaction.
- Reduce pharmacodynamic interactions of dementia medication – for example, both beta blockers and AChEI can cause bradycardia, thus increasing the risk of this occurring in a patient taking this combination.
  - This should be checked by all pharmacists at any level, although in reality, specialist old age pharmacists or mental health pharmacists for older people are more aware of this drug interaction.

- Ensure that anticholinergic burden is kept to a minimum and that unnecessary drugs are stopped – if anticholinergic drugs are deemed necessary, pharmacists should seek safer alternatives that have minimal effects on cognitive function (using www.medichec.com or the app).
  - This is usually the role of practice pharmacists in GP surgeries, care home pharmacists, medicines information pharmacists and specialist dementia pharmacists, but should also be considered by all pharmacists of all levels looking after patients with cognitive impairment or patients with a diagnosis of dementia.
- Ensure that antipsychotic drugs are only used as a last resort in people with dementia and that they are reviewed and monitored regularly with a view to stopping them as soon as possible.
  - This is usually an issue in the later stages of dementia and is a role for care home pharmacists or specialist dementia pharmacists.
- All people with dementia receiving psychotropic medicines should have their continuing need for this reviewed at least every three months. Where the benefit of a medicine is not clear, it should be gradually withdrawn with appropriate monitoring of the target symptoms.
  - This is usually an issue in the later stages of dementia and is a role for care home pharmacists or specialist dementia pharmacists.
- Full multidisciplinary reviews should be carried out at least annually; carers should be actively encouraged to participate in these, and pharmacists should be included as a core part of the multidisciplinary team.
  - This role is especially for practice pharmacists in GP surgeries and care home pharmacists.

There are many 'dementia friendly' community pharmacies in the UK. Staff follow a training programme that aims to support all levels of the pharmacy workforce to enable them to develop their pharmacies into 'dementia friendly' environments with an action plan to support this aim. The programme helps raise knowledge and awareness of the disease and equips staff with the skills and behaviours to be able to conduct assessments and early identification of AD with onward referral.

Pharmacy review

Medication reviews by pharmacists are crucial to identify medicines that could worsen cognition or increase the risk of falls. Care home pharmacists and pharmacists working in GP practices may be more suited to carry out these annual medication reviews.

An accurate and up-to-date medication history is vital in people with dementia. This includes medicines prescribed by the GP, but could also include medication prescribed by the memory service, community mental health team or home treatment team (if applicable). It is important to determine whether medication is purchased over the counter in case anticholinergic or sedative drugs are being used. Anticholinergic drugs could worsen cognition and sedative drugs will increase the risk of falls.

Since polypharmacy is more common in older people, pharmacists need to remain extra vigilant for drug interactions in this patient group and to identify any medicines that are no longer required in order to optimise pharmacological therapy. Risk assessment of self-administration of medicines should be part of the care plan in patients with dementia, to assess whether patients are still able to self-administer medicines safely, or whether responsibility should be transferred to a relative or professional carer.

There are a number of different tools for assessing self-administration of medicines (see *Box 8.2*) and these can be very helpful in reducing accidental overdoses or assessing non-adherence of medication in patients with dementia.

> **Box 8.2: Self-administration of medicines tools**
> - The Medication Assessment Tool
> - The Self Administration of Medication (SAM) Assessment Tool
> - The Self-Medication Assessment Tool (SMAT)

Medication counselling can be a challenge in people with memory impairment and successful communication is key, however, the presence of relatives or carers may be necessary. When prescribing and dispensing medication, it is important to keep the medication regimen simple and easy to follow and ensure that dispensed medicines are clearly labelled with straightforward directions for use. Compliance aids should be used where necessary.

Successful communication

There is a great deal of skill involved in communicating well, and training courses are available through the Alzheimer Society. However, we can all learn from the 'ten things to do to improve communication', recommended by Alzheimer Scotland:[20]

1. Believe that communication with the person is possible.
2. Try to focus on the nonverbal signs as well as what is said.
3. Avoid making assumptions; check things out with the person.
4. Make your communication a two-way process that engages the person with dementia.
5. Avoid the use of jargon or complicated explanation – keep your conversation as simple as possible without being patronising or sounding childish.
6. Do not ask questions which have 'why' in them – the person with dementia may find the reasoning involved in answering difficult and become annoyed with themselves.
7. Be a good listener – give the person your full attention and resist the temptation to finish their sentences and talk at the person.
8. Talk at a slower pace so that the person has an opportunity to grasp what is being said.
9. Maintain a calm and unhurried approach.
10. Discover the best time of day to spend time talking with the person.

Covert administration of medicines[21]

Some patients with cognitive disorders may lack capacity to make an informed choice about whether medication will be beneficial to them or not. In these cases, the clinical team may consider whether it would be in the patient's best interests to conceal medication in food or drinks.

A legal framework exists to ensure this practice is not carried out illegally, that the patient does lack capacity to refuse medication, and that it is in their best interests to administer their medication in this way. Pharmacists need to be aware of this to protect patients and to give advice to carers and other health professionals when appropriate.

Medicines

Cognitive enhancers such as AChEIs (donepezil, rivastigmine and galantamine) and memantine may provide some modest cognitive, functional and global benefits in patients with certain types of dementia, mainly Alzheimer's disease.

Donepezil

The starting dose is 5 mg once daily (taken at bedtime). This should be reviewed after one month and if it is tolerated offer to increase the dose to 10 mg. Donepezil is also available in orodispersible tablets and oral solution. Due to the cost, these are only recommended for people who have difficulties swallowing tablets.

Rivastigmine (oral)

The starting dose is 1.5 mg twice daily. It should be reviewed after two weeks and increased in steps of 1.5 mg twice daily at intervals of at least two weeks according to response and tolerance. The maximum dose is 6 mg twice daily.

Rivastigmine (transdermal)

To start, a 4.6 mg/24 hours daily patch should be used and treatment reviewed after four weeks. If this is tolerated it can be increased to 9.5 mg/24 hours daily for a further six months. After six months if well tolerated and cognitive deterioration or functional decline is demonstrated, it can then be increased to 13.3 mg/24 hours daily. Rivastigmine is also available in an oral solution, however, this is currently more expensive then transdermal patches.

Galantamine modified release

The starting dose is 8 mg m/r daily increasing by 8 mg every 4 weeks to a maximum dose of 24 mg m/r.

If an oral AChEI is not tolerated due to gastrointestinal adverse effects, transdermal rivastigmine can be considered.

Memantine

The starting dose is 5 mg once daily. If tolerated this can be increased in steps of 5 mg every week to a maximum 20 mg per day (this is the usual maintenance dose). Memantine is available in a titration pack with one week (7 tablets) each of 5 mg, 10 mg, 15 mg and 20 mg.

Memantine should be avoided if the estimated glomerular filtration rate (eGFR) is less than 5 mL/minute/1.73 m^2. The dose should be reduced to 10 mg daily if eGFR is 5-29 mL/minute/1.73 m^2. If eGFR is 30-49 mL/minute/1.73 m^2 the dose should also be reduced to 10 mg daily, but if it is well tolerated after at least 7 days the dose can be increased in 5 mg steps to 20 mg daily.

Guidelines recommend the use of a combination of AChEI plus memantine rather than AChEI alone in patients with moderate to severe AD.[21]

See *Table 8.1* for a summary of titration schedules.

Table 8.1: *Dementia medication titration schedules*[22]

Medication	Frequency	Week 1	Week 2	Week 3	Week 4	Week 5	Week 7	Week 9
Donepezil (oral)	Once daily	5 mg	5 mg	5 mg	5 mg	10 mg	10 mg	10 mg
Rivastigmine (oral)	Twice daily	1.5 mg	1.5 mg	3 mg	3 mg	4.5 mg	6 mg	6 mg
Rivastigmine (patch)	Once daily	4.6 mg/ 24 hrs	4.6 mg/ 24 hrs	4.6 mg/ 24 hrs	4.6 mg/ 24 hrs	9.5 mg/ 24 hrs	9.5 mg/ 24 hrs	9.5 mg/ 24 hrs
Galantamine m/r (oral)	Once daily	8 mg m/r	8 mg m/r	8 mg m/r	8 mg m/r	16 mg m/r	16 mg m/r	24 mg m/r
Memantine (oral)	Once daily	5 mg	10 mg	15 mg	20 mg	20 mg	20 mg	20 mg

Tolerability may differ between AChEIs. When adverse effects occur with these agents, they are generally predictable from their pharmacology, dose-dependent and tend to be transient. Memantine tends to be well tolerated, but caution should be used in people with epilepsy. See *Table 8.2* for adverse effects and how to manage them.

Table 8.2: *Dementia medication adverse effects and management**

	Adverse effect	Frequency	Management
Acetylcholinesterase inhibitors (AChEIs)	Gastrointestinal symptoms (e.g. anorexia, nausea, vomiting, diarrhoea)	Very common	• Generally mild and transient and disappear within a few days of treatment. • Can be minimised by taking drug after food. • If symptoms persist discuss with/refer to a specialist who may reduce the dose or try an alternative acetylcholinesterase inhibitor or switch to memantine.
	Headache, fatigue, dizziness and muscle cramps	Common	• Generally mild and transient. The ability of the patient to continue driving or operating complex machinery should be evaluated. • Consult a specialist if problematic. May need dose reduction/ discontinuation.
	Agitation, confusion, insomnia, abnormal dreams and nightmares	Common	• Consult a specialist if problematic. May need dose reduction/ discontinuation. • Consider changing once daily dose to an earlier time in the day (e.g. for donepezil) to reduce insomnia, abnormal dreams and nightmares.
	Syncope	Common	• Consult specialist. May need dose reduction/discontinuation. • In investigating seizures, the possibility of heart block or long sinus pauses should be considered.
	Bradycardia	Common/ uncommon**	• Seek urgent review. Stop treatment and consult a specialist. • Caution in sick sinus syndrome, sinoatrial or atrioventricular block, or concomitant treatment with digoxin or beta blockers.
	Enhanced predisposition to peptic ulceration	Uncommon/rare	• Care with active gastric or duodenal ulcers or people with a predisposition to them. Consult a specialist to consider discontinuation of treatment. • Patient should be monitored regularly for symptoms.
	Lowered seizure threshold	Uncommon/rare	• Extreme caution in epilepsy. • Review treatment with a specialist if seizures develop as may be caused by an underlying disease. The possibility of heart block or long sinus pauses should be considered.
	Bronchoconstriction	Unknown	• Caution in COPD or asthma, consult a specialist to review treatment.
	Exacerbation of bladder outflow problems	Unknown	• Caution if history of prostatic conditions, urinary retention. • Avoid galantamine in urinary retention or post bladder surgery.
	Hepatic impairment	Unknown	• Avoid in severe impairment, caution in mild/moderate impairment. • See BNF guidance for each drug and seek advice from consultant hepatologist.
	Renal impairment	Unknown	• Avoid in severe impairment (except donepezil which is not affected by renal impairment). • Caution in mild/moderate impairment. • See BNF guidance for each drug and seek advice from consultant nephrologist.
Memantine	Somnolence Dizziness	Common	• The ability of the patient to continue driving or operating complex machinery should be evaluated. • Consult a specialist if problematic for the patient.
	Hypertension	Common	• Caution in those with uncontrolled hypertension or cardiac disease. • Review treatment with a specialist if this develops. May need dose reduction/discontinuation.

*This information is based on the manufacturer's Summary of Product Characteristics and the British National Formulary.
**Depending on the AChEI.
Very common: > 1/10; Common: >1/100, <1/10; Uncommon: >1/1000, <1/100; Rare: >1/10,000, <1/1000.

Table 8.2: *Dementia medication adverse effects and management* (continued)*

	Adverse effect	Frequency	Management
Memantine (continued)	Dyspnoea	Common	● Caution in people with COPD or asthma. ● Consult a specialist to review treatment.
	Constipation	Common	● Refer back to a specialist if severe or is not self-limiting. ● Consider as required, or regular laxative.
	Headache	Common	● Refer back to a specialist if severe or is not self-limiting.
	Elevated liver function test	Common	● Refer back to the specialist for review.
	Drug hypersensitivity	Common	● Stop and refer back to the specialist.
	Fungal infections	Uncommon	● Refer back to the specialist if severe.
	Gait abnormal	Uncommon	● Refer back to the specialist if severe.
	Venous thrombosis/ thromboembolism (VTE)	Uncommon	● Refer for treatment of VTE, and review memantine with a specialist.
	Confusion, hallucinations, psychosis, fatigue	Uncommon	● Refer back to the specialist for review.
	Pancreatitis	Unknown	● Stop if severe, refer back to the specialist.
	Vomiting	Uncommon	● Stop if severe, refer back to the specialist.
	Cardiac failure	Uncommon	● Stop and refer back to the specialist.
	May lower seizure threshold	Very rare	● Extreme caution in epilepsy. ● Review treatment with a specialist if seizures develop as may be caused by an underlying disease
	Hepatic impairment	No data available	● Caution required in mild to moderate impairment. ● Avoid in severe impairment. ● Seek advice from consultant hepatologist.

	Renal impairment	No data available	● See BNF guidance:
			  – Avoid if eGFR <5 mL/min/1.73 m².
			  – Reduce dose to 10 mg/day if eGFR 5-29 mL/min/1.73 m².
			  – Reduce dose to 10 mg/day if eGFR 30-49 mL/min/1.73 m² and if well tolerated after 7 days increase to 20 mg in 5 mg steps.

*This information is based on the manufacturer's Summary of Product Characteristics and the British National Formulary.
**Depending on the AChEI.
Very common: > 1/10; Common: >1/100, <1/10; Uncommon: >1/1000, <1/100; Rare: >1/10,000, <1/1000.

Switching between drugs used in dementia

The benefits of treatment with AChEIs are rapidly lost when drug administration is interrupted and may not be fully regained when drug treatment is reinitiated, therefore caution should be exercised before stopping treatment. Poor tolerability with one agent does not rule out good tolerability with another.

Trials have failed to consistently demonstrate any significant differences in efficacy between the three AChEIs; the main differences are in frequency and type of adverse events. A significant proportion of patients (up to 50%) appear to both tolerate and benefit from switching between AChEIs if they cannot tolerate one. However, switching to another agent should only be done after complete resolution of adverse effects following discontinuation of the initial agent. Switching to another AChEI is not recommended in people who show no apparent benefit to one, or loss of benefit several years after initiation of therapy.[21]

Monitoring

The pulse should be taken before prescribing AChEIs. While ECG is not routinely required before prescribing AChEIs, further clinical assessment, including ECG, should be undertaken before starting treatment if the patient has unexplained syncope or a pulse <50 bpm; see *Figure 8.1*).

Caution should be exercised in prescribing AChEIs in people with sick sinus syndrome, or other supraventricular cardiac conduction disturbances, such as sinoatrial or atrioventricular block. In these conditions, seek specialist advice (e.g. from a cardiologist).

Figure 8.1: *Pulse check pathway (adapted from Rowland et al, 1997)[23]*

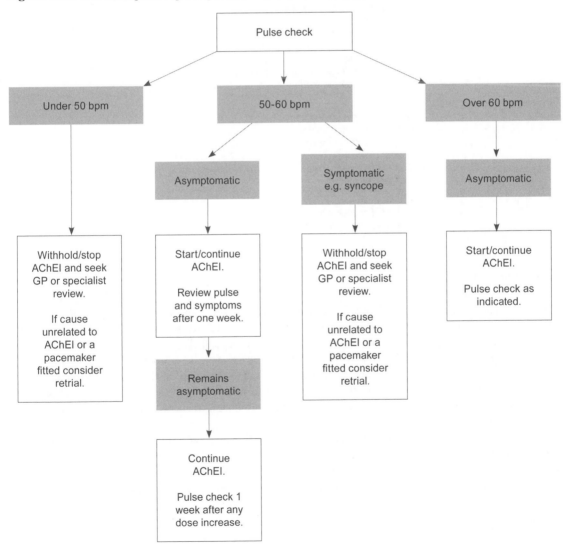

Cautions to consider for dementia medication

While treatment is normally initiated by a specialist, pharmacists should double check that there are no contraindications or cautions that need to be taken into account and that treatment choices are still appropriate. See *Table 8.3* for cautions to be aware of for dementia medication.

Table 8.3: *Cautions for dementia medicines*[22]

Drug	Cautions
Donepezil	• Asthma, chronic obstructive pulmonary disease (COPD) • Sick sinus syndrome, supraventricular conduction abnormalities • Susceptibility to peptic ulcers
Galantamine	• Asthma, COPD, pulmonary infection • Cardiac disease, unstable angina, sick sinus syndrome, supraventricular conduction abnormalities, congestive heart failure • Electrolyte disturbances • History of seizures • Susceptibility to peptic ulcers • Avoid in people: – with gastrointestinal or urinary outflow obstruction – recovering from bladder or gastrointestinal surgery
Rivastigmine	• Asthma, COPD • Bladder outflow obstruction • Conduction abnormalities • Duodenal ulcers or gastric ulcers, or susceptibility to ulcers • History of seizures • Risk of fatal overdose with patch administration errors • Sick sinus syndrome
Memantine	• Epilepsy • History of convulsions • Risk factors for epilepsy

Drug interactions

Donepezil and galantamine are substrates at cytochrome P450 3A4 and 2D6 and therefore plasma levels can be increased or decreased by drugs that either inhibit (e.g. ketoconazole, erythromycin, fluoxetine) or induce (e.g. rifampicin, phenytoin, carbamazepine) these enzymes. Rivastigmine undergoes non-hepatic metabolism and therefore pharmacokinetic drug interactions are unlikely.

Isolated cases of international normalised ratio (INR) increases have been reported in patients on warfarin who commence treatment with memantine. While no causal relationship has been established and this is not listed as a drug interaction in the BNF, it is mentioned in the memantine product information. Close monitoring of prothrombin time or INR is advisable for patients on warfarin during the titration phase of memantine administration.

The effects of antipsychotics may be reduced when administered with memantine, whereas the effects of dopaminergic agonists, selegiline and anticholinergics may be enhanced. For full information on drug interactions, see product information for each drug.

Important pharmacodynamic drug interactions for AChEIs and how to manage them are outlined in *Table 8.4*.

Table 8.4: *Important pharmacodynamic drug interactions with cholinesterase inhibitors*

Drug	Examples	Interaction	Management
Drugs that cause bradycardia	Digoxin Beta blockers Calcium channel blockers Amiodarone	Possible increased risk of bradycardia	• Caution is advised with concomitant use of medicines known to induce QT interval prolongation and/or torsade de pointes • The manufacture of galantamine recommends an ECG if it is taken with any of these medicines
Anticholinergics	Amitriptyline Oxybutynin	Pharmacological antagonism – the effects of AChEIs may be opposed	• Use the Anticholinergic Effect on Cognition (AEC) scale to establish which medicines have an anticholinergic effect on cognition (www.medichec.com)

Note: this is not a comprehensive list of drug interactions. See the individual manufacturers' Summary of Product Characteristics for more information.

Stopping treatment

Dementia medication should not be stopped based on cognitive test scores, discontinuation may lead to worsening cognition and function. Generally, if well tolerated, dementia medication is continued for as long as the patient is able to take it, until near the end of life. Reasons for stopping treatment include:[24]

- the patient/caregiver decides to stop (after being advised on the risks and benefits of stopping treatment)
- the patient refuses to take the medication (take into account local and national covert prescribing guidance)
- there are issues with patient compliance which cannot be reasonably resolved
- the patient's cognitive, functional or behavioural decline is worse on treatment
- there are intolerable adverse effects
- comorbidities make treatment risky or futile (e.g. terminal illness)
- there is no clinically meaningful benefit to continuing therapy (clinical judgement should be used here rather than ceasing treatment when a patient reaches a certain score on a cognitive outcome or when they are institutionalised).

When a decision is made to stop therapy (for reasons other than lack of tolerability), tapering of the dose and monitoring the patient for evidence of significant decline during the next 1-3 months are advised. If such a decline occurs, reinstatement of therapy should be considered.

Management of behavioural and psychological symptoms of dementia (BPSD)

These symptoms provide a significant challenge for patients and their carers and are often difficult to manage. Antipsychotic drugs have been widely used in the past to treat noncognitive symptoms of dementia.

However, in 2004, data emerged linking the use of atypical antipsychotic drugs with an increased risk of stroke and death in patients with dementia.[25] Warnings of these risks have been extended to all antipsychotic drugs, including both typical (also referred to as first-generation, conventional, or older antipsychotics) and atypical or second-generation antipsychotic drugs.[21] Since then, there has been an international drive to limit their use and ensure that they are used appropriately in patients with dementia.

Risperidone (and haloperidol) are the only drugs licensed in the UK for the management of non-cognitive symptoms associated with dementia. Due to the serious adverse effects of haloperidol, risperidone is the agent of choice. It is specifically indicated for short-term treatment (up to 6 weeks) of persistent aggression in patients with moderate to severe AD unresponsive to non-pharmacological approaches and when there is a risk of harm to self or others.[21] Risperidone is licensed up to 1 mg twice a day, although the optimal dose in dementia is 500 micrograms twice a day (1 mg daily).[21]

Other antipsychotic drugs are sometimes used (off-licence) if risperidone is contraindicated or not tolerated. Olanzapine and amisulpride may also be effective and quetiapine (although not as effective as risperidone and olanzapine), may be considered in patients with Parkinson's disease, or Lewy body dementia (at very small doses) because of its propensity for causing movement disorders.[21]

Other groups of psychotropics such as benzodiazepines, anticonvulsants, trazodone and sedating antihistamines such as promethazine have been used widely in the past to manage these symptoms. However, the evidence for any benefit is lacking and tolerability is poor. Therefore, none of these agents are recommended for BPSD.[21]

Box 8.3: Practice point: management of BPSD[21]

- Exclude physical illness which may be precipitating the behavioural symptoms of dementia (e.g. constipation, infection, pain)
- Target the symptoms requiring treatment
- Consider non-pharmacological methods first, individualised to the patient (e.g. aromatherapy, music therapy)
- Carry out a risk/benefit analysis tailored to individual needs when selecting a drug
- Make evidence-based decisions when choosing a drug
- If an antipsychotic is deemed necessary (as a last resort), discuss treatment options and explain the risks to the patient (if they have capacity) and family/carers
- Titrate drug from a low starting dose and maintain at lowest possible dose for the shortest period possible
- Review appropriateness of treatment regularly so that ineffective drug is not continued unnecessarily
- Monitor for adverse effects
- Document all treatment choices and discussions with patients and carers

---

Follow-up

Patients with dementia should be followed up closely in the first 2-3 months of starting cognitive enhancers to assess tolerability and adherence. This is usually done by the memory service, but community pharmacists can play a role as well. Cognitive assessment is no longer required, but blood pressure and pulse and general tolerability are important.

Annual reviews are also necessary and should include medication reviews by pharmacists.

Referral

Community pharmacists who suspect that a person is experiencing memory problems (e.g. forgets to collect medication, appears confused and forgetful) should encourage them to go and see their GP. This is not very urgent but it is important to refer where necessary.

Useful resources

- Alzheimer's Society: 0330 333 0804 / www.alzheimers.org.uk
- National Dementia Helpline: 0300 222 1122
  - Can provide information, support, guidance and signposting to other appropriate organisations
  - The helpline is usually open from:
    - » 9 am - 8 pm Monday to Wednesday
    - » 9 am - 5 pm Thursday and Friday
    - » 10 am - 4 pm Saturday and Sunday
- Age UK: www.ageuk.org.uk

References

1. Alzheimer's Society (2020). www.alzheimers.org.uk

2. National Institute for Health and Care Excellence (2018). Dementia: assessment, management and support for people living with dementia and their carers. www.nice.org.uk/guidance/ng97

3. Dementia UK (2018). www.dementiauk.org/wp-content/uploads/2018/07/What-is-dementia-WEB-June-2018.pdf

4. National Collaborating Centre for Mental Health (2007). Dementia: the NICE-SCIE guideline on supporting people with dementia and their carers in health and social care. www.scie.org.uk/publications/misc/dementia/dementia-fullguideline.pdf

5. Byrne G. Pharmacological treatment of behavioural problems in dementia. *Australian Prescriber* 2011; 28: 67-70.

6. Management of non-cognitive symptoms associated with dementia. *Drug and Therapeutics Bulletin* 2014; 52(10): 114-118.

7. van der Flier WM, Scheltens P. Epidemiology and risk factors of dementia. *Journal of Neurology, Neurosurgery & Psychiatry* 2005; 76(suppl 5): v2-7.

8. Alzheimer's Research UK (2020). www.dementiastatistics.org/statistics/prevalence-by-age-in-the-uk

9. Chen JH *et al*. Risk Factors for Dementia. *Journal of the Formosan Medical Association* 2009; 108(10): 754-764.

10. Baumgart M *et al*. Summary of the evidence on modifiable risk factors for cognitive decline and dementia: a population-based perspective. *Alzheimer's & dementia: the journal of the Alzheimer's Association* 2015; 11(6): 718-726.

11. Ownby RL *et al*. Depression and risk for Alzheimer disease: systematic review, meta-analysis, and metaregression analysis. *Arch Gen Psychiatry* 2006; 63(5): 530-538.

12. Diniz BS *et al*. Late-life depression and risk of vascular dementia and Alzheimer's disease: systematic review and meta-analysis of community-based cohort studies. *British Journal of Psychiatry* 2013; 202(5): 329-335.

13. Fox C *et al*. Anticholinergic medication use and cognitive impairment in the older population: The Medical Research Council cognitive function and ageing study. *Journal of the American Geriatrics Society* 2011; 59(8): 1477-1483.

14. Richardson K *et al*. Anticholinergic drugs and risk of dementia: case-control study. *BMJ* 2018; 361: k1315.

15. Coupland CAC *et al*. Anticholinergic drug exposure and the risk of dementia: a nested case-control study. *JAMA Internal Medicine* 2019; 179(8): 1084-1093.

16. Bishara D *et al*. Anticholinergic effect on cognition (AEC) of drugs commonly used in older people. *International Journal of Geriatric Psychiatry* 2017; 32(6): 650-656.

17. van de Vorst IE *et al*. Prognosis of patients with dementia: results from a prospective nationwide registry linkage study in the Netherlands. *BMJ Open* 2015; 5(10): e008897.

18. Xie J *et al*. Survival times in people with dementia: analysis from population based cohort study with 14 year follow-up. *BMJ* 2008; 336(7638): 258.

19. Matsunaga S *et al*. Memantine monotherapy for Alzheimer's disease: a systematic review and meta-analysis. *PloS One* 2015; 10(4): e0123289.

20. NHS Education for Scotland (2014). The pharmaceutical care of people with dementia. www.nes.scot.nhs.uk/media/ilkd2czp/pharmaceutical-care-of-people-with-dementia-2014.pdf

21. Taylor D *et al*. *The Maudsley Prescribing Guidelines in Psychiatry*, 13th Edition. London: Wiley Blackwell, 2018.

22. British National Formulary (2020). Joint Formulary Committee. British National Formulary (online) London. BMJ Group and Pharmaceutical Press. www.new.medicinescomplete.com

23. Rowland JP *et al*. Cardiovascular monitoring with acetylcholinesterase inhibitors: a clinical protocol. *Advances in Psychiatric Treatment* 2007; 13(3): 178-84.

24. Parsons C. Withdrawal of antidementia drugs in older people: who, when and how? *Drugs & aging* 2016; 33(8): 545-556.

25. Medicines and Healthcare products Regulatory Agency (2004). Atypical antipsychotic drugs and stroke. www.webarchive.nationalarchives.gov.uk/20141205212951tf_/http://www.mhra.gov.uk/Safetyinformation/Safetywarningsalertsandrecalls/Safetywarningsandmessagesformedicines/CON1004298

Case studies

Case study 1

Margo, aged 78 years, has been admitted to your ward. She has started to forget things more frequently. She sometimes doesn't even recognise her husband anymore.

Her husband asks whether she could have some medication for her memory problems.

Points to consider

- What assessments need to be carried out before starting a cholinesterase inhibitor?
- What else should be considered?

A diagnosis of Alzheimer's disease is made. Before starting cholinesterase inhibitors, the following assessments are carried out for Margo:

- The diagnosis is confirmed.
- The pulse is checked (in some cases an ECG may be required if indicated i.e. previous cardiac disease).
- Margo is assessed to see if compliance will be a problem.

In addition to these assessments, you confirm there are no contraindications to cholinesterase inhibitors or cautions which you need to manage. You explain to Margo and her husband about the treatment, when to take it and explain its benefits and limitation. You also ensure that her current medicines do not interact with cholinesterase inhibitors.

Margo is started on donepezil 5 mg daily. A week later, the donepezil is increased to 10 mg daily. At the same time, she is prescribed erythromycin for a chest infection (as she is allergic to penicillin).

Points to consider

- Do you have any concerns regarding her treatment so far?

You are concerned that donepezil has been increased after just one week as normally that should only be done after at least one month, and you know that there is an interaction between donepezil and erythromycin which leads to increased levels of donepezil and a potential increase in adverse effects such as nausea/vomiting and bradycardia.

Points to consider

- How would you manage the interaction and the dose of donepezil?

As the antibiotic course is only for one week it is appropriate that she continues to take this to treat the chest infection. You keep the dose of donepezil at 5 mg once daily and monitor Margo for any adverse effects.

A few weeks later, Margo's husband mentions that she frequently feels sick and has lost her appetite. She went to the chemist and bought some Kwells tablets for the nausea.

Points to consider

- What kind of medication is Kwells?
- Is it appropriate for Margo?

Kwells is hyoscine hydrobromide, an anticholinergic drug used to treat motion sickness and hypersalivation. Donepezil increases acetylcholine in the brain and Kwells inhibits it, so co-administration will negate the effects of donepezil. They should not be used together.

You switch the antiemetic to domperidone which does not cross the blood-brain barrier and does not have central anticholinergic effects. You also advise Margo that taking cholinesterase inhibitors after food can help with these unpleasant symptoms.

If an antiemetic is needed long term, then donepezil should be stopped and switched to another cognitive enhancer less likely to cause nausea/vomiting (e.g. rivastigmine patch or memantine if moderate/severe disease).

Case study 2

Harpreet, aged 72 years, attends the memory clinic for a repeat prescription of donepezil. He has a history of high blood pressure and had a myocardial infarction four years ago. His current medication includes:

- Donepezil 5 mg daily
- Atenolol 50 mg in the morning
- Amlodipine 5 mg in the morning
- Simvastatin 40 mg at night
- Aspirin 75 mg in the morning

Whilst waiting for his prescription, a nurse measures his blood pressure and pulse. His blood pressure reading was 118/79 and pulse was 49 bpm.

Points to consider

- Is this medicines regimen suitable for Harpreet?
- What issues, if any have you identified?
- Are his blood pressure and pulse within the normal range?
- What action, if any would you take?

You know that donepezil and other cholinesterase inhibitors can cause bradycardia and that atenolol is a beta blocker which can also cause bradycardia. You are aware that a pulse <50 bpm is dangerously low.

Cholinesterase inhibitors should be used with caution when they are given with other drugs that can also cause bradycardia as there is an increased risk of bradycardia occurring. Symptoms associated with bradycardia include 'funny turns' and syncope.

You advise Harpreet to stop donepezil and refer him to his GP to have his other treatments reviewed. The GP may switch beta blocker to another antihypertensive that does not interact with donepezil.

CHAPTER 9

Diabetes

Philip Newland-Jones and Nabil Boulos

Overview

Diabetes mellitus is a diverse group of metabolic disorders characterised by defects in insulin secretion, insulin action, or both, resulting in hyperglycaemia as the central feature.[1]

As understanding of the disease has broadened – with a greater appreciation of its distinct etiological subtypes and the complex interplay of concomitant metabolic abnormalities, genetics, and lifestyle – so have the management strategies. Modern diabetes care necessitates a multidisciplinary approach, and the roles of pharmacists across all healthcare settings have become indispensable.

As of 2019, 3.8 million people in the UK are formally diagnosed with diabetes, with an estimated additional 1 million undiagnosed. Together they make up 6.5% of the population (or 1 in 15 people).[2]

Type 2 diabetes mellitus (T2DM) poses a global health problem that is rising dramatically. The trend has slowly started to impact children and young people, with the first child diagnosed with T2DM in the UK in 2000.[2] The overwhelming risk factor for developing T2DM is obesity, contributing to more than 80% of the overall risk.[2,3] Other risk factors are increased age, sedentary lifestyle, hypertension, dyslipidaemia, and (for women) previous diagnosis of gestational diabetes mellitus (GDM). Non-modifiable risk factors include certain ethnicities and genetic factors, although the complexity of genetics involved is still not fully understood. Remarkably, genetic predisposition has a stronger influence on the development of T2DM compared to type 1 diabetes mellitus (T1DM).[4,5]

Diagnosis

The onset of T1DM is characterised by polyuria, polydipsia, fatigue and weight loss, which in most cases tend to occur over a short period of days to weeks.[1,6,7] These symptoms were popularised by Diabetes UK's *4 Ts campaign* (toilet, thirsty, tired, thinner), and diabetes should be suspected if these symptoms present at any age.[8] Symptoms of T2DM tend to be similar albeit much more subtle, and often a picture of obesity will overshadow any possible weight loss. Indeed, most people would have lived with unnoticed hyperglycaemia for years before being diagnosed with T2DM. Other clues may include blurred vision, genital and urinary tract infections and slow-healing wounds.[1,6]

The World Health Organization (WHO) has set widely-adopted criteria for the diagnosis of diabetes (see *Box 9.1*).[9,10] Note that stricter criteria apply for the diagnosis of GDM,[11,12] and additional investigations are required to confirm a diagnosis of the exact type of diabetes, such as C-peptide levels, presence of autoantibodies and genetic tests.[13]

Box 9.1: Practice point: diagnostic criteria for diagnosing diabetes

- HbA1c ≥48 mmol/mol (6.5%), or
- Fasting plasma glucose* of ≥7.0 mmol/L, or
- Random plasma glucose of ≥11.1 mmol/L AND presence of signs and symptoms of diabetes, or
- 2-hour post-load plasma glucose** of ≥11.1 mmol/L

*Fasting is defined as no caloric intake for at least 8 hours.
**This is the blood glucose level 2 hours after ingestion of a standard amount of 75 g glucose. Also known as an Oral Glucose Tolerance Test (OGTT).

Types and aetiology

The two most common types of diabetes are T2DM, forming over 90% of all cases, and T1DM, comprising another 8%, while other less common types form the remaining 2% of cases.[1,2] Both the WHO and the American Diabetes Association (ADA) have issued comprehensive systems for modern classification of diabetes.[1,14] The most common types are summarised in *Table 9.1*, and the specialist reader is advised to refer to the original documents for a full review.

Table 9.1: *Common types of diabetes*

Type	Aetiology	Pharmacological management
T1DM	Pancreatic β-cell destruction (mostly autoimmune)	Insulin Metformin (adjunct) Dapagliflozin (adjunct)
T2DM	Insulin resistance and relative insulin deficiency	Glucose-lowering medicines Insulin
Type 3c	Disease affecting pancreatic exocrine function (e.g. pancreatitis, pancreatectomy, cystic fibrosis)	Insulin (depending on extent of residual insulin secretion) Glucose-lowering medicines
GDM	Metabolic and endocrine changes, leading to impaired insulin response during pregnancy	Metformin Insulin Glibenclamide
MODY	Genetic abnormalities leading to defects in insulin production or release	Depends on subtype – commonly sulfonylureas and metformin
Drug-induced diabetes	Depends on drug. Most commonly due to increased insulin resistance in tissues	Glucose-lowering medicines – mainly sulfonylureas Insulin

T1DM, type 1 diabetes mellitus; T2DM, type 2 diabetes mellitus; GDM, gestational diabetes mellitus; MODY, maturity-onset diabetes of the young.

Type 1 diabetes mellitus (T1DM)

T1DM is characterised by the destruction of pancreatic β-cells responsible for secreting insulin. In most cases, this is an antibody-mediated autoimmune process against pancreatic proteins. Pathogenesis is poorly understood but is likely triggered by genetic and environmental factors.[1,6,14] It should be noted that T1DM can occur at virtually any stage of life, and should not be associated only with a childhood diagnosis. In fact, a recent statistical analysis found that 42% of all diagnoses of T1DM occurred in patients aged over 30 years.[15]

Type 2 diabetes mellitus (T2DM)

T2DM is the most predominant type worldwide.[1,2] The condition exists on a spectrum of insulin resistance and relative insulin deficiency – one factor tends to dominate, although the degree to which each factor contributes may change over the person's lifetime. The trend of rising obesity and lifestyle changes in developed countries has led to T2DM being increasingly diagnosed in children.[16]

Type 3c diabetes

Type 3c (named after the ADA classification of diabetes subtypes), sometimes simply referred to as 'type 3', is diabetes caused by diseases of the exocrine pancreas.[14] The most common causes include pancreatitis, pancreatectomy and cystic fibrosis, all of which can impair insulin secretion, and each present their own characteristic management requirements.

This type of diabetes is also associated with deficiency of glucagon, one of the body's natural stress hormones that promote hepatic glucose production, and consequently, these patients are at a higher risk of hypoglycaemic episodes.[17,18] Insufficiency of exogenous pancreatic enzymes, collectively named pancreatin, will often necessitate the need for pharmacological replacement (with Creon®, Nutrizym 22® or Pancrex V®, for example) to ensure meeting adequate nutritional requirements.[17,18]

Gestational diabetes mellitus (GDM)

GDM refers to diabetes that first appears during pregnancy as a result of the special metabolic and endocrine changes that occur during this period, and resolves after delivery.[11,14] Less data are available on the safety of glucose-lowering drugs and insulin types in pregnancy, yet strict glucose control is required to avoid complications during delivery and in the newborn. Women with GDM have a seven-fold increased risk of developing T2DM later in life.[19] Therefore, follow-up blood tests should be done in the postnatal period and annually thereafter.[12]

Other types

Whereas T1DM and T2DM are polygenic in nature, maturity-onset diabetes of the young (MODY) is the most common monogenetic form of diabetes. The rare condition usually presents before the age of 25 and is often misdiagnosed as T2DM.[1,14,20] Correct genetic diagnosis allows for optimal choice of treatment. Depending on the exact subtype, treatment ranges from sulfonylureas and metformin to simple lifestyle changes.[14,20,21]

Drug-induced diabetes is worth considering for patients with conditions requiring long-term use of drugs that impair insulin secretion or increase insulin resistance.[14] The most common example is long-term use of glucocorticoids such as prednisolone and dexamethasone.

Prognosis

Diabetes is a disorder with implications that go beyond defects in glucose control: the clinical picture involves disturbance in carbohydrate, fat, and protein metabolism, with direct deleterious consequences to the cardiovascular, cerebrovascular, renal and nervous systems. Consequently, people with diabetes are at risk of three microvascular complications and three macrovascular complications (see *Table 9.2*).[6,9,22]

Simply the diagnosis of diabetes increases the risk of developing myocardial infarction, heart failure and stroke by more than two-fold.[2] Unsurprisingly, diabetes remains one of the leading causes of non-traumatic amputations, sight loss and end-stage renal disease.[2] The long-term prognosis for uncontrolled diabetes is poor, and patients with diabetes lose on average 7 years of life expectancy, with cardiovascular disease (CVD) accounting for half of all deaths.[23]

The NHS annual spend on diabetes is over £10 billion.[2] Around 80% of this spend is on management of complications,[2] and the current focus is on early prevention and optimal control of the condition.[22]

Table 9.2: *Complications of diabetes*

Microvascular complications	Macrovascular complications
Retinopathy	Myocardial infarction
Nephropathy	Stroke
Peripheral neuropathy	Foot ulceration

Pharmacy input

The expansive nature of the disease presents an opportunity for pharmacists of all degrees of experience and across all healthcare settings to contribute to the care of patients with diabetes. The Royal Pharmaceutical Society has recently issued a diabetes policy on how pharmacists can improve care for people with T2DM, with a focus on prevention, timely detection, treatment and monitoring (see *Table 9.3*).[24]

Community pharmacists are in an ideal position to support patients through healthy lifestyle promotion. Services such as blood glucose testing and blood pressure checks help identify early risk factors. The results, coupled with vigilant attention to signs and symptoms, can lead to early referral and diagnosis. Pharmacists working within GP practices and primary care networks (PCNs) can provide valuable input at population level: improving prescribing habits through local guidelines development and identifying patients who may benefit from a clinical review of their treatment regimen.

People with diabetes are 2-3 times more likely to be admitted to hospital,[2] and diabetes management becomes a secondary priority if it is not the reason for admission. This occasionally leads to iatrogenic adverse events and complications, resulting in an increased length of stay. In this scenario, the hospital pharmacist is in a unique position to review the patient's management: monitoring blood glucose and renal function can identify opportunities for adjusting doses and timing of medicines, and the varying state of the patient may warrant changing the treatment plans entirely.

Table 9.3: *Pharmacist roles in management of diabetes*

Aspect of care	Implementation: community and primary care	Implementation: secondary care
Prevention	• Offer lifestyle advice and health promotion through services such as medicine reviews and Healthy Living Pharmacies (HLPs).	• Offer lifestyle advice and health promotion through bedside counselling.
Detection	• Identify population at risk, and targeted review in GP or specialist pharmacist clinic. • Offer services such as blood pressure, cholesterol, and glucose checks. • Be aware of early symptoms of diabetes and make appropriate referrals.	• Be aware of symptoms. Interpret incidental findings.
Treatment	• Counsel on optimal use of medicines (including insulin and devices) and manage adverse effects through medicine reviews or GP pharmacist-led clinics. • Ensure optimal formulary choices across the population and mitigate 'therapeutic inertia'.	• Develop local guidelines. • Perform specialist pharmacist reviews as part of the diabetes multidisciplinary team. • Identify and explore non-adherence.
Monitoring	• Identify and prevent early complications (appropriate foot care and management of foot ulcers). • Offer blood pressure and cholesterol checks to detect common comorbidities. • Ensure ongoing GP and clinic review of HbA1c to avoid 'therapeutic inertia'.	• Monitor blood glucose levels and other laboratory results (renal function, liver function tests) on the ward. • Identify need to modify therapy during special situations (e.g. perioperative period, critical care setting, nil by mouth).

Application of patient-centred care can significantly improve outcomes for people with diabetes, and pharmacists have the opportunity to play an essential role in this process. A paradigm shift has occurred over recent years in the assessment and management of diabetes, moving away from the 'glucocentric' nature of the condition and focusing much more on reducing the risk of developing microvascular and macrovascular complications.

This has, in part, been attributed to cardiovascular outcome trials (CVOT) of newer medication classes for T2DM such as glucagon-like peptide-1 receptor agonists (GLP-1RA) and sodium-glucose co-transporter 2 inhibitors (SGLT2i), and more recently, studies focused on primary outcomes in heart failure and renal disease.[25,26] The main focus of this chapter will be on T2DM as this encompasses 90% of patients with diabetes, and thus will support pharmacists in developing roles in the clinical management of this specific group.

T1DM is usually assessed and managed by specialists, and eventually, all people with T1DM become experts in the management of their diabetes. Aside from specialist pharmacists who may work clinically with patients with T1DM, the role of pharmacists is to provide support and advice on how other medications may affect their condition or interact with medications for glucose, blood pressure or cholesterol.

In community pharmacies, pharmacists should explain how relevant interactions or adverse effects may affect control of diabetes, and allow patients to ask for further information. Patients should be offered a medicines review, where the benefits of treatments for blood pressure and cholesterol are explained.

The review is also an opportunity to ask if the patient has access to enough glucose monitoring equipment such as test strips, as there is a direct relationship between adequate frequency of glucose testing and patients achieving their target HbA1c. Pharmacists can also signpost in circumstances where patients are experiencing frequent hypoglycaemic episodes, or are behind with their annual eye screening, injection site monitoring or foot checks.

When people with T1DM are admitted to hospital, pharmacists have an essential role in medication safety, supporting insulin self-administration and diabetes management where possible. Recent data shows that 1 in 25 patients with T1DM develop diabetic ketoacidosis during their inpatient stay,[27] and the whole healthcare team needs to develop new strategies to prevent this from happening. Pharmacists are well-placed to provide guidance relating to insulin perioperatively and to support patients and their medical teams by ensuring certain scenarios (such as an acute kidney injury or the initiation of glucocorticoids) act as trigger points for prompt adjustment in insulin dosing.

The national diabetes audit reports both local and national statistics for eight care processes that should be checked and recorded annually to detect both risk factors for developing complications and any evidence of emerging complications.[28] Diabetes UK has a broader list of healthcare essentials which go beyond process and monitoring, considering all essential requirements for good diabetes care (see *Table 9.4*).[29]

Table 9.4: *Diabetes healthcare essentials for monitoring complications*

National Diabetes Audit	Diabetes UK	
Blood pressure	HbA1c	Care from diabetes specialists
Body mass index (BMI)	Blood pressure	Diabetes education courses
Foot check	Cholesterol	Free flu jab
Smoking status	Eye screening	High quality diabetes care in hospital
Laboratory HbA1c	Foot and leg check	Specialist care before, during, and after pregnancy
Laboratory creatinine	Kidney check (blood creatinine and urine ACR)	Support with any sexual health problems
Laboratory cholesterol	Advice on diet	Emotional and psychological support
Laboratory urine albumin:creatinine ratio (ACR)	Stop smoking support if required	

Pharmacy review

Diabetes is a complex condition and requires a detailed initial review to ensure a thorough assessment, correct diagnosis and initial management. This initial review helps extensively with treatment individualisation. Although it may seem very detailed, one must consider that over 50% of people diagnosed with T2DM have a complication present at the time of diagnosis which may impact management decisions.

Personal information

It is important to ascertain what language is spoken to ensure information can be transferred effectively. Consideration of how best to communicate is also important for people with visual, hearing or speech problems. Similarly, whether there are likely to be any comprehension problems due to underlying conditions such as dementia, and whether the person has any physical disabilities or mobility issues that may influence decision-making.

One must ensure the current occupation is recorded as this may impact the risk of hypoglycaemia due to particular medications, as well as the implications should the person develop complications of diabetes. If the person has a health and social worker, it is worthwhile obtaining their name and contact details to ensure the person has support in accessing healthcare.

Clinical information

There are a number of key points that should be covered when taking a clinical history. Although this list is not exhaustive, these include:

- Patient's main concerns – to ensure you can answer these and allow an effective consultation
- Past medical history
  - Previous cardiovascular events or underlying microvascular disease
  - Heart failure
  - Underlying endocrine or autoimmune conditions
  - Comorbidities likely to require steroids such as rheumatoid arthritis, asthma or chronic obstructive pulmonary disease (COPD)
  - Previous pancreatitis, cancer of the pancreas or previous pancreatic surgery
- Family history
  - Diabetes
  - Heart disease
  - Endocrine or autoimmune diseases
- Occupation
  - Armed forces, police or pilot – this may impact certain roles
  - Professional driver (passenger or heavy goods vehicle)
  - Heavy machinery
  - Physically active
  - Shift work
  - Jobs with steel toecaps – feet at risk
- Women of childbearing potential – could they be pregnant, planning pregnancy, or using contraception?
- Diet and exercise – important to ask what the baseline is like to understand what might need changing
- Alcohol – consider alcohol history. If increased intake, consider:
  - Risk of pancreatitis/pancreatic exocrine insufficiency
  - Liver function and triglyceride levels (fatty liver?)
- Smoking history

- Dental care – is the patient having adequate dental reviews?
- Prescribed medications
  - Steroids
  - Atypical antipsychotics
  - Antiretrovirals
  - Oral contraceptives
  - Beta blockers or thiazide diuretics
  - Tricyclic antidepressants
- Street/gym drugs
  - Injectables – risk of hepatitis B/C or HIV
  - Anabolic steroids
  - Growth hormone
  - Testosterone

Annual review

All patients with diabetes should have an annual review undertaken by a trained healthcare professional who is capable of fully assessing all aspects of diabetes care in line with the Diabetes UK 15 Healthcare Essentials.[29]

Undertaken correctly, an annual review is an in-depth process which is individualised in its approach and information provided. Increasingly in primary care, the annual review is undertaken by multiple healthcare professionals in general practice with pharmacists being utilised for medicines optimisation to support treatment targets for HbA1c, blood pressure and cholesterol. General treatment goals are discussed below and summarised in *Box 9.2*.

Box 9.2: Practice point: treatment goals in diabetes care

- BMI: 18.5-24.9 kg/m^2*
- Exercise: 150 min moderate intensity exercise per week
- HbA1c: 48-53 mmol/L** – without hypoglycaemia
- Blood pressure: 130/80 mmHg (or 120-129/75-80 mmHg if eye, kidney or cerebrovascular disease)
- Total cholesterol: <4 mmol/L or 25% reduction (LDL <2 mmol/L; TG <2.3 mmol/L)
- Lipid lowering: prescribe a statin if QRISK ≥10%, or for all patients with T1DM >40 years old
- Smoking cessation
- Urine ACR <3 mg/mmol

*Note BMI is significantly less useful in individuals with high muscle mass.
**HbA1c targets should be individualised, tailored to needs. Consider frailty, benefits versus risks of tight glucose control, risk of hypoglycaemia, and impact on quality of life (general range 48-70 mmol/L).
ACR, albumin:creatinine ratio; BMI, body mass index; LDL, low density lipoprotein; TG, triglycerides.

HbA1c

HbA1c, or glycated haemoglobin, is a parameter that correlates with average blood glucose level over the past 3 months, slightly weighted towards the most recent 4 weeks. The aim in treating glucose levels in diabetes is to revert the levels to as close to the non-diabetes range that is practicable and safe. The HbA1c target has to be made on an individual basis, but some simple considerations are suggested by the ADA to help with this assessment:[30]

- Risks associated with hypoglycaemia or medicine adverse effects
- Disease duration

- Life expectancy
- Important comorbidities
- Established vascular complications
- Patient attitude and expectant treatment efforts (potentially modifiable)
- Resources and support system (potentially modifiable)

HbA1c has limitations, and its accuracy is dependent on a normal red blood cell turnover and absence of any haemoglobinopathies. Anaemia, chronic kidney disease, recent blood transfusions, medicines which stimulate erythropoiesis, alcoholism and pregnancy may all result in a discrepancy between HbA1c and the actual mean plasma glucose.

Two landmark studies demonstrated the impact of HbA1c reduction: the Diabetes Control and Complications Trial (DCCT) for T1DM[31] and the UK Prospective Diabetes Study (UKPDS) for T2DM[32]. The trials showed significant reduction in the risk of microvascular and macrovascular complications, with a legacy effect persisting beyond the trial period.

With the advent of continuous glucose monitors, which are now used more as standard care for those with T1DM, there is a move towards more meaningful indicators of quality of life by looking at the time in range (TIR) alongside HbA1c. Using TIR as a target for insulin and behaviour adjustment looks to reduce day-to-day variability and swings of low and high glucose levels, resulting in less severe hypoglycaemia, higher day-to-day predictability and increased confidence in people with T1DM.

Blood pressure (BP)

CVD is the leading cause of death in patients with diabetes, thus reducing BP in this population demonstrates significant evidence of benefit through a reduction in risk of both fatal and non-fatal cardiovascular (CV) events. For those aged under 80 years, antihypertensive therapy should be initiated if BP is ≥140/90 mmHg (or ≥130/80 mmHg with a previous history of kidney, eye or cerebrovascular disease).

Essential adjuvant interventions alongside medication should be encouraged, including lifestyle measures such as reducing dietary sodium, moderating alcohol intake, weight loss and regular exercise. In T1DM, target BP should be 130/80mmHg, with consideration for a target of 120/75-80 mmHg for those under the age of 40 years with microalbuminuria.[33]

Most patients will need several medications to control BP, although for those with diabetes, angiotensin-converting enzyme inhibitors (ACEI) or angiotensin-II receptor blockers (ARB) should be considered first-line, followed by a calcium channel blocker or indapamide (especially in the context of heart failure). For patients of black African or African-Caribbean family origin, an ARB should be chosen over an ACEI. Women of childbearing age should be counselled on the increased risk of congenital abnormalities with ACEI and ARB use in the first trimester.

Lipid lowering

The evidence for the use of statins in reducing CV risk in diabetes is significant, even in those without overt vascular disease or with what would be considered normal cholesterol level.[34,35,36] *Table 9.5* summarises recommendations around statin use in diabetes.

Ensure patients on statins are counselled on drug interactions and given advice to follow a low fat, high fibre diet, aiming to normalise weight, reduce alcohol consumption and improve blood glucose levels, all of which will help to reduce lipid levels. The aim of treatment is to reduce non-HDL cholesterol by 40% initially using atorvastatin 20 mg. If this is not achieved, discuss adherence, rediscuss lifestyle measures and consider increasing atorvastatin dose.

Table 9.5: *Initiating statins in diabetes (adapted from Joint British Societies' recommendations)*[33]

T1DM: Do NOT use a QRISK calculator. High-intensity statins should be offered for:	T2DM: Use QRISK3 calculator*. High-intensity statins should be offered for:
• Most patients aged over **40 years**, *unless* short duration of diabetes (<5 years) and absence of other CVD risk factors.	• Patients aged over 40 years and QRISK3 score ≥10%.
• Patients of **any age** with long duration of diabetes (>10 years) or *any* of: albuminuria, eGFR <60 mL/min, proliferative retinopathy, treated hypertension, persistent smoker, neuropathy.	• Patients of any age and existing CVD, persistent albuminuria (>3 mg/mmol), or eGFR <60 mL/min.
• Aim is to reduce non-HDL cholesterol by 40%. • Ensure women of childbearing age are counselled on statins appropriately.	

eGFR, estimated glomerular filtration rate; HDL, high-density lipoprotein. *QRISK2 calculator is also acceptable.

Patients should have liver transaminase enzymes measured at baseline, at 3 months and at 12 months of initiating statins – if more than three times the upper limit of normal, consider reducing the dose of atorvastatin or switching to an alternative high-intensity statin with hydrophilic properties, such as rosuvastatin. Patients who feel they have muscular adverse effects of statins should have their creatinine kinase (CK) levels measured to aid decision-making; if on simvastatin, they should be switched to atorvastatin. *Figure 9.1* shows an example of a statin rechallenge pathway for patients reporting adverse effects.

Figure 9.1: *An example statin rechallenge pathway*

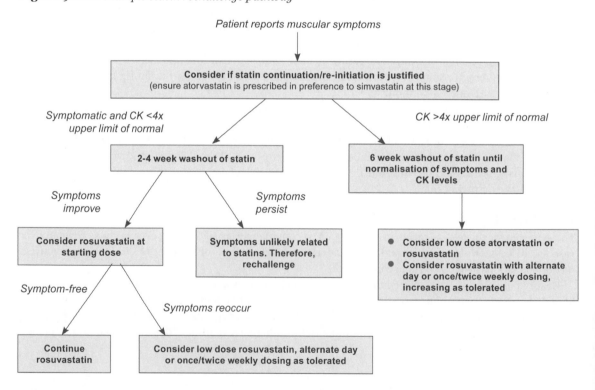

Patients with high triglycerides (>2.3 mmol/L) and low high-density lipoprotein (HDL) also have a high CVD risk regardless of LDL levels. Patients with high triglycerides should be encouraged to reduce alcohol consumption and aim for significant weight loss. It can also be an indication of relative insulin insufficiency, and improved glucose levels will therefore often improve fasting triglycerides. In patients with fasting triglycerides >4.5 mmol/L, fibrates can be used, but if prescribed in combination with statins, the statin dose may need to be reduced due to increased risk of rhabdomyolysis. Patients with triglycerides >10 mmol/L should be referred for specialist review due to the risk of developing pancreatitis.

Smoking

The harm caused to the body by smoking is well recognised, especially in relation to increased risk of cancer and CVD. People with diabetes who smoke have a four-fold greater risk of dying from CVD than those who do not. It is likely that smoking in the context of diabetes increases CVD risk further, but it also shows a link to an earlier onset of microalbuminuria, which in turn increases the risk of microvascular complications.

People with diabetes should be strongly discouraged from smoking and offered smoking cessation advice and support at every opportunity. Nicotine replacement products and varenicline can be used safely in diabetes. However, insulin absorption can be affected by the presence of nicotine, so consider a suggestion of closer monitoring of glucose when there is any increase or decrease in nicotine use.

Renal function and albumin:creatinine ratio (ACR)

Annual urinary ACR monitoring is essential in people with diabetes to be able to detect early nephropathy and prompt steps to slow progression. A raised ACR (>3 mg/mmol) is indicative of increased protein loss through the kidneys due to hyperfiltration, which cannot be detected using an estimated glomerular filtration rate (eGFR). The international guidelines by Kidney Disease: Improving Global Outcomes (KDIGO) outline the degree of chronic kidney disease (CKD) by combined measurement of GFR and ACR to give a classification of A1-A3 and G1-G5 (*Figure 9.2*).[37]

Figure 9.2: *Stages of CKD by GFR and albuminuria categories*

Prognosis of CKD by GFR Albuminuria Categories: KDIGO 2012			Persistent albuminuria categories Description and range		
			A1	**A2**	**A3**
☐ Low risk (if no other markers of kidney disease, no CKD);			Normal to mildly increased	Moderately increased	Severely increased
☐ Moderately increased risk; ☐ High risk; ☐ Very high risk.			<30 mg/g <3 mg/mmol	30-300 mg/g 3-30 mg/mmol	>300 mg/g >30 mg/mmol
GFR categories (mL/min/1.73 m²) Description and range	G1	Normal or high	≥90			
	G2	Mildly decreased	60-89			
	G3a	Mildly to moderately decreased	45-59			
	G3b	Moderately to severely decreased	30-44			
	G4	Severely decreased	15-29			
	G5	Kidney failure	<15			

Reproduced with permission from KDIGO[37]

A number of steps can help slow the progression of nephropathy and reduce microalbuminuria:
- Improve glucose control to target
- Reduce BP to target
- Improve dyslipidaemia to target, and prescribe a statin
- Stop smoking
- Prescribe ramipril or losartan (licenced for use in microalbuminuria with or without hypertension)
- In T2DM, consider a sodium-glucose co-transporter 2 inhibitors (SGLT2i) with evidence of reduction of renal outcomes

For those with diabetes, the risk of renal disease progression determines the frequency of eGFR monitoring: annually for those at low risk, every 6 months for those at high risk, and every 3-4 months for those at very high risk. Ensure local referral pathways to renal specialist services are followed as required.

Education and self-management

It is unrealistic to expect someone to achieve their diabetes goals without receiving education to support self-management.

One would hope that all essential information is conveyed to patients within 12 months of diagnosis, but this is often not the case. When we look at the percentage of patients attending diabetes education courses post-diagnosis, the numbers continue to sit below 15% for England in 2019. At every point of contact, it is essential to consider the level of basic education in diabetes the patient has, referring to local education programmes or online learning, whilst ensuring the patient understands why it is important.

Assessment to help with medication choice

When considering the choice of glucose-lowering medications, one must think laterally and beyond a simple linear treatment algorithm. The paradox of choice is simply that the more treatment options are available, the more difficult it is to choose at all, leading to 'therapeutic inertia'.

When unsure about which is the 'right' choice, prescribers will often revert to what they are comfortable with rather than individualising treatment plans. The list below is not exhaustive, but provides an example of how an overwhelming number of treatment options can be reduced to a suitable number of medication choices to discuss with the patient:

1. Contraindications: rule out what is not suitable.
   - Type of diabetes – if a patient is more likely to have pancreatic insufficiency rather than simply insulin resistance, this will reduce options for treatment, and may indicate that insulin is required.
   - Renal function – the licensing for many medicines in diabetes will limit options and may change the implications for safe use of certain medicines such as sulfonylureas or metformin.
   - Heart failure – the diagnosis of heart failure will rule out the use of pioglitazone, which worsens fluid retention. Also, be vigilant for undiagnosed heart failure when considering pioglitazone.
   - Common adverse effects – for example, glucagon-like peptide-1 receptor agonists (GLP-1RAs) slow down gastric emptying and therefore may not be suitable for people with chronic gastrointestinal conditions where it may exacerbate symptoms.
2. Efficacy: what will achieve target HbA1c?
   - When considering a medicine, consider its likely potency. If the HbA1c drop in clinical trials is too small for the required reduction, then the class can be disregarded.
3. Comorbidities: do the comorbidities affect your options?
   - Cardiovascular disease – a medication that has shown a reduction in major adverse cardiovascular events (MACE), such as a GLP-1RA (liraglutide, semaglutide, dulaglutide) or an SGLT2i, should be used where possible.

- Heart failure – for those with a reduced ejection fraction below 40%, an SGLT2i with proven benefits to heart failure outcomes should be used where possible.
- Diabetic nephropathy – for those with a raised ACR, there is emerging evidence for the use of SGLT2i in reducing eGFR decline and microalbuminuria progression.
- Recurrent steroid use (e.g. asthma, COPD) – patients with T2DM who may require frequent courses of corticosteroids are likely to need insulin earlier in the treatment pathway, especially during times of steroid use to keep blood glucose levels in a safe range. When considering an insulin regimen for this group, use twice-daily regimens to allow the flexibility to increase the morning dose in line with prednisolone dosing.

4. Hypoglycaemia: risk and implications
    - Safety is paramount when considering options. Hypoglycaemia can impact ongoing employment (e.g. professional drivers) and can precipitate cardiovascular events with life-threatening implications in certain circumstances. Hypoglycaemia risk may be high due to reduced capacity for patients' understanding, CKD or frailty. In this context, medications such as sulfonylureas and insulin should only be considered after all other options have been deemed unsuitable.

5. Weight change: benefits of weight loss, implications of weight gain
    - Consider the potential benefits of weight loss or the implications of weight gain when offering medications. Insulin, sulfonylureas and meglitinides will cause weight gain due to the anabolic action of insulin or stimulating the body to produce more insulin.
    - Pioglitazone may cause a small weight increase, dipeptidyl peptidase-4 inhibitors (DPP-4i) are considered weight neutral, whereas metformin will often produce a marginal weight loss. SGLT2i and GLP-1RA can cause beneficial weight loss, although if considering using a GLP-1RA, ensure a drug with robust evidence for weight loss is chosen (semaglutide, liraglutide, dulaglutide).

6. Cost
    - If you have reached a point where there is more than one viable option of equal clinical value for the patient, then consider using the most cost-effective agent. This is especially important where there are minimal clinical differences within a medication class, but a 20-30% price difference between the drugs being considered.

Diet and physical activity

When considering the management of overweight or obese patients with diabetes, it is important that the foundation of management is centred around achieving and maintaining greater than 5% weight loss. Larger improvements in control of diabetes and cardiovascular risk factors can be attained from even greater weight loss. There is no 'one size fits all' approach to dietary advice, and approaches should be individualised whilst considering a number of factors:

- Motivation and readiness to engage
- Life circumstances and comorbidities
- Cultural and religious beliefs
- Financial ability to change diet
- Education/skills in the preparation of foods
- Occupation

If we are to consider interventional trials, a variety of different dietary choices are appropriate for those with pre-diabetes and diabetes, including low fat, low calorie, low carbohydrate and Mediterranean diets. The aim for dietary and physical activity interventions is to achieve a deficit of 500-750 kcal/day, therefore the reduction in calorie intake required has to be balanced with daily energy expenditure from physical activity. As all energy-deficit food and activity interventions will result in weight loss, it is imperative that any change suggested is sustainable in the longer term.

The relationship between carbohydrate and blood glucose levels is cemented in both T1DM and T2DM management. In T1DM, patients with flexible basal-bolus insulin regimens will adjust each mealtime dose of insulin based on the amount of carbohydrate to be eaten utilising an insulin:carbohydrate ratio (the grams of carbohydrates matched to 1 unit of rapid-acting insulin (e.g. 1 unit insulin:10 g carbohydrates).

This ratio is combined with a correction ratio or insulin sensitivity factor (the reduction in blood glucose for every 1 unit of rapid-acting insulin, e.g. 1 unit insulin:3 mmol/L glucose) to calculate the exact dose of mealtime insulin needed. The complexities of this only begin to become fully apparent when considering the glycaemic index of foods, fat content and protein content, all of which change the speed of absorption of carbohydrates and subsequent glycaemic effects in the body.

In T2DM, reducing overall carbohydrate intake has produced robust evidence for improving glycaemia, though absolute reduction needs to be balanced with the individualised factors described above. Importantly, low carbohydrate diets are not no carbohydrate diets, where aiming to keep total carbohydrate less than 130 g/day is a safe approach.

Diabetes UK gives very good, evidence-based advice on low carbohydrate diets with example meal plans for patients. Carbohydrate intake advice should focus on the importance of nutrient-dense, high fibre, minimally-processed options, with a focus on whole grains, non-starchy vegetables and minimising added sugars.

Sugar-sweetened beverages, including fruit juice, should be completely avoided and replaced with water as much as possible. When giving dietary advice around carbohydrates, note that medications such as sulfonylureas or fixed-dose insulin regimens will need to be adjusted accordingly. If you do not adjust insulin in your day-to-day role, specialist advice must be sought for this group of patients to ensure safety against the consequences of hypoglycaemia.

Exercise is an important part of diabetes management. It improves blood glucose levels, increases insulin sensitivity, improves glucose tolerance, reduces cardiovascular risk, aids weight reduction and makes people feel generally happier due to the release of endorphins. Exercise should ideally be regular, with at least 20-30 minutes each day for 5 days of the week. The aim is to maintain the heart rate at 60-85% of the maximum (calculated as '220 minus age'), and a brisk walk is often enough to maintain heart rate in the desired range.

Patients increasing their physical activity should be reviewed to ensure that they are fit to exercise, and those with foot disease, eye disease, heart disease or autonomic neuropathy should be assessed by specialists to give guidance on safe exercise (see *Table 9.6*). Patients on insulin who are embarking on increased physical activity will often need support from a specialist to reduce the risk of hypoglycaemia.

Table 9.6: *Fitness to exercise considerations*

Foot disease	• Check feet – if at risk, contact podiatrist for advice • All patients – ensure appropriate footwear • Charcot feet or foot ulcers – avoid weight-bearing exercise • Neuropathy – ensure no blister or callus formation
Eye disease	• Those with unstable proliferative retinopathy should not exercise until it has been treated by an ophthalmologist and advice sought
Heart disease	• Appropriate exercise indicated after treatment stabilisation • Ask cardiologist for advice if patient symptomatic or known CVD
Autonomic neuropathy	• The ADA recommends that patients with autonomic neuropathy should undergo cardiac investigation before significantly increasing physical activity

Medication

Current evidence suggests that metformin should be initiated at the point of diagnosis of T2DM unless contraindicated. This should be in tandem with diet and physical activity interventions. Monotherapy is suitable for patients diagnosed with an HbA1c of 48-69 mmol/L, as an individualised target is likely to be achieved with metformin alone.

Traditionally, medications in diabetes have been added sequentially to assess each drug's effectiveness and adverse effects. However, most medications utilised in diabetes have distinct common adverse effects and there is merit in more rapid attainment of normalising HbA1c.

A more intensive approach to HbA1c lowering early in the disease process leads to better long-term outcomes. This concept was demonstrated in a recent trial where patients given combination therapy of metformin and a DPP-4i at diagnosis showed slower decline in HbA1c outcomes compared to those given the same drugs in a sequential manner.[38]

Thus, if HbA1c at diagnosis is over 69 mmol/mol, evidence suggests there may be merit in considering dual therapy at diagnosis. The choice of medication used in combination should be based on the approach and assessment detailed in the treatment algorithm produced jointly by the ADA and the European Association for the Study of Diabetes (EASD),[39,40] which considers the presence of CVD, heart failure, CKD, risk of hypoglycaemia and effect on body weight to guide treatment decisions.

For those who present with an initial HbA1c at diagnosis of over 86 mmol/mol or have significant osmotic symptoms, ketosis, weight loss or hypertriglyceridaemia, insulin should be the initial treatment approach. When glucose levels are reduced and the body can return to a less stressful state, there may be an opportunity to convert insulin to oral agents or simplify the regimen to metformin and a potent GLP-1RA (see *Table 9.7*).

Table 9.7: *Therapy choice at diagnosis*[30]

HbA1c (mmol/mol)	Choice of therapy (in tandem with diet and physical activity interventions)
48-69	Monotherapy (metformin)
70-86	Dual therapy (metformin + second agent)
>86 (or significant osmotic symptoms, ketosis, weight loss, hypertriglyceridaemia)	Insulin initially, then when a clear diagnosis of T2DM is made, review opportunity to convert to oral agents or non-insulin injectables if possible

Few other clinical conditions have seen such a diverse influx of pharmacological treatment options in recent years. The unique pharmacodynamic properties and adverse effect profiles of each drug class place the pharmacist in a central role for advising other healthcare professionals on optimal management and individualised patient care.

The guidelines produced by the National Institute for Health and Care Excellence (NICE) for the management of T2DM were published in 2015.[22] Since then, new trial data emphasised the importance of the context of other comorbidities, where drug classes demonstrate different benefits. As a result, NICE guidelines have been superseded by new clinical pathways that consider diabetes in the wider context of its comorbidities.

The guideline produced jointly by the ADA and EASD in 2018 provides an excellent approach to the management of T2DM.[39] Notably, the focus is placed on true patient-centred care: less emphasis on strict step-wise treatment, and more on the individual's needs and comorbidities. The reader is advised to be familiar with this guideline and the 2019 update,[40] which includes a simple diagram summarising approach to treatment. The next section discusses the available treatment options. Some outdated classes have been omitted to allow focus on drugs relevant to current practice.

Metformin

Metformin remains the first-line option for most patients with T2DM. Its established efficacy and high safety profile make it an essential backbone to any treatment plan. Patients with T1DM and a body mass index of ≥25 kg/m^2 may also benefit from the addition of metformin (unlicensed use) to their insulin regimen.[13]

Gastrointestinal adverse effects are the most common problem encountered. These can be alleviated by slow dose titration, taking the drug with mealtimes, and/or switching to the modified-release formulation. For patients who still can't tolerate its adverse effects, a dose reduction is encouraged over discontinuing the drug; as little as 500 mg daily will still provide benefit.[41] Even though doses up to 3 g daily are licensed, there is little clinical benefit for doses above 2 g, but gastrointestinal symptoms become more pronounced.[41]

Lactic acidosis, the most serious complication of metformin, is genuinely rare, and extremely unlikely in patients without other comorbidities (heart failure, hepatic impairment or renal impairment).[42,43] A Cochrane review looking into over 70,000 patient-years of metformin use found no evidence that metformin increases the risk of lactic acidosis compared to other glucose-lowering drugs.[44]

Lactic acidosis may develop in patients who are acutely unwell (e.g. sepsis, dehydration, acute renal impairment, acute heart failure). It's not clear whether, in such cases, metformin may contribute to this complication, but it would be prudent to temporarily withhold the drug until the patient recovers. Similar advice applies in primary care, where patients are counselled on Sick Day Rules,[45] and should withhold metformin if they experience vomiting, diarrhoea or fevers, and only restart it after 24-48 hours of eating and drinking normally.[4]

Sulfonylureas

Acting directly on pancreatic β-cells to stimulate insulin secretion, sulfonylureas can be thought of as having the pharmacological effects and adverse effects of insulins, though to a milder degree. Consequently, they may cause hypoglycaemia and must be taken during mealtimes to match peaks of high plasma glucose. Since insulin is renally degraded, adverse effects are more pronounced in renal impairment and in the elderly. Such patients would benefit from dose reduction or discontinuation of sulfonylureas. Weight gain is another inevitable effect of raising insulin levels, and careful selection of suitable patients must be made before starting therapy. Dietary and lifestyle advice is also essential.

Sulfonylureas have gradually become less favoured in the UK as a therapeutic choice for T2DM since newer classes have an improved adverse effect profile and additional cardiovascular and renal benefits. Sulfonylureas remain a good option for GDM[12] and steroid-induced diabetes.[46]

Pioglitazone

Pioglitazone acts as an 'insulin sensitiser', reducing insulin resistance in the liver and other tissues, with a resulting reduction in hyperglycaemia. It is associated with a small increased risk of heart failure (owing to its effect on fluid retention), bladder cancer, diabetic macular oedema and bone fractures.[39,47] Consequently, it should be avoided in patients with a history of these conditions, and with cautious use in the elderly and frail population. Signs of complications may manifest as weight gain (due to fluid retention), peripheral oedema, dysuria, haematuria and reduced visual acuity. Monitoring of liver functions is recommended.[47]

The complex pharmacology and complications of this drug make it difficult to place on a step-wise treatment approach. Pioglitazone naturally produces most benefit in patients with a dominant picture of insulin resistance. In more specialised settings, its additional metabolic benefits have made it an attractive choice for patients with certain subsets of non-alcoholic fatty liver disease (NAFLD), with or without diabetes.[48,49,50]

Sodium-glucose co-transporter 2 inhibitors (SGLT2i)

SGLT2i ('flozins') inhibit renal reabsorption of glucose and sodium, resulting in a controlled net loss of both. Glucose excretion results in a remarkable weight loss, while sodium excretion results in a small but consistent reduction in blood pressure.[39]

Adverse effects of this class include urinary tract infections and, rarely, diabetic ketoacidosis (DKA). The latter is more likely in the elderly and patients at high risk of dehydration. Consequently, Sick Day Rules apply to SGLT2i as for metformin.[45] Fournier's gangrene (necrotising fasciitis of the perineum) and limb amputations are rare complications, and it is not clear whether the latter is a class effect.[39] Patients who had a previous limb amputation are generally not initiated on SGLT2i.[51]

The remarkable improvement in cardiovascular and renal outcomes imparted by SGLT2i has transformed the approach to diabetes management beyond HbA1c control, adding a new focus on comorbidities. For patients with CVD, CKD or heart failure, SGLT2i and GLP-1RA are extremely beneficial additions to metformin that should be avoided only if a compelling contraindication is present.[51,52] It should be noted that the antihyperglycaemic effect is reduced with renal impairment, yet its other cardiovascular and renal benefits remain pronounced.[39]

In the recent CREDENCE trial, canagliflozin reduced the relative risk of renal complications by 30%,[25] and has recently gained approval for treating diabetic kidney disease in the United States. Similar licensing is expected in the UK in the near future.

Dapagliflozin has recently become the first licensed oral glucose-lowering drug for patients with T1DM (as add-on to insulin),[53] and sotagliflozin is expected to be available in the NHS for the same indication soon.[54] The risk of DKA with SGLT2i means initiating them in this group of patients must only be made by specialists experienced with their use in T1DM.

Dipeptidyl peptidase-4 inhibitors (DPP-4i)

Glucagon-like peptide-1 (GLP-1) is a naturally occurring hormone in the gut, which stimulates pancreatic insulin secretion and inhibits glucagon secretion. DPP-4i (gliptins) inhibit enzymatic degradation of GLP-1, thus prolonging its physiological effect. Since GLP-1 is only secreted in response to food intake, DPP-4i carry no risk of hypoglycaemia, even if the patient is eating less than usual.

DPP-4i have a good safety profile – the main adverse effects are gastrointestinal (nausea and abdominal pain) and transient in nature. Acute pancreatitis is a rare complication, which would manifest as unexpected, severe abdominal pain, and usually requires discontinuation of the drug. Saxagliptin is associated with an increased risk of hospitalisation due to heart failure,[55] although it has been proven that this complication is drug-specific and not a class effect.[39]

The modest reduction of HbA1c imparted by DPP-4i makes them less suitable as first choice when aggressive HbA1c management is the aim. They are ideal for elderly and frail patients when a gentler control of diabetes is desired.[56]

Glucagon-like peptide-1 receptor agonists (GLP-1RA)

GLP-1RA mimic the physiological action of GLP-1, resulting in increased insulin secretion, reduced glucagon secretion and an early feeling of satiety. The pharmacodynamics are similar to those of DPP-4i but are much more augmented. This class produces marked weight loss but is also associated with a higher incidence of gastrointestinal adverse effects than DPP-4i.

The latter effect is transient and seems less noticeable in the longer-acting types of GLP-1RA that require less frequent administration. This is also the reason for the need to initiate GLP-1RA at a low dose, and slowly titrate up. Similar to DPP-4i, they are associated with a small risk of acute pancreatitis, and patients should be advised to stop the drug if they experience severe abdominal pain.

Since both DPP-4i and GLP-1RA produce the same ultimate pharmacodynamic action, a combination of the two provides no added value, and patients on both drugs should always be reviewed to rationalise one or the other.[39]

GLP-1RA is one of two classes (the other being SGLT2i) with strong benefit to cardiovascular and renal outcomes, and again should be strongly considered in patients with relevant comorbidities.

Newer formulations of GLP-1RA have aided in greater patient adherence to therapy. This includes once-weekly injections (dulaglutide and semaglutide), combination injections with insulin (Xultophy®, Suliqua®), and, most recently, an oral form of semaglutide that is expected to become available in the UK in the near future.[57] *Figure 9.3* shows the pharmacokinetic profiles of common GLP-1RA.

Figure 9.3: *Pharmacokinetic profiles of GLP-1RA*

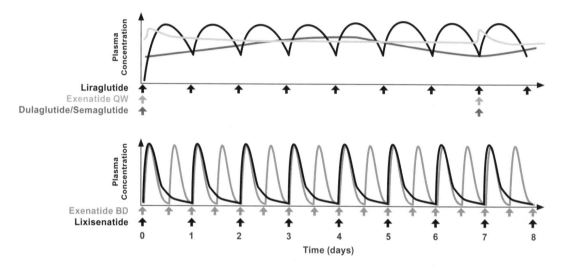

Plasma concentrations of the different GLP-1RA over 8 days. Each arrow represents an administered dose. Top: long-acting GLP-1RA are characterised by continuously elevated plasma concentrations, with half-lives ranging from 13 hours to several days. Examples include liraglutide, once-weekly exenatide (Bydureon®), dulaglutide, and semaglutide. All are given once weekly, with the exception of liraglutide (given once daily). Bottom: short-acting GLP-1RA are characterised by intermittent elevations of drug plasma concentrations, with half-lives between 2 and 3 hours. Examples include twice-daily exenatide (Byetta®) and lixisenatide. BD, twice daily; GLP-1RA, glucagon-like peptide-1 receptor agonist; QW, once weekly.

Insulin

Insulin comprises a critical backbone for management of T1DM and is often required in later stages of T2DM and other types of diabetes. The two key functions of insulin are promoting cellular uptake of glucose (mainly in skeletal and adipose tissues) and inhibiting hepatic glucose production. While endogenous insulin performs these tasks with seamless precision, exogenous insulin is unable to mimic them without associated adverse effects.

Weight gain is an inevitable consequence of the anabolic effects of insulin on lipogenesis, which necessitates counselling on an active lifestyle and a healthy diet. Risk of hypoglycaemia is associated with all types of insulins, although more likely with shorter-acting formulations. Good habits with blood glucose monitoring and learning to recognise early signs of low blood glucose make hypoglycaemia a rare event, and severe hypoglycaemia extremely unlikely.

Pharmacists can provide valuable counselling for patients on insulin. Advice on administration includes rotating injection sites to avoid the development of lipohypertrophy, avoiding injecting insulin into any lumpy areas of skin, mixing certain insulins (intermediate-acting and pre-mixed insulins) by gentle rolling rather than shaking, and changing the needle after every use.

Patients should also be aware of the effect of alcohol, as binge drinking leads to dehydration and often hypoglycaemia.[58] During periods of sickness or fasting, patients should not omit their long-acting insulin but will need more frequent glucose monitoring to adjust their insulin doses.[45,58,59] Specialists in this area should also be familiar with the effect of different types of exercise and diets on insulin requirements.

An understanding of the different types of insulin is key to managing diabetes and providing the right advice for the individual patient. *Figure 9.4* shows the pharmacokinetic profiles of different insulins, and *Figure 9.5* shows two common insulin regimens used in practice.

Figure 9.4: *Pharmacokinetic profiles of insulins*

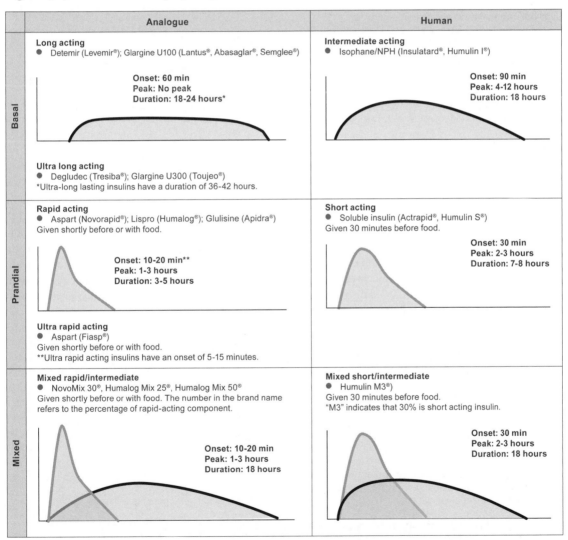

Diagrammatic representation of the extent and duration of action of different insulins over time following a single subcutaneous injection. U100 refers to insulin concentration of 100 units/mL; U300 refers to insulin concentration of 300 units/mL.

Figure 9.5: *Common insulin regimens*

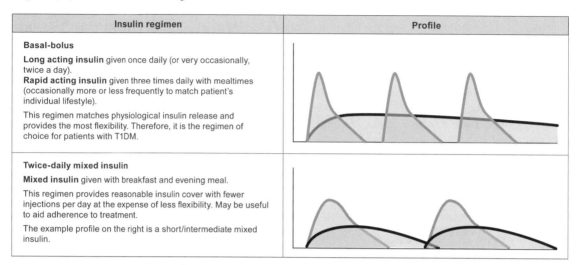

Insulin regimen	Profile
Basal-bolus **Long acting insulin** given once daily (or very occasionally, twice a day). **Rapid acting insulin** given three times daily with mealtimes (occasionally more or less frequently to match patient's individual lifestyle). This regimen matches physiological insulin release and provides the most flexibility. Therefore, it is the regimen of choice for patients with T1DM.	
Twice-daily mixed insulin **Mixed insulin** given with breakfast and evening meal. This regimen provides reasonable insulin cover with fewer injections per day at the expense of less flexibility. May be useful to aid adherence to treatment. The example profile on the right is a short/intermediate mixed insulin.	

Description and pharmacokinetic profiles of basal-bolus and twice-daily mixed insulin regimens. A variety of other regimens can be utilised in practice, depending on the patient's individual circumstances.

Monitoring

Currently, the primary indicator for long-term diabetes control is HbA1c, which should be tested 3-6 monthly, while capillary blood glucose (measured with a glucose meter) helps understand daily fluctuations in glucose with meals and the individual's lifestyle.[22,39] The latter is only useful if the patient is on insulin or a sulfonylurea since other drugs will not need dose adjustment based on the results.[22]

A variety of glucose meters are available on the market. Familiarity with the different features available would allow pharmacists to select the most suitable devices for individual patients or at a population level (see *Box 9.3*). Flash glucose monitors (FGM) and continuous glucose monitors (CGM) involve devices attached to the skin that measure interstitial glucose levels, providing a continuous glucose profile, a particularly useful feature for patients with T1DM. CGM devices can also be set to produce an alarm if blood glucose is too high or too low, adding a layer of safety for patients at risk of such events.

Box 9.3: Practice point: features that influence the choice of a blood glucose meter

- Large screen display (e.g. for patients with visual impairment)
- Talking meter: spoken instructions and reading (e.g. for patients with visual impairment)
- Dual glucose and ketone testing
- Trend and graphical display: 7, 14, or 30 day trend average
- Personalised input: meals (carbohydrate counting), exercise, insulin doses
- Ability to suggest insulin doses based on personalised settings (such as insulin:carbohydrate ratio and insulin sensitivity factor)
- Connectivity with insulin pumps (e.g. via Bluetooth)
- Connectivity with computers or smartphones
- Long test strip expiry (e.g. for patients who test infrequently)
- Features of accompanying lancet (e.g. preloaded drum lancets are suitable for patients with poor dexterity, needle phobia, or visual impairment)
- Integrated barcode scanning and data upload (secondary care only)
- Cost

The wider management of diabetes involves monitoring a multitude of other parameters. These include monitoring for common comorbidities (blood pressure, cholesterol), possible complications (eye screening, foot check, renal function tests) and lifestyle (dietary management, psychological support). Tools such as QRISK3[60,61] are useful to predict the 10-year risk of developing myocardial infarction or stroke, and statins should be initiated if appropriate.

Diabetes UK's 15 Healthcare Essentials is a useful checklist for patients and professionals to help ensure patients receive all the support possible (see *Table 9.4*).[29]

Drug interactions

Drug interactions fall into two categories: pharmacokinetic interactions, which alter plasma levels of glucose-lowering drugs, and pharmacodynamic interactions, which alter the pharmacological efficacy. The latter can be subdivided into drugs that can lead to hyperglycaemia and those that can lead to hypoglycaemia.

Table 9.8, *Table 9.9* and *Table 9.10* show the most clinically relevant interactions you may encounter in practice.[62-65] Advice on recommended actions is given where relevant. For many cases, no specific action is needed and monitoring blood glucose with counselling on recognising adverse effects will suffice. Note that the drugs that cause hyperglycaemia have also been implicated, to varying degrees, in causing drug-induced diabetes.

Table 9.8: *Pharmacokinetic drug interactions in diabetes*

Drug	Interaction	Effect	Action
Nephrotoxic drugs (e.g. contrast media, ciclosporin, aminoglycosides)	Metformin	Reduced renal function leading to accumulation of metformin and increased risk of lactic acidosis	Withhold metformin during acute kidney injury Stop metformin 48 hours before, and for 48 hours after, contrast radiography
Cimetidine	Metformin	Competes with metformin for renal elimination, leading to accumulation of metformin and increased risk of lactic acidosis	Avoid combination if on high dose metformin Watch for signs of lactic acidosis (abdominal pain, deep heavy breathing, altered level of consciousness)
CYP2C9 inhibitors (e.g. fluconazole, trimethoprim, amiodarone)	Sulfonylureas	Increased level of sulfonylureas (CYP2C9 substrates). Risk of hypoglycaemia	Monitor blood glucose closely Adjust dose or switch to alternative class if not controlled
CYP2C9 inducers (e.g. rifampicin, phenobarbital)	Sulfonylureas	Reduced level of sulfonylureas (CYP2C9 substrates). Risk of hyperglycaemia	Monitor blood glucose closely Adjust dose or switch to alternative class if not controlled
UGT enzyme inducers (e.g. rifampicin, phenytoin, carbamazepine, ritonavir)	Canagliflozin	Reduced level of canagliflozin (UGT substrate)	Increase canagliflozin dose to 300 mg (if renal function permits)

Table 9.9: *Pharmacodynamic drug interactions in diabetes*

Drug causing hypoglycaemia	Mechanism
Alcohol	Inhibits hepatic gluconeogenesis
Aspirin (high doses only)	Unclear – possible mechanisms include inhibition of hepatic glucose production and increasing insulin secretion
Quinine	Promotes insulin secretion
Drug causing hyperglycaemia	**Mechanism**
Atypical antipsychotics (most commonly clozapine and olanzapine)	Unclear. Possible mechanisms include inhibition of insulin action on skeletal muscles, and direct damage to pancreatic β-cells
Beta blockers* (most commonly atenolol, metoprolol and propranolol)	Possibly impairing pancreatic insulin secretion. This does not appear to be a class effect of all beta blockers
Calcineurin inhibitors (e.g. ciclosporin, tacrolimus)	Inhibition of pancreatic β-cells growth (a process regulated by calcineurin)
Corticosteroids	Increase insulin resistance in tissues and promote hepatic gluconeogenesis
Protease inhibitors (e.g. ritonavir)	Direct inhibition of cellular glucose transporters, thus promoting insulin resistance
Thiazide diuretics	Unclear. Possible mechanisms include inhibition of cellular glucose uptake and decreasing insulin secretion

*Of more clinical significance is the fact that beta blockers mask the warning signs of hypoglycaemia (which are triggered by the sympathetic system). Non-selective beta blockers may also impair the normal physiological response of the liver to hypoglycaemia (driven by β2-receptors). There is little evidence, however, that beta blockers themselves cause hypoglycaemia.

Table 9.10: *Significant interactions by glucose-lowering medications*

Drug	Effect	Action
Acarbose	Reduces digoxin absorption	Space administration of the two drugs Monitor digoxin levels
GLP-1RA	Reduce gastric motility, slowing drug absorption	Withhold GLP-1RA when there is need to ensure optimal absorption (e.g. administering analgesia and establishing enteral feeds in the postoperative period)
Metformin	Vitamin B12 depletion due to malabsorption, possibly leading to megaloblastic anaemia	Monitor vitamin B12 levels annually, and replace if needed
SGLT2i	Increased glucose and sodium excretion leads to additive diuretic effect with concomitant diuretics	Dose reduction of diuretics may be needed

Special groups

Certain patient characteristics and comorbidities require careful considerations in diabetes management. Resources at the end of this chapter provide specialist guidance for specific patient groups, but a summary is presented below.

Older age often necessitates simplification of treatment regimens, although this will depend on the degree of frailty and life expectancy rather than a certain age threshold. Generally, short-acting drugs and those that carry a greater risk of hypoglycaemia should be avoided. SGLT2i also pose a risk of DKA in the frail who are prone to dehydration. DPP-4i offer a gentle choice of oral treatment, while once-daily intermediate- or long-acting insulin alone may be preferred over more complex insulin regimens.[56,66]

For children with T2DM, consideration needs to be given for licensed options. Metformin and liraglutide are the only options, alongside insulin, licensed for children aged ≥10 years, although other options may be initiated by specialists.[16] Stricter management of the condition, alongside lifestyle advice, is vital to avoid early development of complications.

Diabetes in pregnancy (a broad term referring to both GDM and pre-existing diabetes before pregnancy) requires balancing the benefits of a certain medication against the risks of foetal exposure to the drug. Owing to its large molecular size, insulin doesn't cross the placenta, and is generally considered safe. Metformin is considered a safe oral option for pregnancy and breastfeeding, as is glibenclamide if a sulfonylurea is required.[11,12]

Useful advice

Other medications may be warranted with a diagnosis of diabetes. QRISK3 should be used to assess the 10-year CVD risk in patients with T2DM,[60,61] and statin therapy initiated if the risk is ≥10%.[67] Detailed advice on statins is presented in the Annual review section.

Long-term treatment with metformin may impair vitamin B12 absorption, which requires annual monitoring and supplementation if deficiency if present.[68] T1DM and T2DM (but not GDM) are risk factors for pre-eclampsia in pregnancy, and women with pre-existing diabetes should be started on aspirin 75 mg from week 12 of pregnancy onwards.[69]

Sick Day Rules include advice on how to adjust medicines during periods of sickness or feeling unwell (vomiting, diarrhoea, fevers). Metformin and SGLT2i should always be stopped, and only restarted after 24-48 hours of eating and drinking normally. Long-acting insulin should never be omitted during sick days (and may even require a dose increase since glucose is often raised during a stress response), while prandial insulin requires adjustment if food intake is reduced.[45]

Follow-up

Follow-up for patients with T2DM should be every 3 to 6 months. This allows for the minimum period for HbA1c to show a meaningful trend, while avoiding a diminishing 'therapeutic inertia', that is, lack of clinical interventions despite glycaemic control remaining poor. Accompanying checks should also be done during these follow-ups.

Patients newly diagnosed or newly started on drugs that require up-titration should be seen again after 3 months (occasionally after 1 month of initiating therapy), while those well controlled on stable therapy can be seen every 6 months. Pharmacists working within clinics or GP practices should also be aware of the local eye screening and podiatry services and refer patients to them at least annually.[22] Patients at high risk of foot complications may require more frequent follow-ups for foot checks.[70]

Patients with T1DM or GDM will always be seen by specialists in these respective areas and may have different follow-up intervals.

Referral

There are opportunities in community pharmacies to identify non-adherence, potential adverse effects or diminished clinical inertia. In these cases, pharmacists should recommend referral to the GP or the diabetes specialist who looks after the patient. Understanding the patient's values is also important, since some patients may not be engaged with aspects of glycaemic control, and the pharmacist should then non-judgementally explore how else they can offer support to this patient on an individual basis.

Pharmacists should also be able to recognise symptoms of serious complications of diabetes and glucose-lowering drugs, as well as symptoms of undiagnosed diabetes. This role is essential in primary care, where urgent referral to a GP or hospital is often needed. Prospectively, patients should also be counselled to recognise symptoms of such complications, depending on their individual therapy. If a drug is involved, the patient should not take any further doses and seek advice from a healthcare professional. A useful summary is presented in *Table 9.11*.

Table 9.11: *Common complications of diabetes and treatment options*

Problem/complication	Symptoms	Possible drug causes
Hypoglycaemia	Early: dizziness, fatigue, sweating, trembling, palpitations, nervousness, pallor Late: weakness, confusion, slurred speech, convulsions	Insulin Sulfonylureas
Hyperglycaemia	Thirst, polyuria, fatigue, nausea, blurred vision	None*
Diabetic ketoacidosis (DKA)	As for hyperglycaemia, plus: abdominal pain, confusion, deep and fast breathing (Kussmaul breathing)	SGLT2i
Lactic acidosis**	Dyspnoea, muscle cramps, weakness (asthenia), nausea, abdominal pain, hypothermia	Metformin
Acute pancreatitis	Abrupt abdominal pain, nausea, vomiting, diarrhoea, fever	GLP-1RA DPP-4i

*But concomitant drugs unrelated to management of diabetes may be contributing.

**Lactic acidosis is extremely rare, particularly in patients without other acute illnesses. It may not be relevant to routinely counsel patients on this complication, but healthcare professionals looking after these patients should be able to recognise the symptoms.

In secondary care, pharmacists should be familiar with local guidelines and triggers for referral to the specialist diabetes team (if available). Example guidance for inpatient referral is shown in *Table 9.12*.

Table 9.12: *When to refer to the specialist diabetes team within a hospital setting**

Problem/scenario in a patient with diabetes	Recommendation
• Newly diagnosed T1DM • Newly starting on insulin • Patient is admitted on an insulin pump • Diabetic ketoacidosis (DKA) or hyperosmolar hyperglycaemic state (HHS) • Severe hypoglycaemia • Starting parenteral or enteral nutrition • Variable-rate intravenous insulin infusion (VRIII) for >48 hours or unable to control wglucose levels	Always refer
• Newly diagnosed T2DM • High-dose or long-term corticosteroid therapy started • Persistent hyperglycaemia or hypoglycaemia • Significant education needs	Consider referral
• Minor hypoglycaemia • Simple education needs or diet advice • Routine diabetes care	Referral not routinely required

*List is not exhaustive, but shows common examples.

Useful resources

Societies and guidelines

- NICE (National Institute for Health and Care Excellence) – national guidelines on diabetes, including T1DM, T2DM, diabetes in children, diabetes in pregnancy, and diabetic foot. www.nice.org.uk
- JBDS (Joint British Diabetes Societies) – guidelines for inpatient care. www.abcd.care/joint-british-diabetes-societies-jbds-inpatient-care-group
- ADA-EASD (American Diabetes Association – European Association for the Study of Diabetes) guidelines – most up-to-date clinical guidelines for management of T2DM, with 2019 update. www.link.springer.com/article/10.1007/s00125-018-4729-5 and www.link.springer.com/article/10.1007/s00125-019-05039-w
- Endocrine Society – American guidelines, including diabetes in pregnancy, elderly and diabetes technology. www.endocrine.org
- Diabetes UK – Type 1 Diabetes Technology. National consensus on use of diabetes technology in T1DM. www.diabetes.org.uk/resources-s3/2019-03/Type%201%20Tech%20pathway%20position%20statement%20FINAL%20MARCH%202019.pdf
- ACDC (Association of Children's Diabetes Clinicians) – guidelines for diabetes in children. www.a-c-d-c.org/endorsed-guidelines
- BSPED (British Society for Paediatric Endocrinology and Diabetes) – guidelines for diabetes in children. www.bsped.org.uk/clinical-resources/guidelines

Professional education and resources

- UKCPA (UK Clinical Pharmacist Association) – dedicated diabetes and endocrinology forums (requires membership). www.ukclinicalpharmacy.org/community/our-forums
- UKCPA Integrated Career and Competency Framework for Pharmacists in Diabetes – comprehensive framework of competencies for pharmacists with interest or specialising in diabetes. www.ukclinicalpharmacy.org/wp-content/uploads/2018/05/An-integrated-career-and-competency-framework-for-pharmacists-in-diabetes-First-Edition-2018.pdf
- RPS (Royal Pharmaceutical Society) Diabetes Policy – document on the role of pharmacists in T2DM. www.rpharms.com/recognition/all-our-campaigns/policy-a-z/diabetes/diabetes-policy
- RPS Diabetes Toolkit and Resources – useful support resources for pharmacists caring for patients with diabetes across all settings of care (requires membership). www.rpharms.com/resources/toolkits/diabetes-toolkit and www.rpharms.com/recognition/all-our-campaigns/policy-a-z/diabetes/diabetes-resources
- Wessex Academic Health Science Network – resources for implementing insulin self-administration in hospital. www.wessexahsn.org.uk/projects/58/self-administration-of-insulin-in-hospital
- EASD e-Learning – free online learning modules on diabetes topics. www.easd-elearning.org
- Diabetes on the Net – online resources, including The Six Steps to Insulin Safety module. www.diabetesonthenet.com and www.diabetesonthenet.com/course/the-six-steps-to-insulin-safety/details
- Medicine Matters – Diabetes – educational platform with the latest news on diabetes, including subscription to a weekly clinical newsletter. www.diabetes.medicinematters.com

Patient education and resources

- Diabetes UK – comprehensive support and resources for patients with diabetes (all types). www.diabetes.org.uk, www.diabetes.org.uk/forum and www.diabetes.org.uk/helpline
- Diabetes UK – 4 Ts Campaign – awareness campaign on symptoms of T1DM, including printable posters. www.diabetes.org.uk/get_involved/campaigning/4-ts-campaign

- Diabetes UK – Type 2 Diabetes and Me – for patients with T2DM. www.diabetes.org.uk/guide-to-diabetes/managing-your-diabetes/education/type-2-diabetes-and-me
- Diabetes UK – 10 tips for healthy eating with diabetes. www.diabetes.org.uk/guide-to-diabetes/enjoy-food/eating-with-diabetes/10-ways-to-eat-well-with-diabetes
- NHS Type 1 Diabetes – comprehensive support and resources for patients with T1DM. www.nhs.uk/conditions/type-1-diabetes/get-support
- T1 Resources – for patients with T1DM. www.t1resources.uk/home
- Bertie – for patients with T1DM. www.bertieonline.org.uk
- DigiBete – for children and young people with diabetes. www.digibete.org
- Women with Gestational Diabetes – for women with GDM. www.womenwithgestationaldiabetes.com
- DVLA (Driver and Vehicle Licensing Agency) – rules and advice on driving and diabetes. www.gov.uk/diabetes-driving

Tools for follow-up and monitoring

- Diabetes UK – 15 Healthcare Essentials – checklist of monitoring and follow up requirements for patients with diabetes. https://www.diabetes.org.uk/guide-to-diabetes/managing-your-diabetes/15-healthcare-essentials
- QRISK3 – validated tool for calculating 10-year myocardial infarction and stroke risk. www.qrisk.org/three
- T1 Resources – Sick Day Rules (T1DM) – algorithm for insulin adjustment during sick days in T1DM. www.t1resources.uk/resources/item/sickday-rules-pdf
- How to... Sick Day Rules (T1DM + T2DM) – advice on sick day rules, including an algorithm for insulin adjustment during sick days in both T1DM and T2DM. www.diabetesonthenet.com/resources/details/how-advise-sick-day-rules

References

1. World Health Organization (WHO). Classification of diabetes mellitus 2019. Geneva: World Health Organization; 2019. www.apps.who.int/iris/rest/bitstreams/1233344/retrieve
2. Diabetes UK. Latest facts and stats. London: Diabetes UK; 2019. www.diabetes.org.uk/resources-s3/2019-02/1362B_Facts%20and%20stats%20Update%20Jan%202019_LOW%20RES_EXTERNAL.pdf
3. Hauner H (2017). Obesity and diabetes. In: Holt RG, Cockram CS, Flyvbjerg A, Goldstein BJ, eds. *Textbook of Diabetes*, 5[th]Edition. Chichester: John Wiley & Sons Ltd, 215-228.
4. Wass K, Owen K, Turner H, eds. Diabetes. *Oxford Handbook of Endocrinology and Diabetes*, 3[rd]Edition. Oxford: Oxford University Press; 2014. 683-821.
5. Prasad RB, Groop L. Genetics of type 2 diabetes – pitfalls and possibilities. *Genes* 2015; 6: 87-123.
6. International Diabetes Federation. IDF Diabetes Atlas. 9[th]Edition [Online]. Brussels, Belgium: 2019. www.diabetesatlas.org
7. Mayer-Davis EJ *et al*. ISPAD Clinical practice consensus guidelines 2018: definition, epidemiology, and classification of diabetes in children and adolescents. *Pediatric Diabetes* 2018; 19(Suppl 27): 7-19.
8. Diabetes UK. Do you know the 4 Ts of type 1 diabetes?. London: Diabetes UK. www.diabetes.org.uk/get_involved/campaigning/4-ts-campaign
9. World Health Organization (WHO). Definition and diagnosis of diabetes mellitus and intermediate hyperglycaemia. Geneva: World Health Organization; 2006. www.who.int/diabetes/publications/Definition%20and%20diagnosis%20of%20diabetes_new.pdf
10. World Health Organization (WHO). Use of glycated haemoglobin (HbA1c) in the diagnosis of diabetes mellitus. Geneva: World Health Organization; 2011. www.who.int/diabetes/publications/report-hba1c_2011.pdf
11. Blumer I *et al*. Diabetes and pregnancy: an Endocrine Society clinical practice guideline. *J Clin Endocrinol Metab* 2013; 98(11): 4227-49.
12. National Institute for Health and Care Excellence (NICE). Diabetes in pregnancy: management from preconception to the postnatal period. London: NICE; 2015 [updated Aug 2015]. www.nice.org.uk/guidance/ng3
13. National Institute for Health and Care Excellence (NICE). Type 1 diabetes in adults: diagnosis and management. London: NICE; 2015 [updated Jul 2016]. www.nice.org.uk/guidance/ng17

14. American Diabetes Association (ADA). Diagnosis and classification of diabetes mellitus. *Diabetes Care* 2014; 37(Suppl 1): S81-90.

15. Thomas NJ *et al*. Frequency and phenotype of type 1 diabetes in the first six decades of life: a cross-sectional, genetically stratified survival analysis from UK Biobank. *Lancet Diabetes Endocrinol* 2018; 6: 122-29.

16. Zeitler P *et al*. ISPAD clinical practice consensus guidelines 2018: type 2 diabetes mellitus in youth. *Pediatric Diabetes* 2018; 19(Suppl 27): 28-46.

17. Cui Y, Andersen DK. Pancreatogenic diabetes: special considerations for management. *Pancreatology* 2011; 11: 279-94.

18. Rickels MR *et al*. Detection, evaluation and treatment of diabetes mellitus in chronic pancreatitis: recommendations from PancreasFest 2012. *Pancreatology* 2013; 13(4): 336-42.

19. Bellamy L *et al*. Type 2 diabetes mellitus after gestational diabetes: a systematic review and meta-analysis. *Lancet* 2009; 373: 1773-9.

20. Hattersley AT *et al*. ISPAD clinical practice consensus guidelines 2018: the diagnosis and management of monogenic diabetes in children and adolescents. *Pediatric Diabetes* 2018; 19(Suppl 27): 47-63.

21. Juszczak A *et al*. When to consider a diagnosis of MODY at the presentation of diabetes: aetiology matters for correct management. *British Journal of General Practice* 2016; 66(647): e457-9.

22. National Institute for Health and Care Excellence (NICE). Type 2 diabetes in adults: management. London: NICE; 2015 [updated Aug 2019]. www.nice.org.uk/guidance/ng28

23. Morgan CL *et al*. Relationship between diabetes and mortality: a population study using record linkage. *Diabetes Care* 2000; 23(8): 1103-7.

24. Royal Pharmaceutical Society (RPS). Using pharmacists to help improve care for people with type 2 diabetes [Online]. London: Royal Pharmaceutical Society. www.rpharms.com/recognition/all-our-campaigns/policy-a-z/diabetes/diabetes-policy

25. Perkovic V *et al*. Canagliflozin and renal outcomes in type 2 diabetes and nephropathy. *N Engl J Med* 2019; 380(24): 2295-306.

26. McMurray JJ *et al*. Dapagliflozin in patients with heart failure and reduced ejection fraction. *N Engl J Med* 2019; 381: 1995-2008.

27. Healthcare Quality Improvement Partnership. National Diabetes Inpatient Audit England and Wales, 2017. NHS Digital; 2018. www.files.digital.nhs.uk/pdf/s/7/nadia-17-rep.pdf

28. Health and Social Care Information Centre. National Diabetes Audit, 2017-18 – Report 1: care processes and treatment targets. NHS Digital; 2019. www.files.digital.nhs.uk/88/F1E544/National%20Diabetes%20Audit%202017-18%20Full%20Report%201%2C%20Care%20Processes%20and%20Treatment%20Targets.pdf

29. Diabetes UK. 15 Healthcare Essentials. London: Diabetes UK; 2018. www.diabetes.org.uk/resources-s3/2018-07/15-Healtcare-essentials.pdf

30. American Diabetes Association (ADA). Standards of medical care in diabetes – 2020. *Diabetes Care* 2020; 43(Suppl 1): S1-212.

31. Diabetes Control and Complications Trial (DCCT)/Epidemiology of Diabetes Interventions and Complications Research Group. Retinopathy and nephropathy in patients with type 1 diabetes four years after a trial of intensive therapy. *N Engl J Med* 2000; 342: 381-9.

32. UK Prospective Diabetes Study Group (UKPDS). Effect of intensive blood-glucose control with metformin on complications in overweight patients with type 2 diabetes (UKPDS 34). *Lancet* 1998; 352(9131): 854-65.

33. JBS3 Board. Joint British Societies' consensus recommendations for the prevention of cardiovascular disease (JBS3). *Heart* 2014; 100 (Suppl 2): ii1-ii67.

34. Collins R *et al*. MRC/BHF Heart Protection Study of cholesterol-lowering with simvastatin in 5963 people with diabetes: a randomised placebo-controlled trial. *Lancet* 2003; 361(9374): 2005-16.

35. Colhoun HM *et al*. Primary prevention of cardiovascular disease with atorvastatin in type 2 diabetes in the Collaborative Atorvastatin Diabetes Study (CARDS): multicentre randomised placebo-controlled trial. *Lancet* 2004; 364(9435): 685-696.

36. Cholesterol Treatment Trialists' (CTT) Collaboration. Efficacy and safety of more intensive lowering of LDL cholesterol: a meta-analysis of data from 170,000 participants in 26 randomised trials. *Lancet* 2010; 376(9753): 1670-1681.

37. Kidney Disease: Improving Global Outcomes (KDIGO). KDIGO 2012 clinical practice guideline for the evaluation and management of chronic kidney disease. *Kidney International Supplements* 2013; 3(1).

38. Matthews DR *et al*. Glycaemic durability of an early combination therapy with vildagliptin and metformin versus sequential metformin monotherapy in newly diagnosed type 2 diabetes (VERIFY): a 5-year, multicentre, randomised, double-blind trial. *Lancet* 2019; 394(10208): 1519-1529.

39. Davies MJ *et al*. Management of hyperglycaemia in type 2 diabetes, 2018. A consensus report by the American Diabetes Association (ADA) and the European Association for the Study of Diabetes (EASD). *Diabetologia* 2018; 61: 2461-2498.

40. Buse JB *et al*. 2019 update to: Management of hyperglycemia in type 2 diabetes, 2018. A consensus report by the American Diabetes Association (ADA) and the European Association for the Study of Diabetes (EASD). *Diabetologia* 2020; 63(2): 221-8.

41. Garber AJ *et al*. Efficacy of metformin in type II diabetes: results of a double-blind, placebo-controlled, dose-response trial. *Am J Med* 1997; 103(6): 491-7.

42. DeFronzo R *et al.* Metformin-associated lactic acidosis: current perspectives on causes and risk. *Metabolism* 2016; 65: 20-9.

43. Pernicova I, Korbonits M. Metformin – mode of action and clinical implications for diabetes and cancer. *Nat Rev Endocrinol* 2014; 10(3): 143-56.

44. Salpeter SR *et al.* Risk of fatal and nonfatal lactic acidosis with metformin use in type 2 diabetes mellitus [Online]. *Cochrane Database of Systematic Reviews* 2010; Issue 1. www.cochranelibrary.com/cdsr/doi/10.1002/14651858.CD002967.pub3/full

45. Down S. How to advise on sick day rules. *Diabetes & Primary Care* 2018; 20(1): 15-6.

46. Joint British Diabetes Societies for Inpatient Care (JBDS-IP). Management of hyperglycaemia and steroid (glucocorticoid) therapy [Online]. Solihull: Association of British Clinical Diabetologists (ABCD); 2014. www.abcd.care/sites/abcd.care/files/resources/JBDS_IP_Steroids.pdf

47. Takeda UK Ltd. Actos tablets – Summary of Product Characteristics [Online]. The electronic Medicines Compendium (eMC); 2019. www.medicines.org.uk/emc/product/1287/smpc

48. National Institute for Health and Care Excellence (NICE). Non-alcoholic fatty liver disease (NAFLD): assessment and management [Online]. London: NICE; 2016. www.nice.org.uk/guidance/ng49

49. Chalasani N *et al.* The diagnosis and management of nonalcoholic fatty liver disease: practice guidance from the American Association for the Study of Liver Disease. *Hepatology* 2018; 67(1): 328-57.

50. Leoni S *et al.* Current guidelines for the management of non-alcoholic fatty liver disease: a systematic review with comparative analysis. *World Journal of Gastroenterology* 2018; 24(30): 3361-73.

51. Wilding J *et al.* SGLT2 inhibitors in type 2 diabetes management: key evidence and implications for clinical practice. *Diabetes Ther* 2018; 9: 1757-73.

52. Ali A *et al.* SGLT2 inhibitors: cardiovascular benefits beyond HbA1c – translating evidence into practice. *Diabetes Ther* 2019; 10: 1595-622.

53. Astrazeneca UK Limited. Forxiga 5 mg film-coated tablets – Summary of Product Characteristics [Online]. The electronic Medicines Compendium (eMC); 2019. www.medicines.org.uk/emc/product/2865/smpc

54. National Institute for Health and Care Excellence (NICE). Sotagliflozin with insulin for treating type 1 diabetes technology appraisal guidance TA622 [Online]. London: NICE; 2020. www.nice.org.uk/guidance/ta622

55. Scirica BM *et al.* Saxagliptin and cardiovascular outcomes in patients with type 2 diabetes mellitus. *N Engl J Med* 2013; 369(14): 1317-26.

56. Strain WD *et al.* Type 2 diabetes mellitus in older people: a brief statement of key principles of modern day management including the assessment of frailty. A national collaborative stakeholder initiative. *Diabet Med* 2018; 35: 838-45.

57. Aroda VR *et al.* PIONEER 1: randomized clinical trial of the efficacy and safety of oral semaglutide monotherapy in comparison with placebo in patients with type 2 diabetes. *Diabetes Care* 2019; 42(9): 1724-32.

58. Joint British Diabetes Societies for Inpatient Care (JBDS-IP). Discharge planning for adult inpatients with diabetes [Online]. Solihull: Association of British Clinical Diabetologists (ABCD); 2017. www.abcd.care/sites/abcd.care/files/resources/JBDS_Discharge_Planning_amendment_RCN_2017.pdf

59. Joint British Diabetes Societies for Inpatient Care (JBDS-IP). Admission avoidance and diabetes: guidance for clinical commissioning groups and clinical teams [Online]. Solihull: Association of British Clinical Diabetologists (ABCD); 2013. www.abcd.care/sites/abcd.care/files/resources/JBDS_IP_Admissions_Avoidance_Diabetes.pdf

60. Hippisley-Cox J *et al.* Development and validation of QRISK3 risk prediction algorithms to estimate future risk of cardiovascular disease: prospective cohort study. *BMJ* 2017; 357: j2099.

61. ClinRisk Ltd. QRISK®3-2018 Risk Calculator [Online]. ClinRisk; 2018. www.qrisk.org/three

62. Shenfield GM. Drug interactions with oral hypoglycaemic drugs. *Australian Prescriber* 2001; 24(4): 83-5.

63. Triplitt C. Drug interactions of medications commonly used in diabetes. *Diabetes Spectrum* 2006; 19(4): 202-11.

64. May M, Schindler C. Clinically and pharmacologically relevant interactions of antidiabetic drugs. *Ther Adv Endocrinol Metab* 2016; 7(2): 69-83.

65. Rehman A *et al.* Drug-induced glucose alterations part 2: drug-induced hyperglycemia. *Diabetes Spectrum* 2011; 24(4): 234-8.

66. Kirkman MS *et al.* Diabetes in older adults: a consensus report. *JAGS* 2012; 60(12): 2342-56.

67. National Institute for Health and Care Excellence (NICE). Cardiovascular disease: risk assessment and reduction, including lipid modification [Online]. London: NICE; 2014 [updated Sep 2016]. www.nice.org.uk/guidance/cg181

68. Aroda V *et al.* Long-term metformin use and vitamin B12 deficiency in the Diabetes Prevention Program Outcomes Study. *J Clin Endocrinol Metab* 2016; 101(4): 1754-61.

69. National Institute for Health and Care Excellence (NICE). Hypertension in pregnancy: diagnosis and management [Online]. London: NICE; 2019. www.nice.org.uk/guidance/ng133

70. National Institute for Health and Care Excellence (NICE). Diabetic foot problems: prevention and management [Online]. London: NICE; 2015 [updated Oct 2019]. www.nice.org.uk/guidance/ng19

Case studies

Case study 1

Beatrice, aged 66 years, attends her routine appointment at a pharmacist-led diabetes clinic within a GP practice. Her past medical history includes type 2 diabetes mellitus (T2DM), heart failure (HF), hypertension, and stage 2 chronic kidney disease (CKD).

Her drug history is as follows:

- Amlodipine tablets 10 mg in the morning
- Bisoprolol tablets 5 mg in the morning
- Linagliptin tablets 5 mg in the morning
- Metformin tablets 1 g twice daily
- Ramipril capsules 2.5 mg in the morning

Her most recent blood results and measurements are as follows:

Result	This appointment	12 months ago
HbA1c (mmol/mol)	75	69
HbA1c (%)	9	8.5
eGFR (mL/min/1.73 m^2)	70	74
Albumin:creatinine ratio (mg/mmol)	7	6
Total cholesterol (mmol/L)	5.5	5.4
LDL cholesterol (mmol/L)	3.5	3.2
Blood pressure (mmHg)	148/92	144/90
Weight (kg)	89	85
Body mass index (kg/m^2)	31	30

She lives independently with her husband in their own house and has two adult children who do not live with her. Beatrice has never smoked, but drinks an occasional glass of wine in the evening or at weekends. She is otherwise fit and healthy, and reports that she had been trying to lose weight recently.

As the GP pharmacist within the practice, you decide Beatrice would benefit from intensifying her current therapy for diabetes.

Points to consider

- What general factors do you need to consider before initiating new treatment?
- Assess the possible treatment options for Beatrice.
  - Consider how you would arrive at a choice, how to introduce the new treatment, and what drug-specific considerations you would have to think of.
- What necessary monitoring and follow-up would be needed moving forward?
  - How would you assess benefit from treatment?
- What non-pharmacological advice would you give Beatrice as part of a consultation (as her GP pharmacist or her community pharmacist)?

The first step in a clinical assessment of a patient with diabetes is agreeing on an appropriate HbA1c target.

The American Diabetes Association (ADA) recommends a target of ≤53 mmol/mol (7%), while the National Institute for Health and Care Excellence (NICE) guidelines on T2DM recommend 53 mmol/mol (7%) for patients on drugs that may cause hypoglycaemia, and 48 mmol/mol (6.5%) for patients not on such drugs.

Higher glycaemic targets may be acceptable in frail patients or those with a lower life expectancy. Patients with complex comorbidities or care needs, especially those who may not show awareness or are unable to communicate symptoms of hypoglycaemia, may also require higher targets for safety. In all cases, an individualised target needs to be decided upon in agreement with the patient, and a pragmatic approach taken with those who are non-adherent or disengaged with the management of their condition.

Assessing the social situation and lifestyle will similarly help decide which glucose-lowering drugs are less appropriate. A person who lacks capacity to self-administer injectable medicines will require either a relative living with them to be trained, a regular visit from a district nurse for drug administration (if this can be arranged), or avoidance of that drug altogether.

Intensive insulin regimen may not be suitable for a patient who is disengaged with their treatment and is not likely to monitor their blood glucose. Patients with chronic alcoholism or who are known to binge drink may not be good candidates for starting SGLT2i due to their increased risk of dehydration and developing diabetic ketoacidosis (DKA).

Despite her comorbidities, Beatrice lives independently and has a reasonable life expectancy, thus it is appropriate to aim for a tight target of 53 mmol/mol or lower.

The joint guidelines published by the ADA and European Association for the Study of Diabetes (EASD) in 2018 (and the accompanying 2019 update) provide the most up-to-date guidelines relevant to current practice. In making your decisions, follow the flowchart within the guidelines.

Metformin remains the first-line option for all patients with T2DM, but Beatrice is already established on metformin. While the maximum licensed dose is 3 g/day, the clinical benefit from doses above 2 g is minimal, and gastrointestinal adverse effects become more prominent with higher doses. Additionally, a higher dose may pose a higher risk of lactic acidosis in light of Beatrice's CKD and heart failure. Therefore, it is reasonable to continue at 2 g/day currently.

The choice of additional drugs depends on the patient's comorbidities; namely, whether they have established atherosclerotic cardiovascular disease (ASCVD) or CKD. If they do, SGLT2i and GLP-1RA would provide significantly more benefit over any other class at this stage, and there must be compelling reasons not to choose either of these classes at this point. Both classes also result in considerable weight loss, which is a desirable feature for many patients.

Beatrice has no history of ASCVD, but has established HF and stage G2A2 CKD. Her eGFR is above 60 mL/min/1.73 m^2, but her albumin:creatinine ratio (ACR) is 7 mg/mmol (or 70 mg/g). Following the guidelines, this would make SGLT2i the class of choice for her. Canagliflozin and empagliflozin are the two drugs with evidence of benefit in HF and CKD. The second option would be a GLP-1RA, since it has evidence of cardiovascular disease (CVD) benefit (although no direct evidence of benefit in HF). The evidence is strongest for liraglutide and semaglutide, with the latter offering a convenient once-weekly administration that would aid adherence.

Points to consider

- What are the other treatment options?
- Why are some of them not appropriate in these circumstances?

Beatrice is initiated on canagliflozin 100 mg.

Points to consider

- What information and advice would you give her?

You counsel Beatrice on its small risk of causing urinary tract infections (UTIs), and on recognising signs of DKA. You also explain the Sick Day Rules, including stopping metformin and canagliflozin when she experiences vomiting, diarrhoea, or a fever, and resuming them only when she recovers and is eating and drinking normally for at least 48 hours.

Linagliptin is stopped as it will not provide significant HbA1c reduction over canagliflozin, and this will also help reduce Beatrice's tablet burden.

Points to consider

- What monitoring and follow-up is required?
- Is it appropriate to carry out a cardiovascular risk assessment?
  - Given the information you have already have, use the QRISK3 assessment tool to calculate Beatrice's 10-year risk.
  - What are the implications, if any, on Beatrice's treatment?

In addition to regular routine monitoring every 3-6 months, in Beatrice's case, canagliflozin should be reviewed after 3 months and increased to 300 mg daily if tolerated, and because she is taking metformin, which may reduce vitamin B12 absorption, vitamin B12 levels should also be checked annually – if low, replacement with hydroxocobalamin may be necessary.

Consideration should be given to increasing the dose of ramipril to 5 mg daily. This would provide benefit for her blood pressure and declining renal function, especially given her microalbuminuria.

Points to consider

- What non-pharmacological advice can you give Beatrice?
- What sources of information would be useful?

You direct Beatrice to the Diabetes UK 10 tips for healthy eating with diabetes and advise her that canagliflozin can only produce weight loss if used in conjunction with lifestyle changes in diet and physical activity.

You also advise her to reduce her salt intake to a maximum of one teaspoonful (6 g) per day, provide advice about drinking alcohol and signpost her to a number of additional online resources on the Diabetes UK website.

Case study 2

Richard, aged 85 years, was admitted to hospital with confusion and an acute kidney injury (AKI) secondary to dehydration. He had been increasingly less independent during the period leading to his admission, and had been eating and drinking minimally for the past 48 hours. His past medical history includes type 2 diabetes mellitus (T2DM) that was diagnosed 20 years ago, myocardial infarction (MI), chronic kidney disease (CKD), and atrial fibrillation (AF). He also has diabetic retinopathy, and his vision has deteriorated in recent years.

His drug history and hospital prescription chart are as follows:

Drug	Pre-admission	Hospital chart
Aspirin dispersible tablets	75 mg in the morning	75 mg in the morning
Atorvastatin tablets	80 mg at night	Withheld
Bisoprolol tablets	2.5 mg in the morning	2.5 mg in the morning
Canagliflozin tablets	300 mg in the morning	300 mg in the morning
Metformin tablets	1 g twice daily	1 g twice daily
Novomix 30 prefilled pen	32 units with breakfast and evening meal	32 units with breakfast and evening meal
Ramipril capsules	5 mg in the morning	Withheld
Rivaroxaban tablets	15 mg in the morning	15 mg in the morning

His blood results on this admission (Day 1, 16:00) are as follows:

Test	Result	Test	Result
Sodium (mmol/L)	142	eGFR (mL/min/1.73 m²)	22
Potassium (mmol/L)	3.7	Glucose, random (mmol/L)	26
Urea (mmol/L)	9	HbA1c (mmol/mol)	71
Creatinine (micromole/L)	223	HbA1c (%)	8.5

He weighs 62 kg, and his baseline creatinine from five months previously was 99 micromoles/L (eGFR is 42 mL/min/1.73 m²). He lives alone at his own house.

It was also found that Richard had been confused and forgetful with using his insulin at home, and had omitted it in the days prior to admission. His regular insulin was restarted, and his glucose profile on day 2 was as follows:

Time (Day 2)	Glucose (mmol/L)
07:00	5.4
12:00	3.9
15:00	3.6
18:00	7.8

As the ward pharmacist, you are asked to review Richard's medications on day 2 of admission.

Points to consider

- What immediate actions would you need to take regarding his medications?
- What further information would you need to collect to make these decisions?

The most acute problems for Richard are his AKI and hypoglycaemia.

Metformin is renally cleared, and an AKI will lead to drug accumulation. While the resultant effect on blood glucose is negligible, the risk of lactic acidosis increases. Lactic acidosis with metformin is extremely rare but even with the low risk of complications, the benefits of continuing metformin during an AKI are minimal.

Canagliflozin is partly cleared renally. Its accumulation in this case is not likely to contribute to hypoglycaemia during an AKI, but nor will it have any glycaemic benefits. However, there is a risk of euglycaemic DKA with dehydration.

Richard has been omitting his insulin at home – this would have also contributed to his dehydrated state. Restarting his regular insulin at the same pre-admission dose in this case was not appropriate. Kidneys play a role in insulin degradation, and renal impairment often results in accumulation of insulin. Stopping insulin completely is rarely warranted, but dose reduction will often help optimise treatment during this period, with the main objective of avoiding hypoglycaemia.

Richard is usually on Novomix 30, a mixed insulin with 30% rapid acting component and 70% intermediate acting component – the decision on the appropriate dose will also depend on how much he is eating currently compared to his usual meals at home. Given his AKI, dehydration and hypoglycaemia, a dose reduction by 20-50% may be warranted, then up-titrating the dose as he starts to improve.

Alternatively, Novomix 30 can be temporarily switched to an intermediate-acting insulin (e.g. Insulatard) while he is not eating or drinking as much. Insulatard can be given twice daily at an equivalent dose to the intermediate-acting component (which makes up 70% of Novomix 30). Insulatard can also be cautiously introduced at 60% of total dose during this acute situation until a better trend in Richard's glucose is available.

You decide to withhold metformin and canagliflozin, stop Novomix 30 and start Insulatard 18 units twice a day in the morning and evening (avoiding nighttime administration).

Richard's AKI slowly resolved, with results trending back towards his baseline:

Test	Result (Day 5)	Result (Day 6)	Result (Day 7)
Sodium (mmol/L)	136	136	134
Potassium (mmol/L)	4.1	3.8	4.0
Urea (mmol/L)	7	6	6
Creatinine (micromoles/L)	160	144	141
eGFR (mL/min/1.73 m^2)	33	38	39

Richard is no longer able to live independently and a package of care is arranged. As the ward pharmacist (or specialist diabetes pharmacist) you are asked to review and optimise his diabetes medications in preparation for discharge.

Points to consider

- What treatment targets would you set for Richard given his current state?
- Assess the treatment options for Richard, and consider a management plan for his diabetes.
- What additional considerations and monitoring need to be taken into account following discharge?

The recommended HbA1c targets for most adults do not apply in the frail elderly population – higher targets are often necessary as the benefits of tight glycaemic control are overshadowed by clinical risks.

A decision on an appropriate target is guided by the degree of frailty, life expectancy, number of comorbidities and extent of microvascular and macrovascular complications. Frailty may be one of the more difficult factors to quantify for the non-specialist, and sometimes a discussion with a geriatric specialist can help assess this.

Consensus recommendations on suitable targets are:

HbA1c targets (adapted from Strain et al, 2018)

Degree of frailty	HbA1c target
Fit older adult	58 mmol/mol (7.5%)
Moderate-severe frailty	64 mmol/mol (8.0%)
Very severe frailty	70 mmol/mol (8.5%)

HbA1c targets (adapted from Kirkman et al, 2012)

Extent of complication and life expectancy	HbA1c target
• No or very mild microvascular complications • Life expectancy >10-15 years	<53 mmol/mol (7.0%)
• Complex comorbidities • Diabetes duration >10 years and requiring insulin	<64 mmol/mol (8.0%)
• Advanced microvascular complications • Major comorbidities • Life expectancy <5 years	64-75 mmol/mol (8.0-9.0%)

Following a discussion with the geriatrician, Richard was assessed to be severely frail. He has had a diagnosis of T2DM for over 20 years, and is showing evidence of both microvascular (retinopathy, CKD) and macrovascular (MI) complications. A reasonable HbA1c target in his case would be 64-70 mmol/mol (8.0-8.5%).

It appears that his current HbA1c already falls within this target. However, given his recent admission with AKI and reduced level of independence, a review of his treatment prior to discharge is needed, removing drugs with higher risk of complications with his comorbidities, and adding safer drugs if the treatment target is not yet reached.

Points to consider

- What are the most suitable treatment options for Richard?
- Which drugs are not suitable and why?

As a general rule, metformin, DPP-4i, and long-acting insulins provide three safe options for the very frail population, although this should not replace individualised assessment.

- Metformin – as his eGFR is trending towards his baseline value and is now 39 mL/min/1.73 m^2, the dose should be reduced to 500 mg twice daily.
- DPP-4i – a rule of thumb is that DPP-4i would reduce HbA1c by 11 mmol/mol (1%), therefore if a higher reduction is needed, additional options should be added. Richard would benefit from a DPP-4i suitable for his degree of renal impairment, as per the manufacturer's recommendations. Linagliptin is minimally excreted in urine, so is an optimal choice for patients with variable or borderline creatinine levels. Saxagliptin is the only DPP-4i associated with increased risk of hospital admissions due to heart failure, and should be especially avoided in the elderly and frail.
- Insulin remains a useful option, although with careful consideration for choice of regimen. The aim should be to reduce the risk of hypoglycaemia (i.e. avoiding rapid-acting insulins if possible). Long-acting insulin is an optimal choice when eGFR is above 30 mL/min/1.73 m^2, while intermediate-acting (isophane/NPH) insulin may be useful in severe renal impairment as its shorter duration of action reduces the risk of its accumulation, and minimises the risk of nocturnal hypoglycaemia.

The treatment plan for Richard is to stop canagliflozin due to risk of dehydration and DKA, restart metformin at a lower dose of 500 mg twice daily with meals, stop Novomix 30, and start insulin glargine (e.g. Lantus) once a day in the morning.

Points to consider

- What other options are available for Richard?
- What monitoring is required?

It is clear that Richard's independence has critically diminished following this admission. His memory and his deteriorating vision make timely insulin self-administration impractical and potentially unsafe. Some options to consider are presented here:

1. Stop insulin completely – this may be the simplest option at the expense of achieving the desired glycaemic control. If this option is chosen, it must be made at the point of diabetes assessment rather than retrospectively at the point of discharge. As a general rule, patients with T2DM on ≥20 units of insulin daily will still require some form of insulin on discharge, and discontinuation in this case might lead to readmission with dehydration or complications such as hyperosmolar hyperglycaemic state (HHS). For patients with T1DM, the regimen can be greatly simplified, but should never be discontinued completely, regardless of their insulin requirement.

2. Administration by a relative or next of kin – a patient's partner or next of kin, if they live with them or are willing to visit to administer insulin, may be considered. This would depend on the next of kin's motivation and own ability to do this regularly, and they would require proper training prior to discharge.

3. Administration by a district nurse – although carers can prompt and help the patient take oral medicines, they are not trained to assist with injectable drugs. A trained community nurse can help with this through daily visits, although this needs prior arrangement, and in most cases it is not feasible for visits more frequent than once daily. Whenever possible, the regimen should be accommodated to fit this visit. For example, a basal-bolus regimen can be simplified (if appropriate) to once-daily rapid-acting insulin and once-daily long-acting insulin, both administered in the morning.

4. Nursing home or other care setting – if unavoidable, and the patient's medication regimen is deemed too complex for once-daily nursing support, a higher care setting may need to be arranged where the patient is offered more frequent nursing support.

As Richard is established on a long-acting insulin, a pre-breakfast glucose level (measured by the district nurse, for example) is sufficient to allow dose adjustment. If the patient has some capacity to self-monitor blood glucose, consider a suitable glucose meter; for patients with visual impairment, meters with large display or 'talking meters' are valuable.

CHAPTER 10

Epilepsy

Ann Dougan

Overview

Epilepsy is defined by the International League Against Epilepsy (ILAE)[1] as a disorder of the brain characterised by any of the following conditions:

- At least two unprovoked (or reflex) seizures occurring more than 24 hours apart
- One unprovoked (or reflex) seizure and a probability of further seizures similar to the general recurrence risk (at least 60%) after two unprovoked seizures, occurring over the next 10 years
- Diagnosis of an epilepsy syndrome[1]

An epileptic seizure is defined as a transient occurrence of signs and/or symptoms due to abnormal excessive or synchronous neuronal activity in the brain.[1]

Seizures are classified into either:

- Generalised seizures – characterised by beginning synchronously in bilaterally distributed networks in both hemispheres and include tonic-clonic, absence, myoclonic, clonic, atonic and tonic seizures.
- Focal seizures – these originate within networks limited to one hemisphere and may, or may not, propagate to the contralateral hemisphere.[2] These vary depending on the location of origin and may manifest as motor, sensory, psychic or autonomic.

Overall epilepsy affects 1% of the population,[3] and 1 in 4 patients with learning disabilities.[4] Certain types of epilepsy are genetic in origin and often associated with other symptoms, forming syndromes, which frequently include learning disabilities.

The majority of epilepsies are idiopathic, although in time advances in medical science may reveal a genetic cause or genetic tendency for many. Other causes include structural lesions, such as hippocampal sclerosis, brain tumour, traumatic brain injury, stroke or focal cortical dysplasias. Some individuals have a predisposition for seizures which can be triggered by, for example, photic, auditory or tactile stimuli, termed reflex epilepsy.[1] Hormonal fluctuations (e.g. a rise in oestrogen levels) can affect the seizure threshold, such that some women experience an increase in seizure frequency at the time of their menstrual period, known as catamenial epilepsy.

Two-thirds of people with epilepsy can be successfully treated, usually with one or two drugs and rarely require intervention by a pharmacist. The remaining third are classified as refractory, or drug-resistant, epilepsy, defined as 'failure to achieve sustained seizure freedom after adequate trials of two tolerated and appropriately chosen and used antiepileptic drugs (AEDs)'.[1,5,6] The ILAE defines seizure freedom as three times the longest previous seizure free interval, or one year, whichever is the greater.[1] Drug resistance is more common in those with focal than with generalised epilepsy.[7]

For people who have been seizure free for 10 years, the last five of which without AEDs, or have passed the age of an age-dependent epilepsy syndrome, epilepsy is deemed to have resolved.[1]

In the long term, epilepsy affects memory and cognitive function, which is exacerbated by prolonged use of AEDs. Life expectancy may be reduced as a direct consequence of epilepsy, such as status epilepticus, accidents with or without head injury, drowning, bronchopneumonia or Sudden Unexpected Death in Epilepsy (SUDEP). Indirect causes of mortality include suicide and cardiovascular disease.

Diagnosis

The diagnosis of epilepsy is made on clinical grounds and should be made by a specialist.[8,9] The two most common investigations are routine electroencephalogram (EEG) and brain magnetic resonance imaging (MRI). These test results may be normal, but this does not exclude a diagnosis of epilepsy. In some cases, abnormalities may be seen in the EEG which can help to distinguish between the type of epilepsy (generalised or focal) and localise the seizure onset.

Brain MRI may show structural lesions which can be indicative of a cause.[8,10] Video-telemetry can be useful to determine seizure semiology, or exclude other causes, and forms part of the work-up for surgery to evaluate the probability of success.[10] Other investigations may serve to exclude differential diagnoses such as hypoglycaemia, syncope or migraine.

Treatment

In general, a broad-spectrum agent (e.g. valproate, carbamazepine, lamotrigine or levetiracetam) forms the foundation of epilepsy therapy, with the choice of medication depending on the seizure type or clinical syndrome.[8]

Sodium valproate is the most effective agent for generalised seizures and epilepsy syndromes involving generalised seizures (tonic-clonic, myoclonic, absence), and is used first line in the absence of contraindications, such as women of childbearing potential.

Carbamazepine or lamotrigine are the drugs of choice for focal seizures.[8] Lamotrigine is as effective as carbamazepine for focal seizures but may be better tolerated, have fewer adverse effects and a lower potential for drug interactions. In cases where carbamazepine is proving effective but adverse effects are intolerable, consideration may be given to substitution by one of its derivatives, oxcarbazepine or eslicarbazepine.

Levetiracetam has few adverse effects and low interaction potential and is widely used for many types of epilepsy.

For absence seizures, valproate and/or ethosuximide are the drugs of choice[8] – this is the main indication for ethosuximide.

Adjunctive therapy is used when seizure freedom is not achieved with monotherapy. Any of the aforementioned drugs can be added – lacosamide or zonisamide are commonly used. Other options include oxcarbazepine, eslicarbazepine, perampanel, topiramate, gabapentin, pregabalin or tiagabine.

Perampanel and topiramate are licensed for adjunctive therapy only and must be used in conjunction with one of the foundation drugs. These two drugs are poorly tolerated so tend to be reserved for refractory epilepsy.

Gabapentin and pregabalin can be useful as adjunctive therapy but are rarely used as monotherapy. They can cause significant sedation and weight gain which limits their use.

Benzodiazepines are effective, but their continued use is limited initially by sedation, and later by tolerance. A 3-5 day course of clobazam can be effective in limiting cluster seizures. Buccal midazolam is indicated to terminate prolonged seizures in children. It is used off-license in adults.

For some epilepsy syndromes, specific drugs or combination of drugs demonstrate particular efficacy. Rufinamide is licensed as adjunctive therapy for Lennox-Gastaut syndrome. Vigabatrin, although licensed as adjunctive therapy, is primarily used to treat West syndrome, for which the benefits are considered to outweigh the risk of visual field defects. The combination of valproate, stiripentol and clobazam has a synergistic effect in Dravet syndrome. In November 2018, cannabidiol was reclassified into schedule 2 of the controlled drugs regulations, and subsequently into schedule 5, and may now be employed in the treatment of Dravet syndrome or Lennox-Gastaut syndrome.

By contrast, drugs which act by prolonging the refractory period of the sodium channel, such as lamotrigine, may worsen myoclonic seizures and should be avoided in Dravet syndrome, epilepsy with continuous spike-waves during sleep and atypical benign focal epilepsy. In these conditions, valproate is the drug of choice.[8]

Older drugs, such as phenytoin and phenobarbital, with narrow therapeutic windows, many interactions and long-term adverse effects are rarely used routinely, but are usually reserved for the treatment of status epilepticus. However, for long-established patients well controlled on one of these agents, no attempt should be made to switch them without a compelling reason.

See *Table 10.1* for a summary of commonly used drugs and indications.

Table 10.1: *Commonly used drugs*

Drug	Starting dose	Maximum daily dose	Type of epilepsy
Acetazolamide	250 mg twice daily	1 g in two divided doses	Catamenial epilepsy
Brivaracetam	25 mg once daily	200 mg in two divided doses	Focal ± to bilateral Adjunctive therapy
Carbamazepine MR	200 mg twice daily	2 g in two divided doses	Generalised, focal
Clobazam	10 mg once daily	60 mg in two or three divided doses	Cluster seizures Adjunctive therapy
Clonazepam	0.5 mg at night	8 mg in one to four divided doses	All forms of epilepsy Adjunctive therapy
Eslicarbazepine	400 mg at night	1.6 g at night	Focal ± to bilateral
Ethosuxamide	250 mg twice daily	2 g in two divided doses	Absence seizures, myoclonic
Gabapentin	300 mg once daily	3.6 g in three divided doses	Focal ± to bilateral
Lacosamide	50 mg twice daily	400 mg in two divided doses	Focal ± to bilateral Adjunctive therapy
Lamotrigine	25 mg once daily	500 mg in two divided doses	Monotherapy for focal, LGS Adjunctive therapy for generalised
Levetiracetam	250 mg twice daily	3 g in two divided doses	Generalised, focal
Oxcarbazepine	300 mg twice daily	2.4 g in two divided doses	Generalised, focal
Perampanel	2 mg at night	12 mg (16 mg off-licence) at night	Focal ± to bilateral Adjunctive therapy
Phenobarbital	15 mg at night	180 mg at night	All forms except absence seizures
Phenytoin	3-4 mg/kg in one to three doses	Depends on levels	Generalised, focal Status epilepticus
Pregabalin	25 mg twice daily	600 mg in two divided doses	Adjunctive therapy
Primidone	125 mg at night	1.5 g at night	All forms except absence seizures
Rufinamide	200 mg twice daily	1.8-3.2 g in two divided doses	Lennox-Gastaut
Sodium valproate MR	300 mg twice daily	2.5 g in two divided doses	All forms of epilepsy
Stiripentol	20 mg/kg/day	3 g in two or three divided doses	Dravet syndrome
Tiagabine	5 mg once daily	45 mg in two or three divided doses	Focal ± to bilateral Adjunctive therapy
Topiramate	25 mg once daily	500 mg in two divided doses	Generalised, focal
Vigabatrin	1 g in one or two doses	3 g in one or two divided doses	West syndrome (infantile spasms)
Zonisamide	50 mg at night	500 mg in one or two divided doses	Focal ± to bilateral

Other specialist options for treatment include vagus nerve stimulation (VNS), ketogenic diet or surgery. For people with a unilateral structural lesion, such as hippocampal sclerosis, surgery offers a much greater chance of seizure freedom than drug therapy, up to 90% for non-dominant temporal lobe cavernoma.[10] VNS is used as an adjunct to medication. By sensing the onset of a seizure it electrically stimulates the vagus nerve to terminate it, producing a 50% reduction in seizure frequency in over 60% of recipients.[11]

Pharmacy input

Pharmacists play an important role in the management of epilepsy by supporting patients through medication changes and assisting to optimise their medication. They can offer advice and assistance to aid compliance, or to follow titration plans. Thorough knowledge of pharmacokinetics enables pharmacists to predict the likelihood of interactions when data is lacking.

In addition, pharmacists can help reduce the risk of rebound seizures by maintaining continuity of brand and formulation and can advise on prescription charge exemptions. Pharmacists accessibility, either in a community pharmacy or by the provision of contact details in the clinic, enables patients to obtain advice between appointments, while hospital pharmacists may provide a useful gateway to consultants, nurses, secretaries and clinic staff.

Pharmacy review

People with well-controlled epilepsy should be reviewed annually, ideally by a neurologist.[8]

In the event of deterioration in seizure-control, community pharmacists should:

- enquire about general health and sleep patterns and recent changes in the patient's home or work life that may be affecting seizure control – various factors may produce deterioration in seizure control, including:
  - illness
  - anxiety
  - stress
  - lack of sleep
  - other causes – a good rapport with the patient and sensitive questioning may elicit the influence of other factors that lower the seizure threshold, such as alcohol, cocaine or amphetamines.
- ask about compliance and suggest means of reducing the number of missed doses.
- ask about any concurrent medication, including herbal products, and check for interactions.
  - St. John's wort reduces the plasma concentration of many AEDs and should be avoided.

Pharmacists working in GP surgeries can also order appropriate blood tests if electrolyte or metabolic disturbances such as hyponatraemia, hypomagnesaemia or hypoglycaemia are suspected – these can adversely influence seizure control.

People with drug-resistant epilepsy may be referred to a specialist pharmacist clinic by their consultant neurologist to help optimise their antiepileptic medication to improve seizure control. It is helpful if the patient is accompanied by a relative or carer who can give an account of the seizures, as patients themselves are generally unable to recall these events.

Specialist pharmacists should:

- ask about seizure pattern, including frequency, severity, duration, and recovery time – patients, or their carers, are encouraged to keep a seizure diary and to bring it to each consultation to facilitate evaluation of drug changes. Seizure diaries are available free to patients from the Epilepsy Society or as mobile phone apps.

- take an accurate drug history, including details about the formulation, dosage and brand names.

So-called AEDs are really anti-seizure drugs because they do not reverse the condition, but reduce the seizure burden and ideally confer seizure freedom.

Monotherapy is preferable to combination therapy to limit side effects, toxicity and interactions, and facilitate compliance. Combination therapy is reserved for failure of two successive trials using single drugs to achieve seizure freedom.[8,9]

Management

Brand continuity

Whenever possible, patients should be maintained on the same brand of their medication to avoid confusion and dosing errors. However, not at the expense of missed doses.

The brand is particularly important for drugs with a narrow therapeutic index or variability in solubility or absorption, such as carbamazepine, phenytoin, phenobarbital and primidone, for which differences in bioavailability between manufacturers' products may cause adverse effects or loss of seizure control.[12]

These factors are less important for:

- clobazam and clonazepam
- eslicarbazepine
- lamotrigine
- oxcarbazepine
- perampanel
- rufinamide
- topiramate
- valproate
- zonisamide.

Pharmacists should base the need for a consistent brand on clinical judgement and consultation with the patient and/or carer. For drugs with a wide therapeutic index, almost complete absorption and high solubility across a range of pH, any brand may be prescribed. Drugs in this category include:

- ethosuximide
- gabapentin and pregabalin
- lacosamide
- levetiracetam and brivaracetam
- tiagabine and vigabatrin.

However, consideration should be given to negative perceptions of patients/carers towards certain products. A different colour or shape of a tablet may induce anxiety in some people, for instance, those with learning difficulties, which is in itself a trigger factor for seizures. If a different product has to be supplied patients should be informed. Any breakthrough seizures suspected of occurring as a result of a brand change should be reported to the MHRA using the Yellow Card Scheme.

Care should also be taken when switching between formulations that are not bioequivalent. For instance, when switching from phenytoin capsules to suspension the dose must be reduced by 10%.

Adverse effects

Certain adverse effects, such as somnolence, dizziness and visual disturbances, are common to all AEDs, with headache and nausea being less common. They are mainly dose-related, becoming more troublesome at higher doses, and usually wearing off over a few days, only to return at the next dose increase.

These effects can be minimised by starting low and gradually increasing the dose to an optimal level over weeks or months. Slow-release formulations are used preferentially to minimise peaks and troughs in concentration, thus providing more consistent seizure-control and minimising adverse effects. Perampanel has a long half-life and should be taken within 15 minutes of going to bed to minimise such adverse effects.

Persistent adverse effects can often be managed by a slower titration; firstly by dropping back one step to the previously tolerated dose and then increasing either more slowly or by smaller increments. However, in some cases, even these approaches may not be successful and the patient is maintained on the highest tolerated dose, or the drug gradually withdrawn and substituted with another.

Any AED can cause a rash, but particular attention should be paid to rashes developing within 3 months of the initiation of phenytoin, lamotrigine or rufinamide. These drugs can cause serious hypersensitivity reactions, involving widespread rash, fever, eosinophilia, facial oedema, lymphadenopathy and possibly splenomegaly. The offending drug should be stopped immediately, and the patient referred to A&E.

The aromatic AEDs (carbamazepine, oxcarbazepine and eslicarbazepine) have a genetic association with severe cutaneous reactions such as toxic epidermal necrolysis. It is recommended that individuals at risk, most commonly people of Far Eastern origin, are tested for HLA-B*1502 polymorphism before commencing one of these agents.

Individual drugs may be associated with specific adverse effects (see *Table 10.2*):

- Topiramate – a common adverse effect is paraesthesia of fingers and toes (this also occurs more rarely with phenytoin, carbamazepine, gabapentin or pregabalin). Topiramate is also associated with weight loss.
- Valproate may cause tremor, alopecia, weight gain, obesity, and metabolic syndrome, all of which are reversible on discontinuation. Thrombocytopenia is a rarer adverse effect.
- Vigabatrin can cause visual field defects, and patients should undergo regular eye examinations. In the event of any visual disturbance, this drug should be weaned off.
- Perampanel, levetiracetam and probably brivaracetam can affect mood and behaviour – this usually takes the form of irritability, anxiety, agitation or aggression. Other people exhibit a labile mood or emotions, euphoria, hallucinations, mania, and rarely suicidal ideation. These effects may or may not be dose-related but they do not resolve with time.
  - The patient should be weaned off the offending drug or the dose reduced to an acceptable level. Those with a tendency for such behaviours are at higher risk and these medications are preferably avoided in them when alternatives are available.

Please consult the Summary of Product Characteristics for a full list of adverse effects: www.medicines.org.uk/emc

In the long term, AED therapy leads to cognitive impairment and memory problems which can impair concentration and the ability to study. This exacerbates that already caused by the natural progression of epilepsy itself.

Evidence suggests that long-term use of enzyme inducers (phenytoin, phenobarbital, carbamazepine, oxcarbazepine or topiramate) can predispose patients to osteoporosis by increasing vitamin D clearance, leading to secondary hyperparathyroidism, increased bone turnover and reduced bone density. The explanation for valproate is less clear. Consideration should be given to calcium and vitamin D supplementation for those at high risk, such as those with long-term immobility, inadequate sun exposure or low vitamin D levels.

Box 10.1: Practice point: adverse effects

- Rashes that develop after initiation of lamotrigine, phenytoin or rufinamide should be taken seriously.
- Patients taking carbamazepine, oxcarbazepine or eslicarbazepine should be monitored for hyponatraemia.
- Somnolence, dizziness and visual disturbances are common to all AEDs and are mainly dose-related – they usually wear off over a few days, but may return at the next dose increase.

Table 10.2: *Adverse effects*

Drug	Common ADRs	Serious ADRs
All AEDs	Drowsiness, dizziness, visual disturbances	Cognitive impairment, memory loss
Brivaracetam, levetiracetam	Diarrhoea, headache	Behavioural changes
Carbamazepine, eslicarbazepine, oxcarbazepine	Hyponatraemia	Hypersensitivity syndromes
Clobazam, clonazepam	Sedation, tolerance	
Ethosuximide	Nausea, vomiting, hiccups	Haematological toxicity
Gabapentin, pregabalin	Weight gain	
Lacosamide	Dry mouth, flatulence	Prolonged PR interval
Lamotrigine	Diarrhoea, fatigue, nausea	Hypersensitivity syndromes
Perampanel	Irritability, agitation	Aggression, psychoses
Phenobarbital		Hypersensitivity syndromes
Phenytoin	Nystagmus, ataxia, dysarthria	Hypersensitivity syndromes
Rufinamide	Nausea, diarrhoea	Hypersensitivity syndromes
Sodium valproate	Tremor, weight gain, alopecia	
Stiripentol	Nausea, vomiting, weight loss	Aggression, irritability
Tiagabine	Tremor, nausea, diarrhoea	Emotional lability
Topiramate	Paraesthesia, weight loss	
Vigabatrin	Abdominal pain	Visual field defects
Zonisamide	Weight loss	Irritability

Drug-resistant epilepsy

For patients with drug-resistant epilepsy, successive drug trials are carried out to achieve optimisation. The consultant usually specifies a drug, or a series of drugs, based on the patient's previous drug history. Drug changes are made one at a time to facilitate the accurate evaluation of each for beneficial and/or adverse effects.

Medication changes can be achieved by a switch from one drug to another using an overlap method (see *Table 10.3*), whereby the dosage of one drug is gradually reduced at the same time as the other is increased, or by an addition to the regimen, which might be followed at a later date by gradual withdrawal of a drug thought to be making little contribution to seizure control. Naturally, a crossover switch involves two drugs but the drug being withdrawn has already been evaluated as ineffective or intolerable.

If at some point during a switch seizure control improves, the patient should stay on the combined dosage that has been reached, i.e. low dosage of both drugs. The switch can be resumed at a future date if the improvement is not maintained.

It is important that patients understand and can follow the titration procedure, especially when it involves a gradual switch from one drug to another. Clear dosage instructions and a written titration plan are helpful in view of memory and cognitive deficits. Patients should be instructed to ignore dosage instructions in the PIL but to follow the personalised dosing regimen they have been given by their specialist and continue in this way until either the seizures stop, or the maximum tolerated dose is reached, or the target dose reached, whichever happens first. In the event of adverse effects becoming intolerable, or prolonged, patients are instructed to reduce the dose to the previous step in the plan.

Table 10.3: *Plan for gradual decrease in perampanel dosage and gradual increase in brivaracetam dosage*

		Morning	Night
Current dose	Perampanel		10 mg
	Brivaracetam		
Weeks 1 and 2	Perampanel		8 mg
	Brivaracetam		25 mg
Weeks 3 and 4	Perampanel		8 mg
	Brivaracetam	25 mg	25 mg
Weeks 5 and 6	Perampanel		6 mg
	Brivaracetam	25 mg	50 mg
Weeks 7 and 8	Perampanel		6 mg
	Brivaracetam	50 mg	50 mg
Weeks 9 and 10	Perampanel		4 mg
	Brivaracetam	50 mg	75 mg
Weeks 11 and 12	Perampanel		4 mg
	Brivaracetam	75 mg	75 mg
Weeks 13 and 14	Perampanel		2 mg
	Brivaracetam	75mg	100 mg
Weeks 15 and 16	Perampanel		2 mg
	Brivaracetam	75 mg	100 mg
Weeks 17 onwards	Perampanel		Stopped
	Brivaracetam	100 mg	100 mg

Continue increasing dosage of brivaracetam as above until either:
* the seizures stop or,
* the maximum tolerated dose is reached or,
* the target dose is reached, whichever happens first.
Note: other antiepileptic medication to remain at current dosage.

When a new drug is being added to the regimen, rather than a switch, it is important to point out that common adverse effects such as sedation and dizziness are cumulative. If the new drug appears beneficial but such adverse effects persist, it may be possible to offset this by making a slight reduction in one of the other drugs.

Decisions regarding the introduction or switching of AEDs should always be made in conjunction with the patient's neurologist or specialist team.

Drug interactions

When dispensing antiepileptic medication, pharmacists should check for interactions and drugs that may lower the seizure threshold, of which quinolones or tramadol are usually the main culprits.[13] Others include:

* antibiotics – consider the choice of antibiotic carefully. Imipenem has been known to lower the seizure threshold by virtue of the cilastatin component. Penicillins, cephalosporins and isoniazid are only problematic in overdose
* buproprion
* diphenhydramine – this is an ingredient in some cough and cold products and sleep aids

— If the person needs sleep aid products they may require additional support – lack of sleep can lead to deterioration of seizure control
— In the first instance, you should provide advice on sleep hygiene measures
- mefenamic acid
- opiates
- theophylline.

See *Table 10.4* for a summary of common drug interactions to look out for.

Table 10.4: *Interactions with antiepileptic drugs*

Drug	Enzyme inducers (e.g. phenytoin, phenobarbital, carbamazepine)	Enzyme inhibitors (e.g. valproate)	High-dose oxcarbazepine, eslicarbazepine, topiramate	Perampanel, lamotrigine
Other AEDs	↓ Valproate ↓ Lamotrigine ↓ Topiramate ↓ Oxcarbazepine ↓ Perampanel ↓ Zonisamide ↓ Ethosuximide	↑ Lamotrigine ↑ Phenytoin ↑ Phenobarbital ↑ Tiagabine	↓ Carbamazepine ↑ Phenytoin ↑ Phenobarbital	
Antidepressants	↓ Antidepressants (especially tricyclics) ↑ Carbamazepine ↑ Phenytoin	↓ Tricyclics ↑ Valproate		↑ Lamotrigine
Antipsychotics	↓ Antipsychotics			
Oral contraceptives	Contraceptive failure	↓ Valproate	Contraceptive failure	Contraceptive failure ↓ Lamotrigine
Azole antifungals	↑ Carbamazepine ↑ Phenytoin (toxicity)			
Carbapenems	↑ Carbamazepine (toxicity)	↓ Valproate		
Warfarin	Labile INR	Increases bleeding risk		
Statins	Rosuvastatin or pravastatin preferred with carbamazepine			
Antihypertensives	Avoid dihydropyridines			
Ciclosporin, tacrolimus	↓ Ciclosporin ↓ Tacrolimus	↑ Ciclosporin ↑ Tacrolimus		

This is not a complete list of possible interactions. Consult the individual drug monographs (www.medicines.org.uk/emc) and/or Stockley's Interactions Checker, via MedicinesComplete.

↓ = levels of drugs are reduced as a result of the interaction; ↑ = levels of drugs are increased as a result of the interaction.

If treatment is required for the management of psychotic symptoms, for example, postictal psychosis, risperidone or olanzapine are the preferred antipsychotics. Clozapine has a higher risk of lowering the seizure threshold.

The potential for interactions involving AEDs is high because phenytoin, phenobarbital and carbamazepine are some of the strongest drug-metabolising-enzyme (DME) inducers. Whilst oxcarbazepine, eslicarbazepine and topiramate have also been found to possess inducing properties, the majority of newer AEDs have a lower potential for interactions, along with fewer adverse effects, which accounts for the increasingly widespread use of levetiracetam, lamotrigine and lacosamide in recent times.

Interactions can occur between AEDs themselves. However, these are only clinically significant on starting or stopping one of the drugs. Once treatment is established on a combination of drugs, a state of balance will exist.

Enzyme inducers stimulate the rate of metabolism of most co-administered AEDs, including valproate, lamotrigine, topiramate, oxcarbazepine, zonisamide, ethosuximide, tiagabine, perampanel and most benzodiazepines.[14,15] However, the interaction is unlikely to be clinically significant because the pharmacological effect of the additional drug tends to offset the loss of activity resulting from the reduction in serum concentration. Dosage adjustments may be required for valproate, lamotrigine and tiagabine after the addition of carbamazepine to counteract the significant reduction in the serum concentration. St. John's wort has the potential to increase the elimination of any AED and should be avoided.

Valproate, on the other hand, is a strong enzyme inhibitor and its addition to a regimen can increase the risk of toxicity of any concomitant other drugs that are substrates for cytochrome P450 (CYP450) enzyme system or glucuronidation. Topiramate and oxcarbazepine at high doses act as inhibitors of CYP2C19, despite being inducers of CYP3A4.

Lamotrigine, in particular, is at higher risk of cutaneous reactions when added to a regimen containing valproate, owing to the doubling of its concentration. For this reason, lamotrigine is introduced at half the usual dose in patients already established on valproate, with slower titration and a lower target dose. For patients already stabilised on lamotrigine, to which valproate is added, the dose of lamotrigine may need to be reduced once valproate reaches higher dosages. Phenobarbital and tiagabine levels may also be increased by valproate, necessitating dosage reduction.

The combination of valproate and phenytoin produces a complex system of interactions. The two drugs compete for protein binding such that the risk of toxicity occurs at lower than expected dosage. Phenytoin metabolism is inhibited by valproate, whilst that of valproate is induced by phenytoin.

Phenytoin toxicity may result from the addition of CYP2C19 inhibitors such as valproate, topiramate or oxcarbazepine, or courses of azole antifungals, chloramphenicol, isoniazid or sulfonamides. Carbamazepine toxicity may result from the introduction of antimicrobials such as macrolides, fluconazole, isoniazid, metronidazole, protease inhibitors, or grapefruit juice.

Aside from drug metabolism interactions, highly protein-bound AEDs, such as valproate, phenytoin and tiagabine compete with other highly-bound drugs for protein binding sites, thus increasing the free (active) fraction with the attendant risk of adverse effects and toxicity. Affected drugs include methotrexate, co-trimoxazole and protease inhibitors. Higher circulating blood levels, in turn, leads to increased elimination, thus reducing the total body concentration. Subsequent removal of the competing drug increases protein binding, thereby lowering the level of activity.

Carbapenems should be avoided in patients established on valproate.[16] Meropenem has been shown to reduce the serum valproate concentration by over 60% within 2 days.

Depression is commonly associated with epilepsy. Enzyme-inducing AEDs may increase the metabolism and thus lower the plasma concentration of many antipsychotics and antidepressants, tricyclics in particular. Whereas valproate has the opposite effect on tricyclic antidepressants, and they, in turn, can increase the plasma concentration of phenytoin, carbamazepine, valproate and lamotrigine.

Concomitant use of drugs that are substrates for the CYP450 enzyme system may require dosage increase, particularly where adequate levels are crucial for efficacy, such as ciclosporin, tacrolimus or sirolimus to prevent transplant rejection.

Cardiovascular drugs that may be affected by carbamazepine include simvastatin, atorvastatin and fluvastatin.[16] Refer the patient to their GP or cardiologist for consideration of switch to an alternative statin not subject to CYP3A4 metabolism, such as rosuvastatin or pravastatin. The efficacy of dihydropyridines is adversely affected by inducers, with considerable inter-patient variability. Alternative antihypertensives are preferred.[16]

Warfarin is not recommended for patients taking phenytoin because a complex interaction produces unpredictable effects on the INR, making it difficult to achieve a stable level of anticoagulation. Barbiturates and carbamazepine reduce the efficacy of warfarin, whereas valproate may increase it, besides interfering with platelet function and coagulation processes. INR should be monitored more closely in patients already stabilised on warfarin, or when starting, stopping or adjusting the dose of any interacting AED.

The most significant interactions between AEDs and steroids involve the oral contraceptive pill. Enzyme-inducing AEDs, including high-dose oxcarbazepine (900 mg/day), lamotrigine (300 mg/day), perampanel (12 mg/day), topiramate (200 mg/day) and rufinamide stimulate the metabolism of both the combined oral contraceptive pill and the progesterone-only pill, leading to a failure rate of 3%, three-fold higher than the national average (1%).[16]

Options for reliable contraception include a high-dose oestrogen pill, a minimum of 50 micrograms ethinylestradiol, or higher if breakthrough bleeding occurs, with or without spermicidal gel or a barrier method. Alternatively, three packs can be taken back-to-back, known as 'tricycling', followed by a short 4-day break every three months. These methods are more reliable than barrier methods but may not be completely fail safe. Levonorgestrel intrauterine devices (IUD) provide more reliable contraception, being based on local hormone release rather than serum levels. When lamotrigine is used at doses lower than 300 mg per day, 30 micrograms ethinylestradiol is sufficient. Women taking high-dose perampanel (12 mg) should use additional contraception and continue this for 28 days after stopping perampanel. For emergency contraception, an IUD or doubling the levonorgestrel dose (3 mg) is recommended.

Conversely, oestrogens can induce the metabolism of certain AEDs, lamotrigine, valproate, and possibly oxcarbazepine. The plasma concentration of lamotrigine may be halved, rebounding by up to 84% during the pill-free week.[16] Concurrent valproate ameliorates this effect.

Box 10.2: Practice point: drug interactions

- Many common AEDs are potent enzyme inducers or inhibitors, and thus are subject to drug interactions.
- When dispensing antiepileptic drugs, or doing a pharmacy review, check for interactions that may reduce the seizure threshold.
- Interactions between antiepileptic drugs are only clinically significant on starting or stopping drugs.

Special groups

Pregnancy and breastfeeding

The use of an AED during pregnancy increases the risk of major congenital malformations during the first trimester – often before a woman is aware she is pregnant. This highlights the importance of contraceptive advice and planned pregnancies.

Ideally, women with epilepsy should begin to plan for pregnancy at least a year before conception, with a review with their neurologist to discuss the risks and harms of treatment and to allow time for any medication changes to be completed. It is recommended that folic acid 5 mg is commenced three months before conception and continued at least until the end of the first trimester, as it is widely believed to reduce the malformation risk, although, there is no clear evidence to support this.

Valproate carries the highest risk of malformations, up to 10% for neural tube defects and 30-40% risk of neurodevelopment disability, such as low intelligence and autistic spectrum disorders.[17,18,19] Phenytoin is well known to cause craniofacial abnormalities and cardiac defects, but as mentioned previously this drug is rarely used routinely.

Teratogenicity rates with newer AEDs are reported in the region of 2-3%.[17,18,19] The paucity of data relating to the newer AEDs means the risks are less well defined than for older drugs. It is important to encourage women to notify their pregnancy via the online UK and Ireland registry for ongoing surveillance of major congenital malformation risks to enable more information to be gathered (www.epilepsyandpregnancy.co.uk).

Do not suggest changing AEDs during pregnancy, or at any other time, even for valproate, without consultation with a neurologist. The risk of destabilising seizure control may have consequences for the foetus, and the mother, that outweighs the risk of teratogenicity and developmental delay posed by the medication. Any medication changes should be carried out in a controlled manner under close supervision by the neurology team.

Pregnancy itself may destabilise epilepsy owing to the increased volume of distribution and high circulating levels of oestrogens and progestogens, which increase the clearance of some AEDs, for instance, lamotrigine, levetiracetam, phenytoin, phenobarbital, topiramate and oxcarbazepine.[19] Dosages of these drugs may need to be increased, under the close supervision of a neurologist. Levels revert to normal within a few days of delivery and dosage should be gradually decreased accordingly whilst observing for signs of toxicity.

Post-partum women may be at higher risk of seizures due to sleep deprivation, pain, breastfeeding or anxiety. New mothers will require advice on how to safely care for their baby. Recommendations include feeding the baby sitting in a reclined position with pillows either side, changing on a mat on the floor, bathing the baby accompanied and in shallow water, carrying in a car seat to afford protection in the event of falling, using a buggy with a release brake or strap and wearing an ID tag to alert passers-by. Preconception counselling and advice on caring for the baby are available on the Epilepsy Society website.

For breastfeeding mothers, consideration should be given to the likelihood of AEDs affecting the infant. Factors to consider include: Has the baby had prior exposure (i.e. during pregnancy)? Is the drug in the neonatal formulary? Is the infant lethargic or crying inconsolably, or having feeding difficulties? Advice should be sought from a specialist paediatric pharmacist.

Drugs to avoid include ethosuximide, zonisamide and regular benzodiazepines,[20] but pharmacists should be sensitive to the feelings of the mother and avoid sweeping statements to prevent abrupt cessation of therapy. Suggest that she has a discussion with her neurologist as soon as possible.

Encourage new mothers to attend follow-up appointments with their neurologist and obstetrician and plan for their next pregnancy.

Women of childbearing potential

When dispensing AEDs to a woman of childbearing potential, pharmacists could consider enquiring about contraception, and offer advice on appropriate options. If it transpires that she is trying to get pregnant, the pharmacist should emphasise the need for effective planning and suggest she visit her neurologist for a review and her epilepsy management. Women who become pregnant, or think they might be pregnant, should contact their neurologist immediately.

Pharmacists should be alert when dispensing valproate prescriptions for women of childbearing potential, ascertaining if she is aware of the risks of taking valproate should she become pregnant, ensuring she is using effective contraception, and providing her with the Patient Guide. Intrauterine devices (IUDs), progestogen-only implants and sterilisation are the most effective methods, having failure rates of less than 1%. However, the woman's wishes should be respected.

Resources for patients and healthcare professionals on valproate in females is available on the MHRA website.

In view of the risks of teratogenicity in the event of pregnancy, valproate should be avoided in girls and women of childbearing potential if there are other equally effective agents available.[21] When other drugs have not been tolerated or have been deemed ineffective, valproate may be initiated and supervised by a specialist. Women unaware of the risks should make an appointment with their neurologist or GP to discuss their options.

Monitoring

Monitoring of drug efficacy is a clinical judgement based on the patient's, or carer's, observations and a review of the seizure diary.

Therapeutic drug monitoring is not routinely performed, but may be useful in the following circumstances:

- Pregnancy
- Poor compliance or toxicity are suspected
- An interacting drug is introduced
- Adjustments are made to the phenytoin dosage

In view of its saturation kinetics, small changes in phenytoin dosage can produce unexpectedly large jumps in serum concentration, with the risk of toxicity. The cardinal signs of phenytoin toxicity are nystagmus, ataxia and dysarthria. As it is highly protein-bound, interpretation of phenytoin levels should take account of serum protein levels, as only the free fraction is responsible for clinical activity.

When testing for drug compliance, the drug level should be taken the same day, thereby giving the patient no chance to modify their behaviour beforehand. For these patients, long-acting drugs with once-daily dosing may limit the risks posed by missed doses, such as zonisamide, eslicarbazepine, perampanel, phenytoin or phenobarbital.

Carbamazepine is converted to an active metabolite, carbamazepine-10,11-epoxide, and when monitoring the levels of both should be requested.

Serum levels of valproate or levetiracetam are of limited value as they bear little relation to clinical efficacy or toxicity, which are usually diagnosed clinically.

Patients taking carbamazepine, oxcarbazepine and eslicarbazepine should be monitored for hyponatraemia every 6-12 months. If they become symptomatic (nausea, fatigue, headache, muscle weakness, disorientation) they should be encouraged to add salt to their food or to boost their sodium levels with a packet of crisps or salted nuts.

Follow-up and referral

Adults and children with epilepsy should receive an annual review, either by their GP or their specialist.[8] Patients undergoing treatment changes should be followed up more frequently by the specialist team, usually every 2-3 months, but this may be more often depending on the needs of the patient. Between reviews, if there are concerns about adverse effects, deterioration in condition, or changes in seizure-type or pattern, patients should be referred back to their specialist team.

Women who become pregnant or are planning a pregnancy should be referred to their specialist for an urgent review of their epilepsy and re-evaluation of drug therapy. Many hospitals run joint epilepsy antenatal clinics, allowing review by an obstetrician, specialist epilepsy neurologist, epilepsy nurse, midwife, and neuropsychiatrist if required, at the same appointment.

Suspicion of status epilepticus requires emergency ambulance transfer to hospital.

For help with social issues, public transport passes, letters for college/work/travel, financial support documentation or liaison with learning disabilities support teams, local epilepsy nurses should be contacted. Occupational therapists can perform safety assessments in patients' homes to help reduce risks of injury.

Box 10.3: Practice point: medicines

- People with epilepsy should never run out of their medicines.
- All changes to epilepsy drugs or dosages should be made in collaboration with the specialist team.
- Brand continuity is essential for some categories of antiepileptic drugs.
- Valproate should ideally be avoided in females of childbearing potential, but should not be stopped abruptly.

Information and advice

Lifestyle advice can help people with epilepsy reduce the risk of injury and perhaps also of seizures. Those who experience an aura, or warning, prior to a seizure may have time to get to a safe place or sit down to reduce their risk of injury.

People with epilepsy should be encouraged to keep physically and mentally active as it may reduce stress and aid relaxation, all of which reduce the frequency of seizures. However, people with epilepsy should avoid solo sports, for instance, skydiving, climbing and scuba diving. They should not swim or bathe alone. The risk of drowning is more than 15 times higher than the general population.

Advice about travelling is important – when using public transport people should stand well back from the platform edge, and avoid travelling alone following a seizure. Individuals who have had a seizure should inform the DVLA. A single seizure comes under the 1999 Motor Vehicles (Driving Licences) Regulations and such individuals can regain their (group 1) licence after 6 months provided the risk of seizure recurrence is less than 20%. People diagnosed with epilepsy are prohibited from driving until they have been seizure free for 12 months, or 5 years for a heavy goods vehicle (group 2) licence, under the 1998 Road Traffic Act.

The DVLA does not recommend driving during periods of drug withdrawal or dose reduction, but patients can apply to be reinstated after 6 months provided there have been no further seizures during that time.[22]

Advice about medication should include:

- Do not stop medication except on medical advice, to reduce the risk of rebound seizures.
- Allow sufficient time when requesting repeats, to avoid running out of medication.
- Take missed doses as soon as they remember, unless the next dose is due. They should not take a double dose. Once-daily dosing can be taken any time on the same day. Those who frequently forget doses may benefit from suggestions to aid memory, such as keeping nighttime doses beside the bed and morning doses with breakfast things.
- Modified release preparations should be swallowed whole and not cut or chewed.

When drug changes are taking place it is important to manage expectations. For patients with drug-resistant epilepsy, the more drugs they have tried which have failed, the less likely they are to achieve seizure freedom.[23,24] Success, however, can be measured by a reduction in seizure frequency or duration, or severity. Emphasise that it is impossible to predict how any individual will respond to a particular drug beforehand.

Box 10.4: Practice point: seizure control

- Seizure control can be adversely affected by stress, infection, lack of sleep or certain drugs.
- Seizure diaries can help monitor the pattern, frequency, severity, duration and recovery time of seizures.
- Electrolyte or metabolic disturbances such as hyponatraemia, hypomagnesaemia or hypoglycaemia can adversely influence seizure control.

Useful resources

- Epilepsy Action. www.epilepsy.org.uk
- Epilepsy Scotland. www.epilepsyscotland.org.uk
- UK epilepsy pregnancy register. www.epilepsyandpregnancy.co.uk
- Epilepsy Society – pre-conception counselling and advice on caring for the baby. www.epilepsysociety. org.uk/pregnancy-and-parenting#.XWU-kdKWz50
- MHRA – resources for patients and health care professionals on valproate in females. www.gov.uk/ guidance/valproate-use-by-women-and-girls
- MHRA – advice on brand switching. www.gov.uk/drug-safety-update/antiepileptic-drugs-updated-advice-on-switching-between-different-manufacturers-products
- MHRA – Yellow Card Scheme. www.yellowcard.mhra.gov.uk
- NICE guidance CG137. www.nice.org.uk/guidance/cg137/chapter/1-Guidance#pharmacological-treatment
- DVLA. www.gov.uk/guidance/neurological-disorders-assessing-fitness-to-drive#epilepsy-and-seizures
- Royal College of Obstetricians and Gynaecologists. (2016) Epilepsy in Pregnancy Green-top Guideline No. 68, June 2016. www.rcog.org.uk/en/guidelines-research-services/guidelines/gtg68

References

1. Fisher RS *et al*. ILAE Official Report: A practical clinical definition of epilepsy. *Epilepsia* 2014; 55(4): 475-482.

2. Fisher RS *et al*. Operational classification of seizure types by the International League Against Epilepsy: Position Paper of the ILAE Commission for Classification and Terminology. *Epilepsia* 2017; 58(4): 522-530.

3. World Health Organization (WHO). "Epilepsy". WHO Factsheet, October 2012: number 999; 2014. www.who.int/mediacentre/factsheets/fs999/en/index.html

4. Beghi M *et al*. Learning Disorders in Epilepsy. *Epilepsia* 2006; 47(Suppl. 2): 14-18.

5. Kwan P, Sander JW. The natural history of epilepsy: an epidemiological view. *J Neurol Neurosurg Psychiatry* 2004; 75(10): 1376-1381.

6. Kwan P *et al*. Definition of drug resistant epilepsy: consensus proposal by the ad hoc Task Force of the ILAE Commission on Therapeutic Strategies. *Epilepsia* 2010; 51(6): 1069-1077.

7. Picot MC *et al*. The prevalence of epilepsy and pharmacoresistant epilepsy in adults: A population-based study in a Western European country. *Epilepsia* 2008; 49(7): 1230-1238.

8. National Institute for Health and Care Excellence (NICE). Epilepsies: diagnosis and management. London: NICE; 2012 [updated 2016]. www.nice.org.uk/guidance/cg137

9. SIGN 143. Diagnosis and management of epilepsy in adults. May 2015 [revised 2018]. www.sign.ac.uk/sign-143-diagnosis-and-management-of-epilepsy-in-adults.html

10. West S *et al*. Surgery for epilepsy. *Cochrane Database of Systematic Reviews* 2015; Issue 7: CD010541.

11. Jeyul Yang MD, Ji Hoon Phi. The Present and Future of Vagus Nerve Stimulation. *J Korean Neurosurg Soc* 2019; 62: 344-352.

12. MHRA (2017). Antiepileptic drugs: updated advice on switching between different manufacturers' products. www.gov.uk/drug-safety-update/antiepileptic-drugs-updated-advice-on-switching-between-different-manufacturers-products

13. Chen HY *et al*. Treatment of drug-induced seizures. *Br J Clin Pharmacol* 2015; 81(3): 412-419.

14. Johannessen SL, Landmark CJ. Antiepileptic Drug Interactions – Principles and Clinical Implications. *Curr Neuropham* 2010; 8(3): 254-267.

15. Patsalos PN, Perucca E. Clinically important drug interactions in epilepsy: general features and interactions between antiepileptic drugs. *Lancet Neurol* 2003; 2(6): 347-356.

16. Patsalos PN, Perucca E. Clinically important drug interactions in epilepsy: interactions between antiepileptic drugs and other drugs. *Lancet Neurol* 2003; 2(8): 473-481.

17. Tomson T *et al*. Comparative risk of major congenital malformations with eight different antiepileptic drugs: a prospective cohort study of the EURAP registry. *Lancet Neurol* 2018; 17(6): 530-538.

18. Hernandez-Díaz S *et al.* Comparative safety of antiepileptic drugs during pregnancy. *Neurology* 2012; 78(21): 1692-1699.

19. Tomson T & Battino D. Teratogenic effects of antiepileptic drugs. *Lancet Neurology* 2012; 11(9): 803-813.

20. Davanzo R *et al.* Antiepileptic drugs and breastfeeding. *Italian Journal of Pediatrics* 2013; 39: 50-61.

21. MHRA (2019). Valproate use by women and girls. www.gov.uk/guidance/valproate-use-by-women-and-girls

22. Driver and Vehicle Licensing Agency. At a glance guide to the current medical standards of fitness to drive. Drivers Medical Group, 2010. www.gov.uk/guidance/neurological-disorders-assessing-fitness-to-drive#epilepsy-and-seizures

23. Kwan P, Brodie MJ. Early identification of refractory epilepsy. *N Engl J Med* 2000; 342(5): 314-319.

24. Schiller Y, Najjar Y. Quantifying the response to antiepileptic drugs: effect of past treatment history. *Neurology* 2008; 70(1): 54-65.

Case studies

Case study 1

Elaine, aged 32 years, presents a prescription for sodium valproate 1 g twice daily.

Points to consider

- What concerns do you have about this prescription?
- What questions should you ask Elaine?
- What suggestions would you make?
- Are there any resources you can recommend?

You know that valproate is highly teratogenic and as such is not recommended in females of childbearing potential. You ask Elaine:

- what condition she is taking sodium valproate for
- if she is using effective contraception
- if she planning to get pregnant.

Elaine tells you that she has epilepsy. She recently stopped taking the contraceptive pill because she and her husband are trying for a baby.

You enquire when she last saw a neurologist. She replies that, since her epilepsy is well controlled, she hasn't seen a specialist for some years.

You ask if she is aware of the risks of taking valproate whilst pregnant. She seems unaware of this. You inform her that valproate can be associated with congenital malformations and advise her to make an appointment with her GP for referral to a neurologist to discuss her options. You emphasise the importance of continuing to take valproate for the time being because the development of seizures could put both the unborn baby and herself at risk.

You suggest that she restarts contraception until she has seen a neurologist, and recommend an IUD as the most effective form of contraception. She is reluctant to have an IUD implanted but agrees to go back on the pill.

You provide her with the MHRA patient guide to valproate and pregnancy (available from Sanofi or via the link below).

Women taking sodium valproate for epilepsy or mood stabilisation should be reviewed by their specialist for alternatives if possible. If no other drug is suitable, she should be made aware of the risks, and counselled on the use of effective contraception. A pregnancy test may be performed at the specialist's discretion. For other indications, such as migraine, refer the person to their GP for alternative treatment.

MHRA guidance and resources for patients and healthcare professionals on valproate in females can be found here: www.gov.uk/guidance/valproate-use-by-women-and-girls.

Case study 2

Patrick, aged 27 years, has epilepsy and learning disabilities. He has been admitted to hospital for a ruptured appendix. Post-operatively he experienced two seizures within 24 hours. His mother reported that normally he rarely has seizures.

Patrick is allergic to penicillin (he develops a rash), he weighs 77 kg and he has normal renal and liver function.

His regular medication is:

- Tegretol MR 800 mg twice daily
- Sodium valproate 1 g twice daily

Post-operatively he has been prescribed:

- Paracetamol 1 g four times daily
- Tramadol 50-100 mg four times daily when required

- Senna 15 mg twice daily
- Ciprofloxacin 500 mg twice daily
- Cyclizine 50 mg three times daily when required (orally or by IV administration)
- Ondansetron 4 mg three times daily when required (orally or by IV administration)

Points to consider

- What do you think may have contributed to the development of the seizures?
- What would you do to reduce the risk of further seizures?

You are aware that stress associated with hospital admission, surgery and infection may trigger seizures. In addition, you know that tramadol and fluoroquinolones, such as ciprofloxacin, lower the seizure threshold.

You decide that it is appropriate to consider alternative opioid such as codeine, dihydrocodeine or oral morphine solution. You prescribe codeine and stop the tramadol.

You also decide that it is best to use an alternative antibiotic such as metronidazole and/or clarithromycin. You consult the local microbiology guidelines and discover that ciprofloxacin is the appropriate alternative for patients with a penicillin allergy. However, in this case there is a drug-disease interaction. Therefore, you contact the microbiology team for advice. They advise you to prescribe metronidazole and clarithromycin.

You document this advice in Patrick's care record and inform the surgical team of the required modifications to his therapy.

You speak to Patrick and his mother to explain the potential contributing factors for his recent seizures and the consequent changes to his medication. You reassure them that the likelihood of further seizures is low but he will be observed closely during his hospital stay.

It is important to recognise factors that can contribute to destabilisation of seizure control at any time: psychological factors such as stress, anxiety, depression or sleep deprivation, or pathological factors including hypoglycaemia, electrolyte disturbance, the presence of infection or flare-up of an inflammatory condition, such as IBD. Seizures may also be triggered by alcohol or recreational drugs, for instance cocaine or amphetamines.

CHAPTER 11

Heart failure

Paul Forsyth

Overview

Heart failure is by definition a complex syndrome of signs and symptoms caused by a functional or structural abnormality of the heart which results in decreased cardiac output.[1] It is not one condition, but is an umbrella diagnosis for various sub-conditions.

The typical symptoms of heart failure include (amongst many others) shortness of breath, fluid overload and fatigue.

Heart failure is categorised into three main types:[2]

- Heart failure with reduced ejection fraction (HF-REF)
- Heart failure with mid-range ejection fraction (HF-mREF)
- Heart failure with preserved ejection fraction (HF-PEF)

Heart failure is often the result of a number of complex, overlapping comorbidities and risk factors. Many patients will have several different risk factors and comorbidities which ultimately culminate in heart failure.

Typical risk factors for heart failure include coronary artery disease, hypertension, atrial fibrillation, diabetes and chronic kidney disease. However, heart failure can be present in the absence of such comorbidities, such as in dilated cardiomyopathy. Identification of exact aetiology and pathology should always form part of the diagnostic phase of the syndrome as this may offer specific therapeutic opportunities (e.g. revascularisation in coronary heart disease or valve replacement in valve disease).[2]

The aetiology and comorbid disease profile of HF-REF, HF-mREF and HF-PEF can vary significantly.[2]

The prevalence of heart failure is approximately 1-2% of the adult population, rising to over 10% in patients aged over 70 years.[3] As the general population lives longer, often with multimorbidities, the prevalence of heart failure is increasing across the world.[3]

In England and Wales in 2016/2017 there were 86,466 primary-cause hospital admissions for heart failure.[4] As such this represents a huge financial and resource burden to the NHS. The median age of patients in the NHS England and Wales national heart failure audit was 80.6 years.[4] In such patients, inpatient mortality for heart failure in this audit was approximately 9.4%.[4] One-year mortality for patients surviving to hospital discharge was 23.3%.[4]

In general, heart failure survival rates are comparable to, or worse than, most common cancers.[5,6]

Diagnosis

The first stage of the diagnosis is confirming the presence of the syndrome (i.e. the presence of signs and symptoms). Symptoms are however often non-specific and do not, therefore, help discriminate well between heart failure and other conditions.[2]

If heart failure is suspected, natriuretic peptides blood tests and electrocardiograms (ECG) are usually carried out to strengthen the diagnostic case.[2] Patients with normal serum natriuretic peptides levels and ECGs are unlikely to have heart failure and do not routinely need diagnostic imaging (i.e. normal natriuretic peptides levels are a good 'rule out' for heart failure).[2]

For patients with clinical signs and symptoms and elevated natriuretic peptides (or abnormal ECGs), diagnostic imaging is essential to confirm and categorise the diagnosis. Echocardiography is the most common and widely available test in patients with suspected heart failure to establish the diagnosis. Other modalities such as cardiac magnetic resonance imaging may also be available in some areas and for some patient types. The assessment of ventricular systolic and diastolic functions, chamber sizes, wall thickness and valve function is necessary to differentiate between HF-REF, HF-mREF, HF-PEF and other forms of heart disease.

Pharmacy input

There is a diverse and long-established evidence base for pharmacists improving care in heart failure patients.[7-10] It is vital, however, that pharmacists are embedded into the multidisciplinary team rather than offering 'stand-alone' services if they are to deliver the biggest improvement.[7]

Key areas where pharmacists can improve care include:
- patient education
- medicines reconciliation
- appropriate use of disease-modifying medication (including target dosing)
- medication adherence support
- safe ongoing medication monitoring
- reduction in drug interactions
- reduction in potentially harmful medication.

Pharmacy review

Heart failure patients typically benefit from regular review at 6-monthly intervals during times of clinical stability and much shorter (e.g. days to weeks) during times of acute worsening. Patients with poor prognostic risk factors may also benefit from more regular review.

The level at which pharmacists get involved in the care of patients with heart failure will vary by job role and levels of experience. For example, expert specialist pharmacists may get involved in ensuring that appropriate patients are considered for advanced treatment options like complex devices and cardiac transplantation and therefore must be able to interpret complex diagnostic and test data.

However, these skills are unlikely to be relevant to community pharmacy. Conversely, community pharmacists may get involved in minor ailment management and 'over-the-counter' treatments, but this may not be relevant to specialist roles.

An extensive guide to specific skills and competencies for different types of pharmacists has been jointly produced by the UKCPA Heart Failure Group and the Royal Pharmaceutical Society.[10] *Table 11.1* is adapted from the Knowledge and Skills domain of practice.[10]

Key questions to ask patients

There are three important common symptoms associated with breathlessness that it is important to check at every review. The severity of shortness of breath and its effect on exercise tolerance is graded according to the New York Heart Association (NYHA) scale:
- Class I = No limitation of physical activity. Ordinary physical activity does not cause undue breathlessness, fatigue or palpitations.
- Class II = Slight limitation of physical activity. Comfortable at rest, but ordinary physical activity results in undue breathlessness, fatigue or palpitations.
- Class III = Marked limitation of physical activity. Comfortable at rest, but less than ordinary physical activity results in undue breathlessness, fatigue or palpitations.
- Class IV = Unable to carry on any physical activity without discomfort. Symptoms at rest can be present. If any physical activity is undertaken, discomfort is increased.

Table 11.1: *Examples of necessary skills and competencies within different pharmacist job roles specific to heart failure (reproduced and summarised from Int J Pharm Pract, 2019; 27: 424-435)*[10]

Pharmacist role	What they should know	What they should be able to do
All pharmacists, irrelevant of setting	Knowledge of: • the need, clinical indication and standard dosing schedules for all medicines • all common and/or clinically significant adverse effects of medicines • all clinically significant interactions • pathophysiology of disease and mechanisms of medication	• Dispense all medicines from a legal prescription • Ensure that a medication is appropriate for the individual patient concerned, including dose, frequency, strength, route, timing, and formulation • Supply information to support the patient in taking their medication as prescribed by more experienced members of the MDT • Provide patient general self-care support to aid medication adherence
Any clinical pharmacist role (e.g. any generalist pharmacist with responsibility for medication optimisation)	Advanced knowledge of: • medications in major clinical conditions • generic lifestyle factors affecting major clinical conditions • routine biochemistry and haematology results affecting pharmacological management of major clinical conditions	• Demonstrate ability to use knowledge and skills to follow guidelines and protocols for all major conditions • Identify medication non-adherence and plan interventions to support improved adherence • Identify medication reconciliation problems between different healthcare providers/healthcare sectors and use knowledge and skills to resolve such issues • Deliver a holistic individualised treatment plan • Perform basic generic physical examination of patients • Communicate effectively with patients, carers and MDT about all aspects of general pharmacological issues • Act as an independent prescriber
Specialist/ advanced clinical pharmacists who routinely care for heart failure patients (e.g. cardiology pharmacist, heart failure pharmacist, GP-based pharmacist with a specialist interest in cardiology)	Expert knowledge of: • pharmacological treatment of chronic HF • the iatrogenic causes of HF, both common and rare • medications for other conditions that can worsen prevalent HF • the pharmacological treatment of acute HF • different aetiologies of HF and the relevance to pharmacological treatments • the clinical significance of comorbidity in HF and relevance to pharmacological decisions • the indication for non-pharmacological management of acute HF • the prognosis of HF, including the relevance of independent predictors of prognosis • the complex pharmacological management of palliative HF/end stages of life, including symptom control and discontinuation of therapy	• Deliver a structured review of published literature to help answer a specific clinical question related to medicine use in heart failure and present the findings to the MDT • Demonstrate ability to use knowledge and skills to autonomously make complex decisions in HF patients (using independent prescribing where needed) where there are several potential treatment options • Provide patient self-care support specific to HF to aid medication adherence, including use of daily weights and diuretic dosing • Undertake a focused clinical history from a HF patient and assess the common HF signs and symptoms • Perform physical examination of HF patients relevant to role, including: manual blood pressure non-radial pulses (rate and rhythm), chest auscultation, JVP assessment, venepuncture • Recognise common triggers of decompensation in HF patients • Assess the common signs and symptoms of other forms of CVD, including: ischaemia, syncope, palpitations • Recognise patients with suspected clinical HF and organise appropriate diagnostic tests via the MDT • Interpret common 12-lead ECG abnormalities affecting pharmacological decisions in HF • Interpret common echocardiogram abnormalities affecting pharmacological decisions in HF • Identify scenarios where non-pharmacological treatment options may be warranted and refer via the MDT as appropriate and understands their relevance to medications • Identify scenarios where specific cardiology tests may be warranted and refer via the MDT as appropriate • Communicate compassionately and effectively with patients and carers about all aspects of pharmacological management of HF, including difficult discussions surrounding prognosis • Liaise with specialist palliative care MDT where necessary

CVD = cardiovascular disease; ECG = electrocardiogram; HF = heart failure; JVP = jugular venous pressure; MDT = multidisciplinary team; NYHA = New York Heart Association; PND = paroxysmal nocturnal dyspnoea.

NYHA class should be checked and recorded at every review as it is used in clinical trials and guidelines to determine the appropriateness of treatments. NYHA scoring is subjective however, and can be complicated by other comorbidities including respiratory disease, poor physical conditioning and angina. Patients with worsening NYHA should seek medical or specialist heart failure team advice as it is a red flag symptom.

Paroxysmal nocturnal dyspnoea (PND) is the presence of shortness of breath at night that wakes the patient; it may indicate pulmonary oedema. The presence or absence of PND should be checked at every review. Patients with PND should seek medical or specialist heart failure team advice as it is a red flag symptom.

Related to PND is the symptom of orthopnoea, where people have to elevate their head (e.g. with extra pillows, or sit up) during the night in order to sleep comfortably. The presence or absence of orthopnoea should be checked at every review. Muscular, back and spine problems can complicate this assessment, so should be taken into account. Patients with orthopnoea should seek medical or specialist heart failure team advice as it is a red flag symptom.

Box 11.1: Red flag signs and symptoms

People with any of the following should seek prompt medical or specialist heart failure team advice:
- Worsening NYHA
- Paroxysmal nocturnal dyspnoea (PND)
- Orthopnoea
- Worsening oedema
- Weight increases of ≥1.5 to 2kg (≥3 to 4lbs) in two days
- Any new heart irregularities

Key basic examination skills

In addition to asking about symptoms of breathlessness, examining the patient is important to identify signs of disease progression. This includes assessing oedema, weight, blood pressure (BP), heart rate (HR), and heart rhythm.

The presence or absence of peripheral oedema should be checked at every review. Typically, this will involve checking the ankle and lower leg for evidence of pitting and then tracking this pitting up the leg to see where the highest evidence of pitting is found. This should then be recorded in the notes. Achieving euvolaemia (i.e. not being able to identify pitting oedema) through the lowest achievable diuretic dose is a key therapeutic target for heart failure.[2] The presence of significant and/or persistent peripheral oedema is a poor prognostic sign.

The monitoring of weight is another key sign related to fluid balance. Every patient should ideally have their 'dry weight' determined when euvolaemic. Patients should then be encouraged to keep daily weights under standard conditions (e.g. first thing in the morning after going to the toilet). Some patients may be educated to self-manage these incidents with a short-term diuretic increase (e.g. for 3 days) and to only seek medical or specialist heart failure team advice if this does not achieve euvolaemia.

BP influences treatment optimisation decisions, including the target dosing of key prognostically important disease-modifying medications. Typically, therefore, BP should be checked at every review.

HR influences treatment optimisation decisions, including the target dosing of key prognostically important disease-modifying medications. Therefore, HR should be checked at every review.

Heart rhythm should be also be checked at every review as cardiac arrhythmias, including atrial fibrillation, are common in patients with heart failure.

Advanced examination skills

Pharmacists in specialist or advanced job roles may also learn additional advanced clinical skills including:

- Chest auscultation – lung auscultation is a vital skill needed for identifying pulmonary oedema (often presenting as fine basal crackles). It also helps distinguish between other causes of shortness of breath such as infection (often presenting as coarse crackles). Chest auscultation is also necessary for listening to heart sounds, which can be useful for determining murmurs related to valve disease amongst other things.
- Jugular venous pressure (JVP) assessment – the JVP is usually visually assessed via observation of the right side of the neck. A raised JVP is a sign of fluid overload and helps in the diagnostic and management plan workup of a patient.
- Venepuncture – medication optimisation in heart failure requires regular blood tests for factors like urea and electrolytes (U&Es). Other blood tests, such as full blood counts (FBC), iron studies, liver function tests (LFTs), thyroid function tests (TFTs), natriuretic peptides levels, glucose control and lipids are also routinely checked in heart failure patients.

Self-care

Lifestyle advice and self-care form an important part of management, but are unfortunately often overlooked.

Self-management programmes should be tailored to individual patient requirements.[11] Patients should be educated on factors including their diagnosis, medicines, what symptoms to look out for in case of deterioration and a process for contacting the specialist heart failure multidisciplinary team if needed.[12]

Patients should *NOT* be *routinely* advised to restrict their sodium or fluid consumption. Ask about salt and fluid consumption and, *only if needed*, tell them to restrict fluids if they have dilutional hyponatraemia or high levels of salt and/or fluid consumption.[12] Patients should stick to usual salt intake thresholds advocated in public health guidelines. If fluid restriction is clinically indicated to help with fluid overload, this may typically involve restricting fluids to less than 1.5-2 litres per day. Continue to review these decisions over time. Patients should, however, be advised to avoid salt substitutes as these often contain potassium.

Patients should have an annual influenza vaccine and a one-off pneumococcal vaccine.[11,12] They should also be reminded and encouraged to attend annual vaccination programmes.[11,12]

Simple routine interventions

There are a few key simple routine interventions that all pharmacists should deliver.

Medicines reconciliation is a vital element of safe and appropriate medication use at the point of hospital admission, hospital discharge and post-discharge follow-up.[9] Pharmacists are known to reduce medication errors at such time points[9], and therefore medicines reconciliation should form a key part of reviews at such stages, involving hospital, community and GP-based pharmacists.

Heart failure patients with suboptimal medication adherence have worse outcomes, and pharmacists are known to improve such outcomes through adherence support.[13,14] Patient education and adherence support should form part of every patient review. Adherence support should not solely focus on patient education but should review the World Health Organization's five categories of barriers to adherence: patient-related factors; condition-related factors; treatment-related factors; healthcare system-related factors and socioeconomic factors.[15]

Medication

This section predominantly focuses on the pharmacological treatment of HF-REF. The treatment of HF-mREF often mirrors the treatment of HF-REF, although the evidence base is very limited. There are currently no evidenced-based treatment options for HF-PEF and treatment simply focuses on the achievement of euvolaemia with diuretics and the standard guideline-based treatment of associated comorbidities and risk factors such as hypertension, diabetes and atrial fibrillation.[2,12]

Note that information about the medicines are summaries of overall class effects and are not exhaustive, so should not be used to guide patient-level clinical decisions. For full details check the Summary of Product Characteristics for individual medicines and refer to current local and national heart failure guidelines.

Angiotensin-converting enzyme inhibitors (ACEIs) or angiotensin receptor blockers (ARBs)[11,16]

ACEIs are used first line in all HF-REF patients NYHA I-IV. ARBs are used second line in these patients, but usually only when ACEI is not tolerated due to persistent dry cough. They improve survival, decrease hospitalisations and improve symptoms. Common evidence-based ACEI options include enalapril, lisinopril, captopril, ramipril and ARB options are candesartan, valsartan and losartan. ACEI and ARB are no longer routinely used together in HF-REF. Patients should be started on a low dose with the aim of reaching a target dose. Titrations can be considered 2 weeks after starting treatment. See *Table 11.2* for the starting doses and target doses of ACEIs and ARBs.

Table 11.2: *Starting doses and target doses of ACEIs and ARBs*[11]

Medication	Typical starting dose	Target dose
Enalapril	2.5 mg twice daily	10-20 mg twice daily
Lisinopril	2.5 mg once daily	20-35 mg once daily
Captopril	6.25 mg three times daily	50 mg three times daily
Ramipril	2.5 mg once daily	5 mg twice daily (or 10 mg daily)
Candesartan	4-8 mg daily	32 mg daily
Valsartan	40 mg twice daily	160 mg twice daily
Losartan	25 mg daily	150 mg daily

It is important to be aware of the contraindications and cautions to ensure they are suitable for the patient.
- Contraindications:
  - History of previous allergy or angioneurotic oedema
  - Bilateral renal artery stenosis
- Cautions:
  - Significant hyperkalaemia
  - Significant renal dysfunction
  - Symptomatic hypotension (i.e. low BP plus symptoms of dizziness) or severe asymptomatic hypotension (systolic BP <90 mmHg)

All people taking an ACEI or ARB should have their U&Es and BP checked before initiation, 1-2 weeks after initiation and 1-2 weeks after each dose increase. Dry cough is a well-known adverse effect of ACEIs. For details on this and other adverse effects of ACEIs and ARBs and how to manage them, see *Table 11.3*.

Box 11.2: Practice point: Sick Day advice

- Sick Day advice about missing heart failure medication, including ACE/ARB/ARNI/diuretics, on days of volume depleting illness (such as diarrhoea or vomiting) should NOT be routinely given to every patient, but should be tailored to the individual patient based on the risk of acute kidney injury vs. heart failure deterioration.[17] Seek specialist heart failure team advice if needed.
- Due to the increased risk of hyperkalaemia[18,19], Sick Day advice is appropriate with mineralocorticoid receptor antagonists (MRAs). However, diarrhoea and/or vomiting can both precipitate hyperkalaemia and can also be a clinical symptom of hyperkalaemia. Patients with diarrhoea and/or vomiting should stop the MRA but should also immediately see a medic or the heart failure team for review and to check U&Es.

Table 11.3: *Adverse effects of ACEIs, ARBs, ARNI and MRA and how to manage them*[11,16]

Adverse effect	Management options
Dry cough (ACEI only)	• Exclude other causes of cough (e.g. pulmonary oedema, COPD, asthma, chest infection) before reviewing ACEI. • If cough is persistent, troublesome to the patient, and dry, consider stopping ACEI for 1-2 weeks. • If cough improves, start ARB as an alternative and if it does not improve then restart ACEI. • In more severe patients seek specialist advice before stopping ACEI.
Symptomatic low BP	• The absolute BP value is not important unless it is <90 mmHg systolic or the patient is symptomatic with dizziness. • If a patient is symptomatic with low BP or systolic <90 mmHg, review the need for other BP-lowering drugs. • If the patient has no signs of congestion/fluid retention then consider reducing diuretic. • Doses may be reduced if all else fails, but seek medical or heart failure team advice if unsure or in patients with severe disease.
Renal dysfunction	• If worsening renal function occurs, check for nephrotoxic drugs such as NSAIDs and stop these first. • Rises in creatinine of >20% but <50% are often acceptable and simply monitor the trend more closely (i.e. is it still rising or has it plateaued?). • If creatinine rises by >50%, half dose and monitor more closely. • If creatinine rises by >100%, stop the drug immediately and monitor more closely. Seek medical or heart failure team advice if unsure.
Hyperkalaemia	• Increases in potassium to ≤5.5 mmol/L are typically acceptable. • Increases in potassium >5.5 mmol/L but <6.0 mmol/L, consider halving dose and retest within a few days. • Increases in potassium >6.0 mmol/L, stop the drug immediately, seek medical or specialist heart failure team advice and monitor very closely (e.g. ideally retesting within a day).

Beta blockers[11,16]

These are used first line in all HF-REF patients NYHA I-IV as they improve survival, decrease hospitalisations and improve symptoms. Common evidence-based options include bisoprolol, carvedilol and nebivolol. Patients should be started on a low dose with the aim of reaching a target dose. Titrations can be considered 2 weeks after starting treatment. See *Table 11.4* for the starting doses and target doses of beta blockers.

Table 11.4: *Starting doses and target doses of beta blockers*[11]

Medication	Starting dose	Target dose
Bisoprolol	1.25 mg daily	10 mg daily
Carvedilol	3.125 mg twice daily	25 mg twice daily (or 50 mg twice daily if >85 kg)
Nebivolol	1.25 mg daily	10 mg daily

It is important to be aware of the contraindications and cautions to ensure they are suitable for the patient.
• Contraindications:
  — Asthma
  — 2nd or 3rd degree heart block
  — Decompensated heart failure (contraindicated for starting or increasing but no routine need to stop or reduce existing beta blockers)
  — Significant bradycardia

- Cautions:
  - NYHA Class IV
  - Recent worsening symptoms (e.g. worsening NYHA class, increasing levels of oedema, recent hospital admission with worsening symptoms etc)

Tight resting heart rate control (e.g. approximately 60 beats per minute) is beneficial in patients with sinus rhythm and HF-REF, and may have prognostic benefit. In sinus rhythm patients, aim for either a tight resting heart rate or the target dose used in clinical trials. Benefits of this aggressive up-titration, however, are less clear in patients with atrial fibrillation and a lenient heart rate target (e.g. 80-90 beats per minute) may be appropriate.

All people taking beta blockers should have their BP, pulse and clinical symptoms checked before therapy is initiated, every 1-2 weeks after starting and every 1-2 weeks after each titration. For information on the adverse effects of beta blockers and how to manage them, see *Table 11.5*.

Table 11.5: *Adverse effects of beta blockers and how to manage them*[11,16]

Adverse effect	Management options
Symptomatic low BP	• The absolute BP value is not important unless it is <90 mmHg systolic or the patient is symptomatic with dizziness. • If a patient is symptomatic with low BP or systolic <90 mmHg, review the need for other BP-lowering drugs. • If the patient has no signs of congestion/fluid retention then consider reducing diuretic. • Doses may be reduced if all else fails, but seek medical or heart failure team advice if unsure or in patients with severe disease.
Bradycardia	• Review other heart rate-lowering drugs (e.g. digoxin, amiodarone etc) and stop these before changing beta blocker if appropriate. • If this is not appropriate and pulse <50 bpm, consider halving dose of beta blocker and review in approximately one week. • If the patient has severe bradycardia then seek specialist heart failure team advice and consider stopping the beta blocker. • In all cases consider arranging an ECG to exclude heart block if the patient has no recent ECG on file.
Clinical worsening	• If there are increasing signs or symptoms of fluid overload (e.g. oedema, PND), increase the dose of loop diuretic for approximately three days and then review. • Doses of beta blocker may need to be reduced if this is unsuccessful. Seek specialist heart failure team advice if unsure. • In cases of significant deterioration always seeks heart failure team advice.

Box 11.3: Practice point: use of beta blockers

- Chronic obstructive pulmonary disease (COPD) is *NOT* an absolute contraindication to beta blockers. If reversibility on spirometry is negative then beta blockers can be trialled with caution.
- Peripheral vascular disease (PVD) is *NOT* an absolute contraindication to beta blockers. Patients with PVD have amongst the highest cardiovascular risk and beta blockers should be cautiously trialled. Seek specialist advice if unsure or in cases of severe PVD.
- It may not be appropriate to drive down the heart rate of patients with a beta blocker and a right ventricular pacemaker to a level where they are routinely dependently-paced as this may eventually worsen their heart failure. Seek specialist heart failure team advice.

Diuretics

Loop diuretics (furosemide, bumetanide) are used first line in all HF-REF patients NYHA I-IV. Thiazide diuretics (metolazone, bendroflumethiazide) may be added on in combination second line if needed – they should only be used under the advice of specialist heart failure teams. Diuretics improve symptoms of heart failure (e.g. shortness of breath, oedema). Typically start with a low-dose furosemide, such as 40 mg daily, and increase in increments of furosemide 40 mg until clinical improvement in symptoms. Patients with severe symptoms at presentation may need a higher initial starting dose or intravenous therapy.

Bumetanide has a better bioavailability than furosemide and it may be appropriate to switch from furosemide to bumetanide if sufficient diuretic response (i.e. euvolaemia) is not achieved.

If a patient needs high dose loop diuretics (e.g. furosemide 80 mg twice daily or bumetanide 2 mg twice daily) and still has signs of congestion, seek specialist heart failure team advice and consider combination diuretics (e.g. addition of thiazide diuretic in combination to loop).

Thiazide diuretics work synergistically with loop diuretics and may only need to be trialled once or twice weekly in the first instance. All these patients usually require specialist heart failure team input and monitoring. All people taking diuretics should have their U&Es and BP checked before initiation, 1-2 weeks after initiation and 1-2 weeks after each dose increase.

It is important to be aware of the contraindications and cautions to ensure they are suitable for the patient.

- Contraindications:
  — Hypovolaemia
  — Severe hypokalaemia
  — Severe hyponatraemia
- Cautions:
  — Hypotension
  — Electrolyte disturbances (particularly hypokalaemia or hyponatraemia)
  — Significant renal dysfunction
  — Gout

Adverse effects include renal worsening – haemoconcentration with diuretics can cause rises in creatinine and urea and therefore such changes are not necessarily a sign of kidney injury.[20] Remember to 'Treat the patient, not the blood test'[20]– appropriate clinical examination is vital before deciding on a management plan, including monitoring for new signs or symptoms of dehydration and/or hypotension.[20] Seek specialist advice from the heart failure team if needed.

Mineralocorticoid receptor antagonists (MRA)[11,16]

These are used second line in all HF-REF patients who remain NYHA II-IV, as they improve survival, decrease hospitalisations and improve symptoms. Common evidence-based options include spironolactone and eplerenone. Patients should be started on a low dose with the aim of reaching a target dose. Titrations can be considered 2 weeks after starting treatment. See *Table 11.6* for the starting doses and target doses of mineralocorticoid receptor antagonist.

Table 11.6: *Starting doses and target doses of mineralocorticoid receptor antagonists[11]*

Medication	Starting dose	Target dose
Spironolactone	25 mg daily	25-50 mg daily
Eplerenone	25 mg daily or 25 mg on alternate days	50 mg daily

It is important to be aware of the contraindications and cautions to ensure they are suitable for the patient.
- Contraindications:
  — Severe hyperkalaemia
  — Strong inhibitors of CYP3A4 (for eplerenone)

- Cautions:
  - Moderate hyperkalaemia (e.g. serum K^+ >5.0 mmol/L at initiation)
  - Previous episodes of severe hyperkalaemia
  - Significant renal dysfunction

All people taking mineralocorticoid receptor antagonists should have their U&Es and BP checked before initiation, 1-2 weeks after initiation and 1-2 weeks after each dose increase.

Adverse effects of mineralocorticoid receptor antagonists (low blood pressure, renal dysfunction and hyperkalaemia) are managed in the same way as ACEIs and ARBS; see *Table 11.3*.

Box 11.4: Practice point: MRAs and hyperkalaemia

There is a well known increased real-life incidence of hyperkalaemia in HF-REF patients taking MRA.[18,19] A longer and more intensive U&Es monitoring programme is needed, especially over the first year of therapy. This may involve checks at baseline, one week, two weeks and four weeks post-initiation and then may sequentially lengthen over the next few months. Seek local specialist heart failure team advice if needed, as local guidelines vary.

In addition, gynaecomastia is common with spironolactone (approximately 10% in clinical studies). These patients should be switched to eplerenone if this occurs and the problem should resolve.

Management of the adverse effects of an MRA (low blood pressure, renal dysfunction and hyperkalaemia) are managed similarly to ACEIs and ARBS, see *Table 11.3*.

Angiotensin receptor neprilsyn blocker (ARNI)

An ARNI is a third-line option in patients with HF-REF who remain NYHA II-IV and have left ventricular ejection fraction ≤40% despite ACEI (or ARB), beta blocker, loop diuretic and MRA as it improves survival, decreases hospitalisations and improves symptoms.

The Scottish Intercollegiate Guidelines Network (SIGN) has approved use in left ventricular ejection fraction ≤40%, but the National Institute for Health and Care Excellence (NICE) has only approved use for left ventricular systolic dysfunction ≤35%.[11,12] There is currently only one evidence-based option: sacubitril/valsartan. It is a single molecule with both an ARB (valsartan) and a neprilsyn blocker (sacubitril) attached.

Patients should be started on a low dose with the aim of reaching a target dose of 97/103 mg twice daily. Titrations can be considered 2 weeks after starting treatment. See *Table 11.7* for the starting doses depending on current therapy and other clinical considerations.

It is important to be aware of the contraindications and cautions to ensure they are suitable for the patient.

- Contraindications:
  - Concomitant use of ACEI
  - End-stage renal disease
  - Bilateral renal artery stenosis
  - Known history of angioedema related to previous ACEI or ARB/hereditary or idiopathic angioedema
  - Concomitant use with aliskiren
  - Severe hepatic impairment, biliary cirrhosis or cholestasis
  - Blood pressure <100 mmHg at initiation
- Cautions:
  - Unilateral renal artery stenosis
  - Hyperkalaemia
  - NYHA IV
  - Moderate hepatic impairment (e.g. AST/ALT values more than twice the upper limit of the normal range)

Table 11.7: *Sacubitril/valsartan starting doses*

Previous therapy	Additional considerations	Typical sacubitril/valsartan starting dose
Patients tolerating medium to high dose ACEI or ARB before switch		
ACEI or ARB prior to initiation ≥50% ESC target dose	SBP* >110 mmHg AND eGFR[†] >60 mL/min/1.73 m^2	49/51 mg twice daily[‡]
	SBP ≥100-110 mmHg AND/OR eGFR ≥30-60 mL/min/1.73 m^2	49/51 mg twice daily[‡] OR 24/26 mg twice daily at clinician discretion
	SBP ≥100 mmHg AND eGFR <30 mL/min/1.73 m^2	No safety data in this population, so extreme caution needed Bespoke local heart failure team decision needed before starting
Patients tolerating low dose ACEI or ARB before switch		
ACEI or ARB prior to initiation <50% ESC target dose	SBP ≥100 mmHg AND eGFR ≥30 mL/min/1.73 m^2	24/26 mg twice daily
	SBP ≥100 mmHg AND eGFR <30 mL/min/1.73 m^2	No safety data in this population, so extreme caution needed Bespoke local heart failure team decision needed before starting

*systolic blood pressure.
[†] estimated glomerular filtration rate.
[‡] patients with AST/ALT more than twice the normal reference range should be started on 24/26 mg twice daily.

Box 11.5: Practice point: ARNI

- An ARNI is used instead of an ACEI or ARB, not in addition to it.
- Wash-out period: if the patient is already prescribed an ACEI, the ACEI *MUST* be stopped 36 hours prior to initiation of sacubitril/valsartan to minimise the risk of angioedema. The importance of this wash-out period must *ALWAYS* be communicated directly to the patient. No wash-out period is needed with an ARB.

All people taking an ARNI should have their U&Es, BP and LFTs checked before initiation, and the BP and U&Es rechecked 1-2 weeks after initiation and 1-2 weeks after each dose increase.

Management of the adverse effects of an ARNI (low blood pressure, renal dysfunction and hyperkalaemia) are managed similarly to ACEIs and ARBS; see *Table 11.3*. Any significant adverse drug reactions should have a Yellow Card completed.

I$_f$ channel blockers

These are used third line in HF-REF patients NYHA II-IV and left ventricular ejection fraction ≤35% and sinus rhythm who are not adequately heart-rate controlled (i.e. ≥75 bpm) despite optimal background therapy of ACEI (or ARB or ARNI), beta blocker, loop diuretic and MRA.

They reduce heart failure hospital admission mainly but do not affect mortality. Ivabradine is currently the only licensed evidence-based option.

The patient's heart rate should be checked before starting, and ivabradine therapy only initiated if it is ≥75 bpm. The normal starting dose is 5 mg twice daily. This can be increased to 7.5 mg twice daily if the resting heart rate is persistently above 60 bpm and decreased to 2.5 mg twice daily (one half 5 mg tablet twice daily) if resting heart rate is persistently below 50 bpm. If the heart rate is between 50 and 60 bpm, the dose of 5 mg twice daily should be maintained.

It is important to be aware of the contraindications and cautions to ensure they are suitable for the patient.

- Contraindications:
  - Atrial fibrillation
  - Pacemaker dependent
  - Acute phase of myocardial infarction
  - Unstable angina
  - Acute phase of heart failure
  - Severe hypotension (<90/50 mmHg)
  - Severe hepatic insufficiency
  - Resting heart rate below 70 beats per minute prior to treatment
  - Sick sinus syndrome/sino-atrial block/2nd and 3rd degree AV block
  - Strong cytochrome P450 3A4 inhibitors
- Cautions:
  - Prolonged QT interval

The risk of developing atrial fibrillation is increased in ivabradine patients. Patients should be clinically monitored regularly for the occurrence of atrial fibrillation. This should include ECG if new palpitations or irregular pulses occur. Adverse effects of ivabradine and how to manage them are detailed in *Table 11.8*.

Table 11.8: *Adverse effects of ivabradine and how to manage them*

Adverse effect	Management options
Bradycardia	• If heart rate decreases below 50 bpm at rest, the dose must be reduced to the next lower dose. • Treatment must be discontinued if heart rate remains below 50 bpm or symptoms of bradycardia persist. Seek specialist heart failure team advice if needed.
Visual disturbances	• Ivabradine can influence retinal function. If visual flares or blurring (or other visual disturbance) occurs, consider stopping treatment.

Drug interactions

Details of important drug interactions with heart failure medicines are outlined in *Table 11.9*.

Table 11.9: *Common drug interactions and how to manage them*

Drug	Interactions and how to manage them
ACEI or ARB	• Potassium salts (including dietary 'low salt' substitutes) – these should generally be avoided due to risk of hyperkalaemia • Sacubitril/valsartan – ACEI should <u>never</u> be used in combination • Triple therapy – ACEI + ARB + MRA is not recommended • NSAIDs – increased risk of hyperkalaemia; consider monitoring urea and electrolytes
Beta blocker	• Rate limiting calcium channel blockers like verapamil and diltiazem – stop these as they are harmful in HF-REF • Digoxin/amiodarone – review for ongoing need; these are less beneficial in HF-REF
Diuretics	• NSAIDs
Mineralocorticoid receptor antagonist	• Potassium salts (including dietary 'low salt' substitutes) – these should generally be avoided due to risk of hyperkalaemia • Triple therapy (ACEI + ARB + MRA) is not recommended • NSAIDs – antihypertensive effect may be antagonised and there is a risk of hyperkalaemia; monitor diuretic effect, renal function and potassium levels • Inhibitors/inducers of CYP3A4 (for eplerenone) – amiodarone is commonly used in combination and is a mild to moderate CYP3A4 inhibitors; in such cases the eplerenone dose should not exceed 25 mg daily

Table 11.9: *Common drug interactions and how to manage them (continued)*

Drug	Interactions and how to manage them
ARNI	• Atorvastatin – sacubitril/valsartan can increase peak serum concentrations of atorvastatin by up to two fold and total exposure by up to 1.3 fold; monitor liver function tests and monitor for myalgia; doses of atorvastatin may need to be reduced if problems are encountered • Potassium salts (including dietary 'low salt' substitutes) – these should generally be avoided due to risk of hyperkalaemia • NSAIDs – increased risk of hyperkalaemia; consider monitoring urea and electrolytes
I_f channel blockers	• Verapamil or diltiazem should be avoided – both are moderate CYP3A4 inhibitors

Other treatment options and considerations

Fourth-line treatment options

These are rarely used, but include:

- Cardiac glycosides (digoxin) – HF-REF sinus rhythm patients NYHA II-IV despite optimal background therapy of ACEI or ARB or ARNI, beta blocker, loop diuretic and MRA (reduces the risk of all-cause and heart failure hospitalisations).[2]
- Vasodilators (hydralazine, isosorbide dinitrate) – HF-REF patients with:
  - left ventricular ejection fraction ≤35% (or <45% and a dilated left ventricle) and NYHA III-IV despite treatment with an ACEI or ARB or ARNI, beta blocker, loop diuretic and MRA (reduces risk of HF hospitalisation and death).[2]
  - NYHA II-IV that cannot tolerate ACEI or ARB or ARNI, typically due to renal function (reduce the risk of death).[2]

New treatments (not licensed yet)

At the time of writing (November 2019), the DAPA-HF study had just been published showing mortality and morbidity benefit for the use of dapagliflozin (a sodium-glucose transport protein 2 (SGLT2)) in HF-REF and NYHA II-IV with or without diabetes.[21] However, so far this is not licensed or guideline-based, but this will likely change in the future.

Common drugs to avoid in heart failure

These are numerous medications that are known to either cause or worsen heart failure, so these are not recommended in patients with HF-REF, including:

- NSAIDs or COX-2 inhibitors – they increase the risk of worsening heart failure and hospitalisation.[11,12]
- Thiazolidinediones (glitazones) – they increase the risk of worsening heart failure and hospitalisation.[11,12]
- Rate-limiting calcium channel blockers (e.g. diltiazem or verapamil) – they increase the risk of worsening heart failure and hospitalisation.[11,12]

Special groups

Pregnancy and breastfeeding[22]

All pregnant patients with HF should be managed by a specialist multidisciplinary team. Drugs which should be avoided in pregnancy include ACEIs, ARBs, MRAs, ARNI and I_f channel blockers. Beta blockers and diuretics can be used with caution after specialist advice. In women who are breastfeeding ARNI, ARBs and I_f channel blockers should be avoided, while MRAs (usually spironolactone), ACEIs, beta blockers and diuretics can be used with caution after specialist advice.

Non-pharmacological treatments: complex devices

Heart failure is not just treated with medicine, complex cardiac devices may be appropriate in some patients, including:

- Implantable cardioverter-defibrillator (ICD) – ICDs may be suitable for primary prevention of sudden cardiac death for patients who remain symptomatic (NYHA II-III) despite optimal medical therapy with a left ventricular ejection fraction ≤35% to reduce the risk of sudden cardiac death. ICD is also indicated for secondary prevention of sudden cardiac death (i.e. those with previous cardiac arrest) in NYHA I-III.[2]
- Cardiac resynchronisation therapy (CRT) – CRT with a defibrillator (CRT-D) or without (CRT-P) may be suitable to improve symptoms and reduce morbidity and mortality in HF-REF patients with left ventricular ejection fraction ≤35% and NYHA I-IV despite optimal medical therapy and a broad QRS on ECG (depending on exact QRS width and morphology).[11]

Advanced treatment options

Left ventricular assist devices (LVADS) and cardiac transplant may be appropriate in very small numbers of patients only. These interventions require assessment at sub-specialist tertiary hospitals. All such decisions should be taken by the heart failure team.

Follow-up and onward referral

Primary care follow-up

The primary care team should take over routine management of heart failure as soon as it has been stabilised and its management optimised.[12] This may involve general practice, specialist community care teams and/or pharmacy and varies across the UK.

The primary care team should carry out the following for people with heart failure at all times, including periods when the person is also receiving specialist heart failure care from the specialist team:[12]

- Ensure effective communication links between different care settings and clinical services involved in the person's care.
- Lead a full review of the person's heart failure care, which may form part of a long-term conditions review.
- Recall the person at least every 6 months and update the clinical record (this period should be shortened during times of clinical instability).
- Ensure that changes to the clinical record are understood and agreed by the person with heart failure and shared with the specialist heart failure team.
- Arrange access to specialist heart failure services if needed (i.e. at diagnosis or after a heart failure-related hospitalisation).

Secondary care input

People should be referred, or managed, by secondary care in the following circumstances:

- Suspected heart failure: because very high levels of NT-proBNP (natriuretic peptide) carry a poor prognosis. People with suspected heart failure and an NT-proBNP level above 2,000 ng/litre (236 pmol/litre) should be referred urgently to have specialist assessment and echo within 2 weeks.[12] People with suspected heart failure and an NT-proBNP level between 400 and 2,000 ng/litre (47 to 236 pmol/litre) should be referred to have specialist assessment and echo within 6 weeks.[12]

- Post diagnosis: the specialist heart failure team should offer people newly diagnosed with heart failure an extended first consultation within 2 weeks of confirming the diagnosis.[12]
- Post heart failure hospitalisation: any patient who has been admitted to hospital with worsening heart failure – both patients with a new diagnosis (i.e. incident) or already known to have heart failure (i.e. prevalent) – should be followed up by the heart failure team. Patients who are not followed up by the specialist team are known to have worse mortality at one-year post-discharge.[4] This can commonly occur when patients are admitted to a non-cardiology ward during their inpatient stay.[4] Primary care teams should be encouraged to actively refer these patients to specialist teams if this has not happened.

Palliative care

Despite the mortality benefits of modern pharmacological and device therapies, heart failure has a worse prognosis than many cancers.[5,6] Patients with heart failure often have less access to social and palliative support and are less informed about their condition, and symptom relief is often inadequate. Ways to improve this picture include:

- If the symptoms of a person with heart failure are worsening despite optimal specialist treatment, discuss their palliative care needs with the specialist heart failure multidisciplinary team and consider a needs assessment for palliative care.[12]
- Do not use prognostic risk tools to determine whether to refer a person with heart failure to palliative care services.[12]
- Patients' and carers' needs should be addressed by an early and phased implementation of palliative care support by all healthcare professionals involved in their care, in combination with active conventional treatment.[11]
- A shared care approach between primary care, including pharmacy, and cardiology and specialist palliative support services should be adopted.[11]

Useful resources

This chapter was written in November 2019 but heart failure is a clinical field with lots of innovation and research and therefore advice may change in the future.

Suggested additional reading

- For advanced guidance on the use of diuretics in heart failure:
  - The use of diuretics in heart failure with congestion – a position statement from the Heart Failure Association of the European Society of Cardiology. *Eur J Heart Fail* 2019; 21(2): 137-155[23]
  - 2016 ESC Guidelines for the diagnosis and treatment of acute and chronic heart failure. *Eur Heart J* 2016; 37(27): 2129-2200[2]
  - Dapagliflozin in patients with heart failure and reduced ejection fraction. *N Engl J Med* 2019; Epub ahead of print[21]
- For an in-depth list of medications known to cause of worsen heart failure:
  - Drugs That May Cause or Exacerbate Heart Failure: A Scientific Statement From the American Heart Association. *Circulation* 2016; 134: e32-e69[24]
  - Indications for Cardiac Resynchronization Therapy: A Comparison of the Major International Guidelines. *JACC Heart Fail* 2018; 6(4): 308-316[25]

- Advanced heart failure: a position statement of the Heart Failure Association of the European Society of Cardiology. *Eur J Heart Fail* 2018; 20(11): 1505-1535[26]
- Palliative care in patients with heart failure. *BMJ* 2016; 353: i1010[27]

Guidelines

Up-to-date clinical guidelines for heart failure can be found on the websites of the following organisations and societies:

- National Institute for Health and Care Excellence
- Scottish Intercollegiate Guidelines Network
- European Society of Cardiology
- American Heart Association

Key patient resources

- British Heart Foundation
- Pumping Marvellous
- Chest Heart & Stroke Scotland (Charity)
- Cardiomyopathy UK (Charity)

References

1. McMurray JJV *et al*. ESC Committee for Practice Guidelines. ESC guidelines for the diagnosis and treatment of acute and chronic heart failure 2012: the task force for the diagnosis and treatment of acute and chronic heart failure 2012 of the European Society of Cardiology. Developed in collaboration with the Heart Failure Association (HFA) of the ESC. *Eur Heart J* 2012; 33(14): 1787-1847.

2. Ponikowski P *et al*. 2016 ESC Guidelines for the diagnosis and treatment of acute and chronic heart failure. *Eur Heart J* 2016; 37(27): 2129-2200.

3. Mosterd A, Hoes AW. Clinical epidemiology of heart failure. *Heart* 2007; 93(9): 1137-1146.

4. National Institute for Cardiovascular Outcomes Research (2018). National cardiac audit programme national heart failure audit 2016/17 summary report. www.nicor.org.uk/wp-content/uploads/2018/11/Heart-Failure-Summary-Report-2016-17.pdf

5. Stewart S *et al*. More 'malignant' than cancer? Five-year survival following a first admission for heart failure. *Eur J Heart Fail* 2001; 3(3): 315-22.

6. Mamas MA *et al*. Do patients have worse outcomes in heart failure than in cancer? A primary care-based cohort study with 10-year follow-up in Scotland. *Eur J Heart Fail* 2017; 19: 1095-1104.

7. Koshman S *et al*. Pharmacist care of patients with heart failure a systematic review of randomized trials. *Arch Intern Med* 2008; 168: 687-694.

8. Parajuli DR *et al*. Effectiveness of the pharmacist-involved multidisciplinary management of heart failure to improve hospitalizations and mortality rates in 4630 patients: a systematic review and meta-analysis of randomized controlled trials. *J Card Fail* 2019; 25(9):744-756.

9. Milfred-LaForest SK *et al*. Clinical pharmacy services in heart failure: an opinion paper from the Heart Failure Society of America and American College of Clinical Pharmacy Cardiology Practice and Research Network. *Pharmacotherapy* 2013; 33(5): 529-548.

10. Forsyth P *et al*. A competency framework for clinical pharmacists and heart failure. *Int J Pharm Pract* 2019; 27: 424-435.

11. Scottish Intercollegiate Guidelines Network (2016). SIGN 147 Management of chronic heart failure: a national clinical guideline. www.sign.ac.uk/assets/sign147.pdf

12. National Institute for Health and Care Excellence (2018). Chronic heart failure in adults: diagnosis and management. www.nice.org.uk/guidance/ng106

13. Murray MD *et al*. Pharmacist intervention to improve medication adherence in heart failure: a randomized trial. *Ann Intern Med* 2007; 146(10): 714-25.

14. Schulz M *et al*. PHARM-CHF Investigators. Pharmacy-based interdisciplinary intervention for patients with chronic heart failure: results of the PHARM-CHF randomized controlled trial. *Eur J Heart Fail* 2019; 21(8): 1012-1021.

15. Sabaté E ed. Adherence to Long-Term Therapies: Evidence for Action. Geneva, Switzerland: World Health Organization, 2003. www.apps.who.int/iris/bitstream/10665/42682/1/9241545992.pdf

16. McMurray J *et al*. Practical recommendations for the use of ACE inhibitors, beta blockers, aldosterone antagonists and angiotensin receptor blockers in heart failure: putting guidelines into practice. *Eur J Heart Fail* 2005; 7(5): 710-21.

17. Think Kidneys (2018). "Sick day" guidance in patients at risk of acute kidney injury: a position statement from the Think Kidneys board. www.thinkkidneys.nhs.uk/aki/wp-content/uploads/sites/2/2018/01/Think-Kidneys-Sick-Day-Guidance-2018.pdf

18. Juurlink DN *et al*. Rates of hyperkalemia after publication of the Randomized Aldactone Evaluation Study. *N Engl J Med* 2004; 351(6): 543-51.

19. Medicines and Healthcare products Regulatory Agency (MHRA) (2016). Spironolactone and renin-angiotensin system drugs in heart failure: risk of potentially fatal hyperkalaemia—clarification. www.gov.uk/drug-safety-update/spironolactone-and-renin-angiotensin-system-drugs-in-heart-failure-risk-of-potentially-fatal-hyperkalaemia-clarification

20. Think Kidneys (2017). Changes in kidney function and serum potassium during ACEI/ARB/diuretic treatment in primary care: a position statement from Think Kidneys, the Renal Association, and the British Society for Heart Failure. www.thinkkidneys.nhs.uk/aki/wp-content/uploads/sites/2/2019/07/RA-BSH-2019-Changes-in-Kidney-Function-FINAL.pdf

21. McMurray JJV *et al*. DAPA-HF Trial Committees and Investigators. Dapagliflozin patients with heart failure and reduced ejection fraction. *N Engl J Med* 2019: epub ahead of print.

22. Bauersachs J *et al*. Pathophysiology, diagnosis and management of peripartum cardiomyopathy: a position statement from the Heart Failure Association of the European Society of Cardiology Study Group on peripartum cardiomyopathy. *Eur J Heart Fail* 2019; 21(7): 827-843.

23. Mullens W *et al*. The use of diuretics in heart failure with congestion - a position statement from the Heart Failure Association of the European Society of Cardiology. *Eur J Heart Fail* 2019; 21(2): 137-155.

24. Page PL *et al*. Drugs that may cause or exacerbate heart failure: a scientific statement from the American Heart Association. *Circulation* 2016; 134: e32-e69.

25. Normand C *et al*. Indications for cardiac resynchronization therapy: a comparison of the major international guidelines. *JACC Heart Fail* 2018; 6(4): 308-316.

26. Crespo-Leiro MG *et al*. Advanced heart failure: a position statement of the Heart Failure Association of the European Society of Cardiology. *Eur J Heart Fail* 2018; 20(11): 1505-1535.

27. McIlvennan CK, Allen LA. Palliative care in patients with heart failure. *BMJ* 2016; 353: i1010.

Case studies

Case study 1

George, aged 70 years, has heart failure with reduced ejection fraction (LVEF 35%), coronary heart disease (previous myocardial infarction eight years ago), type 2 diabetes and hypertension. He is a retired plumber, enjoys playing golf and lives with his wife, Agnes.

His regular medication is as follows:

- Enalapril 10 mg twice daily
- Bisoprolol 5 mg daily
- Furosemide 40 mg morning
- Aspirin 75 mg morning
- Atorvastatin 80 mg night
- Amlodipine 5 mg morning
- Metformin 500 mg twice daily

He has come to the surgery for review at your cardiovascular clinic.

Points to consider

- Are these drugs and doses suitable?
- What questions would you ask?
- What assessments would you carry out?
- What investigations would you undertake?

You measure his blood pressure (BP) and pulse. His BP is 155/90 mmHg and pulse 70 bpm (regular). He is NYHA II, which is a slight decline over the last six months. He is now struggling a little more with breathlessness when he plays golf – previously he managed 18 holes without limitation. He has no peripheral oedema and no PND/orthopnoea. His chest sounds were clear and he reports no chest pain. U&Es were normal (creatinine 90 micromols/L, eGFR >60 mL/min, potassium 4.4 mmol/L), HbA1C 45 mmol/mol, total cholesterol 3.4 mmol/L and LDL-cholesterol 1.4 mmol/L.

Points to consider

- What issues do you think need to be addressed?
- What are the priorities?
- What are the possible options?

After discussion with George you decide to start spironolactone 25 mg daily – this improves prognosis (e.g. mortality and hospitalisation risk). It may also improve his symptoms of breathlessness and consequently his quality of life.

Points to consider

- What is a suitable follow-up period for the next appointment?
- What benefits would you expect to see and how would you measure them?
- Are there any adverse effects or interactions you need to consider?

You arrange a follow-up review in 1-2 weeks to check on his progress and to update his bloods.

> **Points to consider**
>
> - What other changes to George's current medicines would be appropriate?
> - Are there any additional treatment options to consider?

After discussion with George you agree on a medium-term plan to optimise the beta blocker if he remains clinically stable, and aim for a resting pulse of approximately 60 bpm. Other plans include optimising the enalapril dose to 20 mg twice daily if blood pressure and renal function allow. Blood pressure should improve with spironolactone initiation and ACE inhibitor/beta blocker optimisation, but this should be kept under close review.

If George remains NYHA II he may also be suitable for sacubitril/valsartan and other advanced measures like complex devices – if this happens you will need to liaise with local specialist heart failure teams.

Case study 2

Betty, aged 82 years, has heart failure with reduced ejection fraction (LVEF 40%), atrial fibrillation, stroke, and depression. She is a widow who lives alone, with little social or family support.

Her regular medication is as follows:

- Candesartan 8 mg morning
- Bisoprolol 1.25 mg daily
- Furosemide 20 mg morning
- Apixaban 5 mg twice daily
- Bendroflumethiazide 2.5 mg morning
- Atorvastatin 40 mg night
- Paracetamol 500 mg four times daily
- Sertraline 50 mg daily

She has come to the community pharmacy and seems to be getting mixed up with her medicines. She also admits to increasing forgetfulness. When you check the PMR you notice that all her medicines are running out of sync and her ordering history is erratic which suggests that she is non-adherent with her medicines. She is NYHA I and has bilateral pitting oedema to the high ankle. She reports no PND or orthopnoea, and her BP was 106/50 mmHg and pulse 79 bpm and irregular.

> **Points to consider**
>
> - Do you have any concerns about Betty's medicine regimen?
> - What can you do to help with current problems?
> - What would you discuss with Betty?

You ask Betty to bring all her medicines into the pharmacy and she goes home and returns with them. You look at all her medicines to work out what she has and how many of each.

You confirm her understanding of why she is taking the medication and how it should be taken – she has a good understanding of this. She also has no problems opening the packets, reading the labels or swallowing the preparations.

> **Points to consider**
>
> - What steps could you take to help Betty?
> - Is there anything you need to consider if Betty suddenly starts to take her tablets as intended?

After a discussion with Betty you agree an action plan, phone her GP surgery and organise the following:

- New prescriptions for her medication to allow everything to run in sync.
- Discuss with the GP that a cognition assessment may be appropriate as she seems to be increasingly forgetful.
- Organise a follow-up check with the practice nurse for blood pressure, pulse and blood tests (U&E, liver function tests, cholesterol and full blood count), as you are concerned that these factors should be monitored if her medication adherence improves over time. If her renal function (creatinine clearance) changes then this may also impact on what apixaban dose is appropriate for her, and this should be reviewed once this test is updated.

You develop a follow-up plan to monitor medication adherence at every review. This may involve liaising with social care, helping her manage her repeat ordering of prescriptions and potentially organising a weekly compliance aid if things do not improve over time.

CHAPTER 12

Hypertension

Helen Williams

Overview

Hypertension, also known as high or raised blood pressure (BP), is a condition in which the pressure in the blood vessels is elevated to a degree which could cause adverse outcomes. Hypertension is defined as a clinic systolic blood pressure ≥140 mmHg and/or clinic diastolic blood pressure ≥90 mmHg, with lower diagnostic thresholds if hypertension is diagnosed by ambulatory blood pressure morning (ABPM) or home blood pressure monitoring (HBPM).

The World Health Organization has identified hypertension as the leading risk factor for death worldwide.[1] It occurs very commonly, affecting over one in four of the adult population in the UK, increasing to one in every two people aged over 60 years.[2,3]

In 90-95% of cases of hypertension, there is no underlying medical illness to cause high blood pressure. The remaining 5-10% of cases are secondary to some other diseases – see *Box 12.1*.

Box 12.1: Secondary causes of hypertension[4]

- Kidney disease
- Adrenal diseases (e.g. pheochromocytoma, Conn's syndrome or primary aldosteronism and Cushing's syndrome)
- Hyperparathyroidism
- Thyroid dysfunction
- Coarctation (constriction or tightening) of the aorta
- Obstructive sleep apnoea
  - Adverse effects from certain medicines can also contribute to secondary hypertension – e.g. hormonal contraceptives, non-steroidal anti-inflammatory agents (NSAIDs), stimulants, some antidepressants, immune system suppressants and decongestants

---

A number of factors increase the risk of developing high blood pressure including smoking, being overweight or obese, excess dietary salt, lack of physical activity, excess alcohol consumption, stress, increasing age, family history and chronic kidney disease.

Hypertension is more common in black people of African or Caribbean family origin, who are also at particular risk of stroke and renal failure.[5] Persistently raised blood pressure increases the risk of an individual experiencing a cardiovascular event, such as a stroke or myocardial infarction, or developing heart failure or chronic kidney disease. The risk associated with increasing blood pressure is continuous with each 2 mmHg rise in systolic blood pressure associated with a 7% increased risk of mortality from ischaemic heart disease and a 10% increased risk of mortality from stroke.[1]

High blood pressure is one of the three main modifiable risk factors for cardiovascular disease (CVD) which accounts for 80% of all cases of premature coronary heart disease.[1] Lowering BP reduces cardiovascular morbidity and mortality – the more the BP is lowered, the greater the benefit. Studies have shown that a 10 mmHg (systolic) or 5 mmHg (diastolic) reduction in BP results in a 22% reduction in the risk of coronary heart disease and 41% reduction in the risk of stroke.[6] Currently in England, only about 70% of those expected to have high blood pressure are diagnosed with the condition and only 67% of adults below the age of 80 years with a hypertension diagnosis are achieving a target blood pressure of <140/90 mmHg.[7,8]

Diagnosis

Hypertension is asymptomatic in most cases and is often, therefore, an incidental finding when people present with unrelated conditions, or it may be identified during a cardiovascular risk assessment. If blood pressure is very high (systolic BP >180 mmHg), patients may complain of headaches or visual disturbances. Prolonged high blood pressure will lead to the development of target organ damage – for example, stroke or transient ischaemic attack (TIA), ischaemic heart disease, renal failure or retinopathy. Adults, particularly those aged over 40 years, should have their blood pressure checked at least every 5 years, with an annual review for those with high normal values in the range 135-139 mmHg systolic or 85-89 mmHg diastolic.

If a patient presents with a high blood pressure reading (BP <140/90 mmHg), the diagnosis should be confirmed by ABPM with a diagnostic threshold of BP persistently >135/85 mmHg. ABPM should be undertaken as earlier as possible after a one-off high BP reading has been recorded and can be performed in community pharmacy or by pharmacists in other settings.

Box 12.2: Practice point: ambulatory blood pressure monitoring (ABPM)

- ABPM uses a portable automated BP monitoring device to monitor an individual's BP, usually over 24 hours. Readings are taken every 30 minutes during the daytime (or waking) hours and every hour overnight (or whilst asleep). The daytime (or waking hours) average BP should be used to confirm a diagnosis of hypertension. Care should be taken to ensure the daytime average is calculated from at least 14 successful BP readings to give an accurate result.
- ABPM is the most accurate method for confirming a diagnosis of hypertension and it correlates closely with the risk of blood pressure-related clinical events. The use of ABPM reduces the number of patients with white coat hypertension being inappropriately diagnosed and treated for hypertension.

If ABPM is not suitable, not tolerated or the patient declines, HBPM over 7 days can be used as an alternative with the same diagnostic threshold. Clinic-based BP readings should not be used to confirm a hypertension diagnosis due to the increased risk of white coat hypertension. If a very high blood pressure is recorded in the clinic setting (BP >180/120 mmHg) the patient should be assessed and treated without waiting for the results of an ABPM.

Pharmacy input

There is a significant opportunity for pharmacists to improve outcomes for patients by increased detection and better management of hypertension. Ensuring a BP check is undertaken in adults presenting to GP surgeries will improve detection, while opportunistic blood pressure checks within community pharmacy have the potential to reach a cohort of people not currently engaging with GPs.

All adults aged over 40 years should have a CV risk assessment every five years – this should include calculation of the CV risk score. This consultation will allow the patients and clinicians to revisit any lifestyle issues which need to be addressed, as well as identify individuals who may now require intervention with drug therapy to lower their risk. GP practices and, in many areas of England, community pharmacies are commissioned to deliver NHS health checks which is a comprehensive risk assessment programme and is another opportunity to improve detection.

Patients with a diagnosis of hypertension should be supported through lifestyle change and, if appropriate, initiation and escalation of antihypertensive therapies, an ideal role for practice-based pharmacists, while ongoing adherence support can be delivered in both GP practice or via community pharmacy.

Pharmacy review

Once a diagnosis of hypertension has been confirmed, the patient will need a full assessment including examination, investigations including blood tests, assessment of CV risk and then intervention to manage the high BP and, if appropriate, lower the CV risk.

In the clinic setting, BP should be measured using a validated manual or automated sphygmomanometer which should be well maintained and regularly calibrated. When using an automated BP machine, the pulse should be palpated prior to the BP being checked – if the pulse is irregular the BP should be measured manually. Blood pressure should initially be measured in both arms and the arm with the highest BP reading used for subsequent monitoring. If there is a difference of more than 15 mmHg between readings from both arms, this warrants further investigation. If the blood pressure measured in the clinic is 140/90 mmHg or higher, a second measurement should be taken; if the second measurement is substantially different from the first (>5 mmHg), a third measurement should be taken. The lower of the last two readings should be recorded as the clinic BP.

If patients have a clinic BP of 180/120 mmHg or more, care should be taken to identify any red flags which would indicate that same day specialist assessment is warranted. For example, signs of retinal haemorrhage or papilloedema (oedema of the optic disc), life-threatening symptoms such as new-onset confusion, chest pain, signs of heart failure, acute kidney injury or suspected phaeochromocytoma (for example, labile or postural hypotension, headache, palpitations, pallor, abdominal pain or diaphoresis).[9]

Box 12.3: Practice point: identifying postural hypotension

To identify postural hypotension, sitting and standing blood pressure should be measured in people:[9]
- with type 2 diabetes
- symptoms of postural hypotension
- aged 80 years and over.

Patients can be encouraged to purchase a home BP monitor and check their BP at home, for example morning and evening for 3 days at the beginning of every month. The British and Irish Hypertension Society (BIHS) assessed BP monitoring devices for home use and a list of validated devices can be found at www.bihsoc.org/bp-monitors/for-home-use.

Patients home BP readings are often lower than clinic BP readings, and therefore adjusted targets apply.

Clinic BP	Equivalent home BP
140/90 mmHg	135/85 mmHg
150/90 mmHg	145/85 mmHg
160/100 mmHg	150/95 mmHg
180/120 mmHg	170/115 mmHg

Investigations should include blood tests to assess renal function, thyroid function, lipid levels, liver function tests and HbA1c, as well as urine albumin:creatinine ratio (ACR) and an ECG to assess for left ventricular hypertrophy. The presence of any other target organ damage should be identified by reviewing the past medical history, including cardiac (ischaemic heart disease or heart failure), brain (prior stroke or transient ischaemic attack), chronic kidney disease, peripheral arterial disease and retinopathy. Possible contributory factors such as smoking, obesity, excess alcohol or salt intake and lack of exercise should be considered and any family history of premature CV disease in a first-degree relative documented.[9]

Hypertension should not be seen as a risk factor in isolation and decisions on management should not focus on blood pressure alone, but on the total cardiovascular risk for an individual. In the absence of established CV disease, this should be calculated using a validated CV risk calculator.

Box 12.4: Practice point: tools for assessing CVD risk

- England and Wales – NICE recommends the use of the QRISK2® risk calculator (www.qrisk.org)
- Scotland – ASSIGN (www.assign-score.com)
- Europe – SCORE (www.heartscore.org)

The CVD risk assessment tools assess the risk of developing CVD based on multiple risk factors including age, gender, ethnicity, smoking status, lipid profile, systolic blood pressure, BMI, diabetes mellitus and family history of premature CVD.

The presence of established CVD or other target organ damage, diabetes or a moderate to high CV risk (>10% over 10 years) indicate a higher risk of CV events and the need for more aggressive intervention to lower the blood pressure.[9]

Lifestyle modification

Lifestyle modification is a key element of management for all people with hypertension. It is the primary strategy in people with BP between 140/90 mmHg and 160/100 mmHg and who are at low risk of cardiovascular events, and therefore do not meet the threshold for drug treatment. Tailor lifestyle advice to the individual patient, and where appropriate cover:

- smoking cessation
- diet including salt intake (aiming for 6 g per day from all sources)[10]
- physical activity
- weight loss
- alcohol consumption.
  See *Table 12.1* for the impact of lifestyle modifications on blood pressure

Table 12.1: *Impact of lifestyle modifications on blood pressure*

Modification	Recommendation	Approximate systolic blood pressure reduction (mmHg)*
Weight loss	Maintain normal body weight	5-20 per 10 kg weight loss
DASH-type diet (Dietary Approaches to Stop Hypertension)	Consume a diet rich in fruits, vegetables, and low-fat dairy products with reduced saturated and total fat	8-14
Reduced salt intake	Reduce daily dietary sodium intake	2-8
Physical activity	Regular aerobic physical activity (at least 30 min/day, most days of the week)	4-9
Moderation of alcohol intake	Limit consumption to 2 drinks/day in men and 1 drink/day in women and lighter-weight people	2-4

*Effects of implementing these modifications are time and dose dependent and could be greater for some patients.
Adapted from DiPiro JT *et al*. Pharmacotherapy: A Pathophysiologic Approach, 7th Edition.

Encourage the person to identify their priorities in terms of lifestyle changes and set goals for achievement over subsequent weeks and months. Support the discussion with written advice and refer or signpost to relevant local services to support their efforts to address these issues.

For people whose BP is between 140/90 mmHg and 160/100 mmHg and who are at low risk of cardiovascular events, lifestyle approaches to management of high BP are currently the only recommended intervention. In patients with BP >160/100 mmHg or >140/90 mmHg with evidence of target organ damage, or who are at moderate to high risk of CV events (QRISK2® >10% over 10 years), lifestyle modification should occur in parallel with the initiation of drug therapy.[9]

Medication

People with BP >160/100 mmHg or those whose BP >140/90 mmHg with evidence of target organ damage, or high CV risk (>10% over 10 years), will require antihypertensive drug therapy. The optimal blood pressure treatment target has not been established. Current guidance in England, Wales and Northern Ireland recommends that patients below the age of 80 years old should be treated to achieve a target BP <140/90 mmHg, while those of 80 years or over should be treated to achieve a target BP <150/90 mmHg.[9] In Scotland, the target blood pressure for uncomplicated hypertension is BP <140/90 mmHg, with a lower target of <135/85 mmHg for individuals with established CVD and diabetes, chronic renal disease or target organ damage.[11]

Table 12.2: *Target blood pressures in uncomplicated hypertension*[9]

Age	Clinic BP target	ABPM/HBPM target (average daytime BP)
Under 80 years	<140/90 mmHg	<135/85 mmHg
Over 80 years	<150/90 mmHg	<145/85 mmHg

In general, clinic blood pressure readings should be used to monitor blood pressure, unless there is a significant element of white coat hypertension, when HBPM or ABPM should be considered.

Patients with severe hypertension (>180/120 mmHg) confirmed by several readings on the same occasion should be assessed and treated immediately. Some international guidelines suggest that dual therapy should be commenced together in patients with blood pressure >20 mmHg above their target as monotherapy is unlikely to be fully effective.

Drug selection should consider efficacy, safety, convenience to the patient and cost, and UK guidelines recommend that the choice is guided by age and ethnicity of the patient to maximise effectiveness.

- Step 1
  - An initial choice of an angiotensin-converting enzyme inhibitor (ACEI) such as ramipril, or angiotensin II receptor blocker (ARB) such as candesartan is recommended as first-line therapy in younger (aged <55 years) non-black patients. Younger patients often have hypertension associated with high concentrations of circulating renin and therefore drugs that antagonise the renin-angiotensin system are likely to be effective.
  - For patients aged 55 years or older and patients of black African or Caribbean family origin of any age who tend to have hypertension associated with lower renin concentrations, calcium channel blockers (CCBs), such as amlodipine, are advocated first line. A thiazide-type diuretic, such as indapamide, is an alternative if a CCB is not suitable, for example, because of oedema or intolerance, or if there is evidence of heart failure or a high risk of heart failure.
- Step 2 – Younger patients should be offered a CCB or a thiazide-like diuretic in addition to the ACEI/ARB; whilst older patients and those of black African or Caribbean origin of any age should be offered treatment with an ACEI/ARB or a thiazide-type diuretic. ARB is preferred to ACEI in patients of black

African or Caribbean family origin due to the higher risk of angioedema with ACEI seen in this group.

- Step 3 – Patients should be offered all three agents; ACEI/ARB plus CCB plus thiazide-type diuretic.
- Step 4 – Defined as resistant hypertension, recommends the addition of spironolactone if the serum potassium is <4.5 mmol/L. If spironolactone is unsuitable, alpha blockers or beta blockers are recommended. Beta blockers may be used in those patients with a high sympathetic drive, often indicated by an increased heart rate.[9]

See *Figure 12.1* for a summary of this stepwise approach.

Figure 12.1: *Choice of antihypertensive drug*

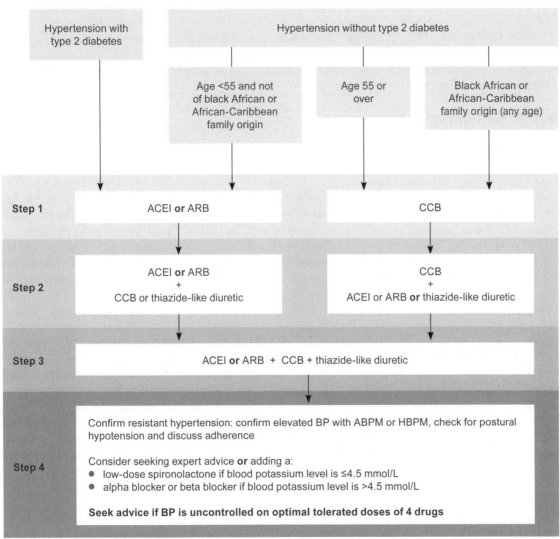

Adapted from the NICE visual summary on recommendations for diagnosing and treating hypertension.
www.nice.org.uk/guidance/ng136/resources/visual-summary-pdf-6899919517

Other international guidelines do not suggest a specific stepwise approach to drug selection but simply present a list of antihypertensive therapies and where they might be most appropriately indicated. Combinations of low doses of antihypertensive drugs are often more effective and better tolerated than single drugs taken in high dose.

There remains uncertainty about the optimal timing for the dosing of antihypertensive drug therapy, with one Cochrane review concluding that evening dosing was associated with a small, but significant reduction in blood pressure when compared to morning dosing, but the quality of the studies included was poor.[12]

A recent large study from Spain reported that nighttime dosing of antihypertensive therapies was associated with a reduction in BP during sleep and an impressive 45% reduction in cardiovascular events over 6 years. However, there were potential flaws in the study design and the analysis used which call in to question these findings.[13]

Further exploration of this effect in blinded studies is warranted, alongside research to assess whether moving to nighttime doses will impact on adherence to therapies. There appear to be few downsides to advising patients who are motivated and adherent to therapy to take their antihypertensive medications at night, until a clear evidence base accrues.

Special patient groups

Ethnicity

People of black African and Caribbean ethnicity are at increased risk of developing hypertension and are at higher risk of stroke and renal failure as a result. ACEIs and ARBs are less effective in this cohort due to lower circulating renin levels. This was illustrated in the ALLHAT study, where stroke and coronary events were more common in black patients randomised to lisinopril compared to those receiving chlortalidone.[14] In this group, NICE recommends CCBs first line with the addition of an ARB or thiazide-type diuretic at step 2.

British Asians also have an increased prevalence of hypertension, diabetes and insulin resistance and are at a particularly high risk of coronary heart disease and stroke. There is currently no evidence to differentiate the response of Asian patients to antihypertensive drug therapies when compared with white Europeans.

Elderly

Very elderly people (aged over 80 years) have a high prevalence of hypertension and are at very high risk of CV events. However, epidemiological data suggest that BP and risk of death are inversely related in older people and, as a result, clinicians have been reticent to treat older people in the past.

The Hypertension in the Very Elderly Trial (HYVET) confirmed that treating hypertension in very elderly people to a systolic BP target of 150 mmHg with indapamide, and if required perindopril, led to a 30% reduction in fatal and non-fatal stroke, 21% reduction in death from all causes, and fewer adverse events in the actively treated group.[15] NICE guidelines endorse treatment of the very elderly to achieve a BP <150/90 mmHg in line with the HYVET study.[9] When prescribing antihypertensives for the very elderly, it is important to remember that they are at increased risk of certain adverse effects, such as postural hypotension. Sitting and standing blood pressure should be used to identify any postural drops in BP at each clinic visit.

Young people

Young people (aged under 30 years) presenting with hypertension should be referred for investigation of secondary causes such as coarctation of the aorta, renal artery stenosis caused by fibromuscular dysplasia, or Cushing's syndrome.

Diabetes

NICE guidance indicates that people with diabetes should be treated in the same way as younger people with ACEI/ARB recommended at step one, ACEI/ARB plus CCB or thiazide-type diuretic at step 2 and all three (ACEI/ARB plus CCB plus thiazide-type diuretic) at step 3.

The NICE BP target for people with diabetes is also 140/90 mmHg, although many specialists will still treat to lower targets if there are other risk factors present, such as albuminuria. After step 3, there is little evidence to support the choice of one drug class over another but NICE recommends the same resistant hypertension strategy for people with diabetes – spironolactone or, where spironolactone is unsuitable, an alpha blocker or a beta blocker.

Renal disease

In patients with chronic renal impairment, blood pressure control slows the progression of renal dysfunction. Renin-angiotensin system antagonists, including ACEIs, ARBs and direct renin inhibitors, reduce the incidence of end-stage renal failure. ACEI/ARBs also reduce protein loss and should be used in patients with hypertension and an albumin:creatinine ratio (ACR) of 30 mg/mmol or more, or rapidly progressive renal dysfunction.

Renin-angiotensin-aldosterone system antagonists may worsen renal impairment in patients with renal vascular disease and careful monitoring of electrolytes and creatinine is mandatory. Salt restriction is particularly important in managing hypertension in renal disease. Thiazide diuretics are ineffective in patients with significant renal dysfunction and loop diuretics should be used in preference when a diuretic is needed.

Stroke

Hypertension is the most important risk factor for stroke in patients with or without previous stroke. There is increasing evidence that in those with a previous stroke, blood pressure reduction reduces the risk of stroke recurrence as well as other cardiovascular events. The UK Royal College of Physicians National clinical guideline for stroke (Intercollegiate Stroke Working Party 2016) recommends that patients post-stroke should be treated to achieve a clinic systolic blood pressure below 130 mmHg, except for people with severe bilateral carotid artery stenosis, for whom a systolic blood pressure target of 140-150 mmHg is appropriate.[16]

For newly identified hypertension in patients post-stroke, blood pressure-lowering treatment should be initiated prior to the transfer of care out of hospital or at 2 weeks, whichever is earliest.

Monitoring

Once initiated on first-line therapy, patients should be reviewed within 4 weeks to:

- Assess effectiveness – if the target BP has not been achieved, then the dose should be increased, or a second agent added in, tailored based on age and ethnicity
- Take bloods for people on ACEI/ARB or thiazide diuretic to check renal function and electrolytes
- Assess adherence and address any issues affecting adherence, including adverse effects

Antihypertensive drug classes

Renin–angiotensin system antagonists

ACEIs, such as ramipril, or ARBs, such as candesartan, are effective antihypertensive agents, particularly in younger patients with higher circulating renin levels. Around 10-20% of patients prescribed ACEIs will report a persistent dry cough – consider an ARB where this occurs.

ACEIs are also associated with a significant incidence of angioedema. This adverse reaction is more common in black people which is why ARBs are preferred to ACEIs in people of black African or Caribbean family origin, although as outlined earlier ACEIs and ARBs are not first-line options for this group.

On initiation, ACEI and ARB can result in a significant initial drop in BP, known as first-dose hypotension, which can be associated with dizziness and lightheadedness. Older people and those on diuretic therapy are at higher risk of experiencing first-dose hypotension. This can be avoided by advising the patient to take their first dose in the evening before bed. Patients prescribed ACEI or ARB should have a blood test to check renal function, potassium and sodium levels at baseline, 2-4 weeks after initiation or any dose change, and annually throughout treatment.

ACEI/ARB should be stopped or reduced to a previously tolerated dose if eGFR falls by ≥25% or serum creatinine increases by 30% or more from baseline after initiation or dose increase. Dose titration may be delayed and blood tests repeated if results indicate a smaller decline in renal function. ACEI/ARB therapy should be stopped if serum potassium rises above 6.0 mmol/L.[17]

Calcium channel blockers (CCBs)
CCBs are used in people aged 55 years or older and in those of black African or Caribbean origin of any age. Dihydropyridine CCBs, such as amlodipine, are commonly used in the treatment of hypertension and are generally well tolerated, although they can be associated with headaches and flushing, which resolve after the first few days treatment, and can also cause ankle swelling and gum hypertrophy, which may necessitate cessation.

Diuretics
NICE recommends thiazide-type diuretics, such as indapamide, in preference to thiazide diuretics in the treatment of hypertension due to a better evidence base confirming a reduction in CV events when used at low doses.

Although generally well tolerated, thiazide-like diuretics may cause hypokalaemia, small increases in LDL-cholesterol and triglyceride and gout associated with impaired urate excretion. Sustained hypokalaemia or gout may necessitate withdrawal of therapy. Erectile dysfunction is also reported, which may affect adherence to treatment.

Spironolactone, an aldosterone antagonist, is recommended as an option at a low dose (25 mg daily) for patients with resistant hypertension. Spironolactone is a potassium-sparing diuretic and should be used with caution, especially if used in combination with ACEI or ARB; it should be avoided in hypertension if the baseline potassium is >4.5 mmol/L. Be cautious in patients with impaired renal function as there is an increased risk of hyperkalaemia.

Check serum creatinine, eGFR and electrolytes (particularly potassium levels) before initiation and recheck within one month of initiation. Monitor monthly for a further 2 months, then every 3 months for a year, then every 6 months thereafter, or more frequently if clinically indicated.

If hyperkalaemia develops (potassium >5 mmol/L), stop spironolactone. If potassium >6 mmol/L, consider treatment to lower the potassium level. If eGFR falls by 25% or serum creatinine increases by >30% from baseline, stop spironolactone.[18]

Aside from renal dysfunction and hyperkalaemia, spironolactone can cause gynaecomastia (enlargement of the breast tissue) and breast or nipple pain in men which may require cessation of treatment, although eplerenone could be considered as an alternative.

Alpha blockers
Long-acting alpha blockers, such as doxazosin, can be considered at step 4, where spironolactone is unsuitable usually due to poor renal function of high baseline potassium. There have been concerns about the

use of alpha blockers in the management of hypertension since the ALLHAT study indicated that doxazosin monotherapy was more often associated with heart failure and stroke than thiazide diuretics.[19]

They may be considered as add-in therapy for patients with resistant hypertension inadequately controlled using other agents. They can frequently cause postural hypotension, so sitting and standing blood pressures should be checked, particularly if the patient reports dizziness or lightheadedness. Postural hypotension may limit the dose of alpha blocker which can be prescribed, or, if symptomatic, necessitate cessation of therapy.

Beta blockers

The use of beta blockers in the management of hypertension has declined over time as a result of evidence that they may be less effective at preventing stroke than other antihypertensive agents. As a result, beta blockers are now only recommended by NICE as an alternative to alpha blockers at step 4. Beta blockers may be useful in hypertensives with other comorbidities, such as coronary heart disease or atrial fibrillation. Additionally, where anxiety is a significant driver of hypertension, beta blockers may have a role.

Beta blockers should be avoided in patients with reversible airways disease. Common adverse effects include bradycardia, tiredness or fatigue, erectile dysfunction, cold extremities, nausea and sleep disturbance or nightmares. Cardioselective agents, such as bisoprolol, should be used to minimise adverse effects but therapy will have to be withdrawn in some patients, particularly where adverse effects are affecting adherence.

Other agents

There are a number of other antihypertensive agents which are not routinely used in clinical practice but may be prescribed occasionally for specific patient groups or in those with resistant hypertension.

Methyldopa, a centrally-acting agent, continues to be used in pregnancy since it does not cause foetal abnormalities, but is not used more widely because it has pronounced central adverse effects including tiredness and depression.

Moxonidine is a newer centrally-acting agent which may be used in resistance hypertension. It can cause dry mouth, headache, fatigue and dizziness, but has fewer central adverse effects than methyldopa.

Minoxidil is a very effective antihypertensive but is associated with severe peripheral oedema and reflex tachycardia and should therefore be reserved for patients with severe hypertension who are also taking beta blockers and diuretics. It causes pronounced hirsutism and is not suitable for use in women.

Hydralazine can be used as add-on therapy for patients with resistant hypertension but is not well tolerated as it is a profound vasodilator.

Aliskiren is a renin antagonist which may be safely added to other inhibitors of the renin-angiotensin-aldosterone system to provide a greater level of inhibition. Its use is limited by cost and a lack of outcome data and can therefore only be recommended as an add-on therapy where other more established treatment options have failed to control BP, or in patients with multiple drug intolerances. It is generally well tolerated but may cause diarrhoea at higher doses.

Reducing cardiovascular risk in people with hypertension

Lipid-lowering therapy

All people with established CV disease should be prescribed a high dose high-intensity statin such as atorvastatin 80 mg daily. Patients with a CV risk score of 10% or more should also be offered a high-intensity statin such as atorvastatin 20 mg daily. The aim should be to lower non-HDL cholesterol (calculated by subtracting the HDL level from the total cholesterol level) by 40% or more from baseline, partly as a marker of adherence to treatment.

Myalgia is the most common adverse effect of statins and can significantly impact on adherence to treatment. In patients with muscle pain, myositis should be excluded by checking the creatine kinase level, and then consideration given to reducing the dose or switching to an alternative statin. A statin intolerance pathway has recently been published by the Accelerated Access Collaborative in England which helps clinicians manage suspected statin-induced muscle pain.[20]

Other adverse effects of statins include GI disturbance, headache, dizziness and insomnia. Rashes and alopecia have been less commonly reported. Depending on the severity of the adverse effects experienced, a lower dose of the same statin may be prescribed, or the patient switched to an alternative statin, for example, a water-soluble agent such as rosuvastatin.

Aspirin

The use of aspirin reduces CV events at the expense of an increase in gastrointestinal complications and it is no longer recommended for primary prevention of cardiovascular events. Its use in hypertensive patients should be restricted to those who have evidence of established cardiovascular disease.

Drug interactions

For important drug interactions and how to manage them, see *Table 12.3*.

Table 12.3: *Drug interactions*

Drug	Interacting drugs	Interaction	Management
Alpha blockers	• Phosphodiesterase-5-inhibitors (e.g. sildenafil, tadalafil, and vardenafil)	• May lead to symptomatic hypotension	• Use with caution, and only in patients on a stable alpha blocker dose • Use lowest possible dose of PDE-5 inhibitor and separate administration of doxazosin and PDE-5 inhibitors by at least 6 hours
	• Potent CYP3A4 inhibitors (e.g. itraconazole, ketoconazole, protease inhibitors, clarithromycin, telithromycin and nefazodone)	• Increased levels of alfuzosin	• Avoid concomitant use
Thiazide diuretics	• Lithium	• Increased plasma lithium with signs of overdosage	• Avoid where possible • If used together, monitor lithium levels and adjust dose as required

	• Class Ia antiarrhythmics (e.g. quinidine, hydroquinidine, disopyramide)
	• Class III antiarrhythmics (e.g. amiodarone, sotalol, dofetilide, ibutilide)
	• Some antipsychotics:
	  – Phenothiazines (e.g. chlorpromazine, thioridazine, trifluoperazine)
	  – Benzamides (e.g. amisulpride, sulpiride)
	  – Butyrophenones (e.g. droperidol, haloperidol)
	• Other drugs include: bepridil, cisapride, diphemanil, erythromycin (IV), halofantrine, mizolastine, pentamidine, sparfloxacin, moxifloxacin, vincamine (IV)
		• Increased risk of ventricular arrhythmias, particularly torsades, if hypokalaemia develops	• Monitor for hypokalaemia and correct, if required, before introducing this combination
			• Clinical, plasma electrolytes and ECG monitoring
			• Or use alternatives not associated with increased risk of torsades

	• Amphotericin B (IV) • Glucocorticoids and mineralcorticoids (systemic route) • Tetracosactide • Stimulant laxatives	• Increased risk of hypokalaemia	• Monitoring plasma potassium and correct if necessary. Caution with digoxin • Use non-stimulant laxatives
	• Other hypertensives	• Increased risk of hypotension	• Monitor BP on initiation and after dose increases

For interactions for beta blockers, ACEIs, ARBs, and aldosterone antagonists, see **Chapter 11**. For interactions for CCBs and statins, see **Chapter 5**.

Advice for patients

People diagnosed with hypertension will need information and advice about the condition and the treatments. *Box 12.5* outlines the important counselling points to consider.

Box 12.5: Practice point: counselling

Patients should be advised that:
- Although they may not have an symptoms of high blood pressure, it is associated with an increased risk of heart attacks, strokes and kidney disease.
- Lowering blood pressure through lifestyle modification and, where appropriate, drug therapy can reduce the risk of these complications occurring.
  - Smoking cessation, improved diet including a reduction in dietary salt intake, increased physical activity, weight loss and alcohol moderation all help to lower blood pressure.
  - Drug therapy can also help to lower BP, but must be taken every day as prescribed to affect BP control.
  - If they are at increased CV risk, they will also need to take a statin.
- The aim should be to achieve a blood pressure of <140/90 mmHg (<150/90 mmHg if over 80 years old).
- They can monitor their BP at home by purchasing a BP monitoring device for around £20.

Useful resources

- Albasri A, Clark CE, Omboni S *et al*. Effective detection and management of hypertension through community pharmacy in England. *Pharmaceutical Journal* 2020 [online].
- BHF resources for home BP monitoring. www.bhf.org.uk/informationsupport/heart-matters-magazine/medical/tests/blood-pressure-measuring-at-home
- ESC. 2018 ESC/ESH Clinical Practice Guidelines for the Management of Arterial Hypertension. www.escardio.org/Guidelines/Clinical-Practice-Guidelines/Arterial-Hypertension-Management-of
- Girvin B *et al*. 2019. Primary care hypertension clinics: tips for pharmacist prescribers. www.prescriber.co.uk/article/primary-care-hypertension-clinics-tips-for-pharmacist-prescribers
- NICE NG136: Hypertension in adults: diagnosis and management. www.nice.org.uk/guidance/ng136
- Rahman MS. 2019. Hypertension: the role of the practice pharmacist. www.guidelinesinpractice.co.uk/cardiovascular/hypertension-the-role-of-the-practice-pharmacist/454832.article

References

1. World Health Organization (WHO). Global health risks. Mortality and burden of disease attributable to selected major risks. Geneva: WHO; 2009. www.who.int/healthinfo/global_burden_disease/GlobalHealthRisks_report_full.pdf?ua
2. Public Health England (PHE). Guidance: Health matters: combating high blood pressure. London: PHE; 2017. www.gov.uk/government/publications/health-matters-combating-high-blood-pressure/health-matters-combating-high-blood-pressure
3. Franklin SS *et al*. Does the relation of blood pressure to coronary heart disease risk change with aging? The Framingham Heart Study. *Circulation* 2001; 103(9): 1245-1249.
4. Rimoldi SF *et al*. Secondary arterial hypertension: when, who, and how to screen? *European Heart Journal* 2014; 35(19): 1245-1254.
5. Lane D *et al*. Ethnic differences in blood pressure and the prevalence of hypertension in England. *Journal of Human Hypertension* 2002; 16(4): 267-273.

6. Law MR *et al*. Use of blood pressure lowering drugs in the prevention of cardiovascular disease: meta-analysis of 147 randomised trials in the context of expectations from prospective epidemiological studies. *BMJ* 2009; 338: b1665.

7. NHS Digital. Quality and Outcomes Framework, 2019-20 Official statistics. London: NHS Digital; 2020. www.digital.nhs.uk/data-and-information/publications/statistical/quality-and-outcomes-framework-achievement-prevalence-and-exceptions-data/2019-20

8. PHE. Hypertension prevalence estimates for local populations. London: PHE; 2020. www.gov.uk/government/publications/hypertension-prevalence-estimates-for-local-populations

9. National Institute for Health and Care Excellence (NICE). Hypertension in adults: diagnosis and management [CG136]. London: NICE; 2019. www.nice.org.uk/guidance/ng136

10. Scientific Advisory Committee on Nutrition. Salt and Health. London: SACN; 2003. www.assets.publishing.service.gov.uk/government/uploads/system/uploads/attachment_data/file/338782/SACN_Salt_and_Health_report.pdf

11. Scottish Intercollegiate Guidelines Network (SIGN). Risk estimation and the prevention of cardiovascular disease (SIGN 149). Edinburgh: SIGN; 2017. www.sign.ac.uk/assets/sign149.pdf

12. Zhao P *et al*. Evening versus morning dosing regimen drug therapy for hypertension. *Cochrane Database of Systematic Reviews* 2011, Issue 10.

13. Hermida RC *et al*. Bedtime hypertension treatment improves cardiovascular risk reduction: the Hygia Chronotherapy Trial. *European Heart Journal* 2019 [online].

14. ALLHAT officers and coordinators for the ALLHAT Collaborative Research Group. Major outcomes in high-risk hypertensive patients randomized to angiotensin-converting enzyme inhibitor or calcium channel blocker vs diuretic: the antihypertensive and lipid-lowering treatment to prevent heart attack trial (ALLHAT). *JAMA* 2002; 288(23): 2981-97.

15. Beckett NS *et al*. Treatment of hypertension in patients 80 years of age or older. *N Engl J Med* 2008; 358: 1887-1898.

16. Royal College of Physicians Intercollegiate Stroke Working Party. Stroke guidelines. London: RCP; 2016. www.rcplondon.ac.uk/guidelines-policy/stroke-guidelines

17. Specialist Pharmacy Services. Suggestions for drug monitoring in adults in primary care. SPS; 2017 [online]. www.sps.nhs.uk/wp-content/uploads/2017/12/Drug-monitoring-October-2017.pdf

18. NICE Clinical Knowledge Summaries. Hypertension - not diabetic: spironolactone. London: NICE; 2020. www.cks.nice.org.uk/topics/hypertension-not-diabetic/prescribing-information/spironolactone

19. ALLHAT Collaborative Research Group. Major cardiovascular events in hypertensive patients randomized to doxazosin vs chlorthalidone: the antihypertensive and lipid-lowering treatment to prevent heart attack trial (ALLHAT). *JAMA* 2000; 283(15): 1967-75.

20. NHS England (NHSE) Accelerated Access Collaborative. Statin intolerance pathway. London: NHSE; 2020. www.england.nhs.uk/aac/publication/statin-intolerance-pathway

Case studies

Case study 1

Alan is a 71-year-old black Caribbean man, married with three grown-up children. He was diagnosed with high blood pressure (BP) two months ago. His untreated BP was 182/110 mmHg and he had no high-risk features. He was started on amlodipine 5 mg daily, which was increased to 10 mg one month ago. He is also on diclofenac 50 mg three timed a day for joint pain, as well as omeprazole 20 mg daily.

You can see from the notes that he is not overweight, has limited mobility due to arthritis, he does not drink or smoke and eats home-cooked food but adds a lot of salt.

In today's clinic review, you measure his BP as 158/94 mmHg. His cardiovascular disease (CVD) risk has previously been calculated as 26.3% (from QRisk2).

He has the following blood results:

- Serum creatinine (SrCr) – 126 mmol/L
- Na$^+$ – 142 mmol/L
- K$^+$ – 4.6 mmol/L
- eGFR – 48 mL/min/1.73 m^2

Points to consider

- What should your objectives be in the consultation?

You decide to address the following areas:

- Reassurance and advice
- Review lifestyle issues
- Review his antihypertensive medication
- Discuss pain control
- Address his CV risk
- Arrange follow-up

Points to consider

- What would you say to reassure Alan?

You reassure Alan that the treatment he has been taking has improved his BP control over the past few weeks, although there is still some way to go. You remind him that lowering his blood pressure is important to reduce his risk of a stroke, heart attack or renal dysfunction. You explain that stroke is more common in people of black African and Caribbean family origin and you consider exploring his understanding of stroke and its consequences and asking about any family experience of stroke he may have. You also highlight that his kidney function is under some strain, which is likely to be related to his high BP.

Points to consider

- What lifestyle issues would you review?

You ask Alan if he has made any changes to his lifestyle, particularly his high salt intake which will be exacerbating his high BP. You suggest herbs and spices rather than salt to improve the flavour of his meals and remind him that it can take 4 to 6 weeks for the taste buds to adjust to a lower salt intake. You direct him to 'Healthy eating The African Caribbean' published by Blood Pressure UK and encourage him to be as physically active as he can be. You suggest chair-based exercise can improve his cardiovascular (CV) health and general wellbeing.

Points to consider
- What aspects of his medication would you review?

Alan is currently only on calcium channel blocker (CCB) monotherapy for his high BP and is not yet at the BP target of <140/90 mmHg. You explore his adherence to this treatment, (although the lower BP measured in clinic today suggests he is taking the medicine) and any adverse effects he might have experienced.

As he is not yet at target, you escalate him to step 2 of antihypertensive therapy and consider either an ARB (in view of his ethnicity) or a thiazide-type diuretic.

Points to consider
- What do you need to consider if starting new medicines?

If you opt for an ARB, such as candesartan, he should be initiated at a dose of 8 mg daily, or if starting a thiazide-type diuretic, such as indapamide, at a dose of 2.5 mg daily. Bloods should be checked in two to three weeks times, and he should be reviewed in four weeks to assess response to therapy, impact on renal function and electrolytes if any, and any adverse effects explored.

Points to consider
- What is the next step if he is not at target after this time?

The candesartan dose can be increased, or if a thiazide-type diuretic was used at step 2 he will need a third agent (e.g. an ARB at step 3).

Points to consider
- What aspects of his pain control medication need to be addressed and why?

Diclofenac will worsen his hypertension and increase his risk of a CV event. You discuss the option of trying a simple analgesic such as paracetamol, with or without codeine, to see if he can manage without a non-steroidal anti-inflammatory (NSAID). If he is not happy to switch from an NSAID, naproxen or ibuprofen are associated with a lower CV risk and should be considered in place of diclofenac.

Points to consider
- What, if anything, needs to be done about Alan's CV risk?

Alan is at high risk of a CV event over the next 10 years. You discuss the addition of a statin, explain that a statin will further reduce his risk of a CV event, and explore his knowledge, attitude and concerns towards statins and adverse effects.

Points to consider

- What should you say about the adverse effects of statins?

You explain that statins are usually well tolerated but reassure him that you are willing to review the statin therapy at any time should adverse effects occur. You may wish to delay initiation until the BP has been controlled and there are no further changes to his antihypertensive therapy planned.

Alan agrees to start a statin and you initiate a high-intensity statin after checking baseline cholesterol and live function tests (LFTs).

Points to consider

- What monitoring and follow-up is required?

You check Alan's cholesterol and LFTs in three months, aiming for a reduction in non-HDL cholesterol of 40% or more (which would indicate adherence to the prescribed treatment), and arrange follow-up visits until his BP has been controlled to target and his statin therapy has been optimised.

Case study 2

Linda is a white British female, aged 54 years. She has had hypertension for more than 10 years, controlled by lifestyle but was recently started on ramipril 2.5 mg daily after the nurse recorded a BP of 153/94 mmHg. She is returning to you today for a review of her BP control.

- Clinic BP today – 151/98 mmHg
- Renal function – SrCr 98 mmol/L
- K^+ – 5.1 mmol/L
- Na^+ – 134 mmol/L
- eGFR – 65 mL/min/1.73 m^2
- TC: HDL ratio was recorded 6 months ago as 5.3
- Her CV risk (QRISK2) is calculated as 6.1%

The patient has indicated in the past that she is not happy to take regular drug therapy as she thinks it is unnatural. She prefers herbal remedies and vitamins and has been taking folic acid and vitamin B6 supplements to try to control her BP. She is overweight with a BMI of 29.

Points to consider

- What should your objectives be in the consultation?

You decide to address the following areas:

- Reiterate key messages
- Address adherence issues

- Review medication
- Discuss lifestyle modification
- Assess cardiovascular (CV) risk

Points to consider

- What key messages would you convey to Linda?

You remind Linda that high BP increases her risk of having a heart attack or stroke and increases the risk of her developing kidney disease, and that lowering the BP with lifestyle and/or drug therapy will reduce her risk of these consequences.

Points to consider

- How would you address adherence issues?

There has been little change in her BP between clinic visits, and therefore you suspect that Linda has not been taking her medication – particularly as she has expressed concerns about medicines in the past. You explore whether this is the case and discuss her attitude to taking medicines.

Points to consider

- What aspects of her medication need to be reviewed?

As Linda is at low CV risk and has no other comorbidities, and her BP is not raised above 160/100 mmHg, she does not require medication changes at this time. Assuming she has not been taking her medications, you could consider stopping her ACEI and focus instead on opportunities to lower her BP with lifestyle.

Points to consider

- What lifestyle issues need to be addressed?

Linda is overweight with a BMI of 29; weight loss would significantly reduce her BP. You explore diet, physical activity and alcohol intake to identify opportunities to lose weight.

You discuss the various options, including referral to an exercise in prescription programme, a weight management programme, dietetics advice or motivational support. Depending on what is commissioned locally, this can include vouchers to access gyms for a number of weeks, or an opportunity to enrol in a local commercial weight management programme such as Slimming World or Weight Watchers. You explain to Linda that it is up to her to decide whether she wants to engage in lifestyle modification and to lower her BP through this route – but stress that if she does it successfully, she could avoid drug therapy long term.

Points to consider

- Should a statin be added to Linda's therapy?

As Linda has a low CV risk, she does not require statin therapy at this time.

Points to consider

- What follow-up is required?

You follow up with Linda over the next few months to support her with her lifestyle modification. You suggest that if she bought a BP monitor she could start to keep an eye on her BP at home and that if she does so, she should seek advice if the BP levels rise over time.

CHAPTER 13

Palliative care

Fiona Dorrington

Overview

The World Health Organization (WHO) defines palliative care as: 'Palliative care improves the quality of life of patients and their families who are facing problems associated with life-threatening illness, whether physical, psychosocial or spiritual.'[1]

Traditionally associated with cancer, palliative care teams now provide support to people with other life-limiting illnesses, including neurological diseases such as multiple sclerosis and motor neurone disease (MND), end stage organ disease and dementia. Palliative care may be applicable at any stage of disease to help with difficult symptoms, but it is usually focused on the last year of life when the aim of care is more about comfort and symptom control rather than life-prolonging interventions.

Early identification of people with palliative care needs has been shown to improve outcomes for patients and their carers, and may even prolong life.[2] For all healthcare professionals, the provision of good, basic palliative care is a core skill.

Palliative care is delivered in acute hospitals, hospices, care homes and in people's own homes. In surveys, 70% of people express a preference to die at home,[3] and there are strong pressures to facilitate this. In the UK, the policy is to enable patients to have choice around their place of care and to avoid the medicalisation of death in an acute hospital setting.

In England in 2018, 45.5% of deaths occurred in hospital and only 5.8% in a hospice.[4] In Scotland, people who died spent 87% of their last 6 months in a community setting.[5] In the community, palliative care is delivered by the primary healthcare team with support from local specialist services. An average UK GP will have 20 deaths in a year, only two of which will be sudden and unexpected.[6] All pharmacists will encounter patients with palliative care needs in their daily practice.

Diagnosis

Lunney *et al* identified three trajectories of illness associated with main causes of death.[6] These are the rapid predictable decline seen in patients with advanced cancer, erratic unpredictable decline seen in organ failure and gradual decline of frailty, dementia and multimorbidity.

The Gold Standards Framework (GSF), Proactive Identification Guidance Tool (PIG),[7] and NHS Scotland Supportive and Palliative Care Indicators Tool (SPICT™)[8] detail a 3-step process to identify patients with advanced or progressive disease who may benefit from additional supportive care. These patients are added to the Gold Standards or End of Life register in the practice.

Step 1: 'The surprise question'

An intuitive response pulling together the whole range of clinical, social and other factors: 'Would you be surprised if the patient were to die in the next 12 months?'

Step 2: General indicators of decline and increasing needs

These include factors which may be evident in community pharmacy such as:

- physical decline
- repeated unplanned hospital admissions
- significant weight loss

- decreasing response to treatments
- significant events (e.g. serious fall, bereavement, or admission to a nursing home).

Access to more detailed clinical factors will be available to pharmacists in GP practice, those providing disease specific clinics or working in secondary care settings (e.g. decreased serum albumin, declining renal and hepatic function, increasing white cell count).

Step 3: Specific clinical indicators

Indicators for cancer, organ failure, neurological diseases, frailty, dementia and multiple comorbidities are detailed in both PIG and SPICT.

Moving towards a palliative approach is likely to be appropriate when the disease is no longer responding to treatment and quality of life is more important than quantity.

For many chronic conditions, prognostication is more difficult as the pattern of decline may include acute episodes which respond to treatment (e.g. infective exacerbation of COPD requiring admission to hospital for intravenous antibiotics). Indications that a patient is nearing end of life include:

- repeated admissions to hospital
- failure to return to the previous level of function following an acute episode
- reduced ability to carry out activities of daily living
- loss of appetite
- increased fatigue.

Treatment

The medicines prescribed will vary depending on the patient's underlying condition – so there is no typical palliative care patient. Typical medicines for common symptoms are detailed in this section and will be seen alongside the disease specific drugs.

A typical regular and PRN medicine list for symptom management in palliative care patients may be similar to those in *Table 13.1* and *Table 13.2*, although they may also be taking a range of additional medicines to manage underlying conditions.

Table 13.1: *Regular medication*

Medication checklist: Sample patient (26/4/1956)

Updated by: Hospice pharmacist 10/4/2019

Medicine	How much to take	What it's for	Morning	Lunchtime	Early evening	Bedtime
Morphine sulfate m/r 30 mg	30 mg (ONE)	Prevent pain	ONE			ONE
Omeprazole 20 mg	20 mg (ONE)	Protect stomach	ONE			
Paracetamol 500 mg	1 g (TWO)	Prevent pain	TWO	TWO	TWO	TWO
Senna 7.5 mg	15 mg (TWO)	Prevent constipation				TWO
Mirtazapine 15 mg	15 mg (ONE)	Help mood				ONE
Dexamethasone 2 mg	6 mg (THREE)	Steroid	THREE			
Lactulose	10 mL	Prevent constipation	10 mL	10 mL		10 mL

Table 13.2: *As required medication: only if needed*

Medicine	Dose	What it's for	Dose interval
Morphine sulfate 10 mg/5 mL	10 mg (5 mL)	Pain	Leave ONE hour between doses
Lorazepam 1 mg	0.5-1 mg	Anxiety – allow to dissolve under the tongue	Leave SIX hours between doses

Pharmacy input

Drug therapy is important in the delivery of palliative care, so there is a role for the pharmacy team whatever the area of practice. For many patients in the community, their local pharmacy will be a trusted source of information and support. Pharmacist knowledge of formulations available, sourcing 'specials', use of alternative routes of administration, medicines review, drug interactions and unlicensed uses provides essential input into the multidisciplinary care of palliative patients. Pharmacists also support symptom management by advising on medicines choice and provision of direct care including prescribing for this patient group. Specialist and consultant pharmacists are an integral part of the multidisciplinary team (MDT) in palliative care teams across primary, secondary and tertiary (hospice or inpatient palliative care units) settings.

Pharmacy review

Many UK GP practices will hold a Gold Standards or End of Life register and this information will be detailed in the patient's medical record. Regular multidisciplinary meetings are held to discuss the patients on the register – this is a good opportunity for GP practice pharmacists to become involved. These are generally held monthly giving the opportunity to review the patients on the list.

Individual patients may require more frequent monitoring, especially after a hospital admission or a significant event (e.g. starting or stopping a chemotherapy regimen, disease progression or changes in symptom management). If you are prescribing medicine for symptoms, agree an acceptable trial period for review with the patient. Management will be dependent on the likely prognosis and specific disease state.

Determining an advanced care plan (ACP) is part of the Gold Standards process and will guide clinicians in their level and intensity of intervention, guided by the wishes of the patient. ACPs may include decisions about admission to hospital versus home-based care, whether intravenous antibiotics are wished, preferred place of care/death and resuscitation status. These plans evolve and are ongoing rather than a one-off set decision.

Careful communication is needed as patients move from an intensive focus on disease management to one based more on comfort and symptom management to avoid feelings of abandonment and that 'nothing can be done'.

As with all patients, a person-centred approach is needed. A typical assessment will require you to:
- Review medicines adherence
- Follow up on any changes to medicines
- Explore any concerns about adverse effects of medicines
- Ask about common symptoms, including:
  — pain
  — nausea
  — constipation
  — breathlessness

Medicines

Ask about adherence to the current regimen and any difficulties.

- Can you swallow all the medicines prescribed?
- Do you always remember when your medicines are due?
- Have your medicines changed since your last prescription?
- Have the medicine changes helped you feel better?
- Would you like any information about the new medicines?
- Ask about potential adverse effects (e.g. nausea, constipation with opioids)
- Do you have any medicines at home you are no longer taking?
  - Offer to take these for safe disposal – stockpiles of discontinued medicines can be a source of confusion

Medicines reconciliation

Patients in the last year of life often experience multiple changes of care settings (e.g. moving between home, hospital and hospice). This is can be a source of unintentional medicine changes and also risks reducing adherence by patients confused by frequent changes.

To help avoid this it is important to:

- reconcile medicines at each change of care setting
- ask patients about medicine changes if they have had an inpatient stay
- discuss any changes with patients or carers
- provide written information to aid adherence and support self-management or to help carers support medicine use
- consider previously dispensed monitored dosage system (MDS) pack at home.

Presentation of medicine is another important aspect to consider. For example, MDS packs are not always the best option for patients at the end of life. Factors which make MDS less suitable include:

- frequent changes of medicine
- packs delivered monthly – 'old' medicines may still be at home and there is a risk of reverting to a previous regimen
- controlled drugs – it is not always practicable to put these in MDS
- liquid or dispersible products to aid compliance – it is not always possible or appropriate to put these in MDS
- MDS is not always possible on discharge from hospital or hospice.

Polypharmacy

As people live longer but with a high burden of disease, polypharmacy is a major issue in the last years of life. People may see multiple medical specialists and accrue large numbers of medicines if regular holistic review is not carried out. An increased number of medicines will also increase the risk of drug-drug interactions. This is where the skills of a pharmacist are required to review and refine drug regimens to include only those medicines which are helpful and actually required. In advanced disease, the risk/benefit of ongoing medicine changes, sensitivity to adverse effects may be increased and goals of therapy change. Polypharmacy is covered in detail in **Chapter 17**.

Difficulty swallowing

Many patients find swallowing medicine becomes a problem with advanced disease and this can be due to a number of factors. Disease-related swallowing problems (e.g. motor neurone disease, or increasing weakness) can make taking medicine by mouth difficult.

Some patients with neurological problems may have medicines given via percutaneous endoscopic gastrostomy (PEG) tube and advice may be necessary to ensure medicines can be given safely and effectively.

The NEWT guidelines[9] are a useful resource and the British Association for Parenteral and Enteral Nutrition has guidance on the practical aspects of administering medicine via feeding tubes.[10]

Fluids and nutrition

As people near the end of life, eating and drinking may become difficult, and as the body slows down the interest and need for food will decline. This can become a source of anxiety for families who will need reassurance and support that this is normal, especially in the last days to weeks of life.

In the last year of life some patients may benefit from the advice of a dietician and speech and language therapist. Where there are swallowing difficulties, these AHPs can advise on choice of food consistency, maintenance of calorie intake and use of supplements and thickeners. Some patients with neurological disease (e.g. MND) may opt for enteral feeding via a PEG tube and this is usually managed via the community dietician, with feed delivered directly from the supplier once a stable regimen is established.[11]

In the last weeks to months of life, particularly in cancer patients, the weight loss is related to disease progression rather than nutritional deficit and these patients are unlikely to benefit from 'building up' with supplements or high calorie foods. People should be encouraged to eat and drink for pleasure and dietary restrictions become less important. Some people enjoy supplement drinks and find them beneficial, while for others, supplements can make them feel full and so unable to enjoy the 'real food' they could be eating and an important element of family life. Presenting food in small appetising portions or eating small snacks throughout the day can help.[12]

In the last days of life comfort is paramount – keeping the mouth moist with sips of fluid or ice chips, use of artificial saliva gels or sprays and maintaining dental hygiene with a soft toothbrush are as beneficial as artificial hydration. Caution is required if the sponges on sticks are used – the sponge tip may become dislodged if the sticks are left immersed in water – use of water in a small oral dose syringe may be more useful to moisten the mouth. There is little evidence that artificial hydration with intravenous or subcutaneous fluids are of benefit at the end of life.

Common symptoms

Pain

Questions to ask when assessing pain are detailed in *Table 13.3*. The answers will allow you to ensure appropriate management: provide advice, change the current prescription, or refer to another healthcare professional as appropriate.

Table 13.3: *Pain assessment questions*

Question	Comment
Where is the pain?	There may be more than one pain – patients need prompting. This information helps establish a baseline and can be used on a pain map in a formal consultation.
Can you describe the pain?	This can guide the choice of analgesic. • Dull aching pain is likely to respond to conventional analgesics (e.g. paracetamol and opioids). • Shooting, burning and abnormal sensation pain may be due to nerve damage and is more likely to respond better to neuropathic agents (e.g. amitriptyline or gabapentin).
Does anything make the pain worse? (e.g. movement or weight bearing)	There could be an acute cause (e.g. fracture, or bone metastases) which requires urgent referral. • If there is pre-existing bone disease, NSAIDs can be helpful.
Does anything make the pain better? (e.g. is the medication effective if taken as needed?)	Chronic pain needs regular medication. • Suggest using regular medication working up the WHO ladder (e.g. paracetamol 1 g every 6 hours). • If addition of weak opioid is helpful, add this regularly. • If additional breakthrough doses of strong opioid are helpful, commence a regular long-acting strong opioid, or review and increase current long-acting preparation doses.

Nausea and vomiting

When assessing nausea and vomiting:

- Differentiate between the feeling of nausea and actual vomiting. Ask:
  - About timing in relation to food/drink
  - About the volume of vomitus
  - If the feeling of nausea is occasional or constant (if there is no vomiting)
- Ask about provoking or relieving factors:
  - Movement
  - Coughing
  - Does vomiting relieve feeling of nausea?
- Ask about potential reversible causes:
  - Constipation
  - Recent medicine changes
  - Recent chemo- or radiotherapy
  - Hypercalcaemia – the patient or carer will describe increasing confusion, sedation, constipation – this will require a blood test to diagnose (calcium, adjusted calcium and albumin) and referral for IV bisphosphonate if hypercalcaemia present
  - Renal insufficiency – uraemia can cause nausea

Breathlessness

Breathlessness is a common symptom even in the absence of underlying respiratory disease.
  Ask the patient if:

- It has come on quickly over the last 24-48 hours
  - Acute onset breathlessness may be due to pulmonary embolus, superior vena cava obstruction (SVCO), or pleural effusion; all of which would require immediate referral
- They have any fluid retention (e.g. puffy ankles, legs, hands)
  - Worsening heart failure can increase breathlessness – check for peripheral oedema; review of diuretics may be required
- They have suffered from any bleeding or been diagnosed with anaemia in the last weeks/months
  - Anaemia can exacerbate breathlessness; a full blood count may help with diagnosis
- The breathlessness worsens if they are anxious
- They have noticed a new cough or felt feverish
  - Antibiotics may be indicated if there is chest infection or aspiration pneumonia
- They have instituted their usual step up plan (e.g. rescue antibiotics/steroids), if they are known to have COPD, as breathlessness may be an infective exacerbation

Constipation

Constipation can lead to nausea, urinary retention, loss of appetite and confusion, especially in patients who are frail or elderly. Always ask about bowel habit if these symptoms present:

- When they last had a good bowel motion
- What is normal for them and if this been maintained
- What type of stool was passed (i.e. was it hard and dry, pellets or soft and clay like?)
- What medicines they are taking – opioids and anticholinergic drugs will contribute to constipation
- About any laxative use

Patients may describe diarrhoea following a period of constipation – this may be overflow where the stool liquefies behind a blockage. The problem then is of constipation, not diarrhoea. Careful assessment is necessary as the addition of anti-diarrhoeal medicine will risk impaction. In these cases, patients will describe the 'diarrhoea' as very liquid – refer these people to a GP or practice nurse; a PR or abdominal examination may be necessary.

Management

Medicines

Medicine review/deprescribing

A number of tools exist to guide deprescribing,[13,14] although most of them do not have an end of life focus. A general principle in the last year of life is to gradually reduce medicines and to focus on medicines contributing to reducing symptoms (e.g. analgesics, antiemetics, diuretics) rather than those for long-term benefit (e.g. statins, bisphosphonates, antihypertensives).[15,16,17] It is important, however, to consider the individual patient's changing risk/benefit and to work with them to achieve an agreed acceptable medicine regimen.

See **Chapter 17** for information on when it is appropriate to deprescribe and how to manage it.

Improving adherence

There may be some changes you can make to help maximise a patient's ability to safely take their medicine. These include:

- large print labels
- replacing childproof caps with screw caps
- cutting tablets at the time of dispensing to aid doses smaller than commercially available tablets (unlicensed, but may be essential to help patient)
- advising on tablet cutters and/or crushers
- changing the preparation (e.g. prescribing morphine sulfate immediate release tablets for breakthrough pain instead of morphine oral solution which needs to be measured)
- providing written information in the form of medicine cards or checklists
- some patients may find smartphone apps helpful, and some families are able to prompt medicine by phone or text.

Swallowing difficulty

Where the patient is finding swallowing solid dosage forms difficult, pharmacists can provide advice or choose to prescribe a more appropriate format. *Table 13.4* provides some possible alternatives to consider. Remember liquid preparations contain sorbitol and large volumes may exceed the dose that promotes diarrhoea.

Table 13.4: *Managing swallowing difficulties*

Consider	Example
Can the tablets be given with soft cold food?	Yoghurt or ice cream can make it easier to swallow, rather than a liquid
Is there a licensed liquid or dispersible formulation suitable for direct switch?	Paracetamol dispersible or suspension
Does the liquid form require a dose adjustment due to increase bioavailability?	Digoxin liquid, phenytoin suspension, citalopram drops
Is an alternative licensed product of the same therapeutic class available as liquid/dispersible?	Switch naproxen tablets to ibuprofen suspension

Table 13.4: *Managing swallowing difficulties (continued)*

Consider	Example
Is there a transdermal preparation?	Fentanyl transdermal patches – check local guidance for appropriate equivalent doses
Is there an equivalent 'special' available?	Gabapentin oral solution – these products are unlicensed, can be expensive, and there may also be a time lag in getting a supply
Is the standard medication crushable? Can the capsules be opened or will it disperse in water?	Gabapentin capsules may be opened and mixed with water – this is an unlicensed use, check NEWT guidelines; this may be an option while waiting for a special to be obtained
Can the injectable form be used enterally?	Glycopyrronium injection – this is an unlicensed use, check NEWT guidelines
Should a syringe pump be considered?	Oral morphine via syringe pump Give 50% of oral total daily dose as 24 hour infusion

Common symptoms

Pain

The WHO analgesic ladder[18] was developed for use in cancer pain and is broadly applicable in malignant pain – the use of opioids in chronic non-malignant pain is less helpful and should be avoided or carefully monitored[19] (you can read about the management of chronic pain in **Chapter 7**). *Figure 13.1* gives examples of drugs suitable for each step of the ladder.

Regular non-opioids are helpful and, wherever possible, patients should take regular paracetamol alongside any opioids and adjuvant medicine.

Figure 13.1: *Pain management step ladder (adapted from the WHO analgesic ladder for cancer pain)*

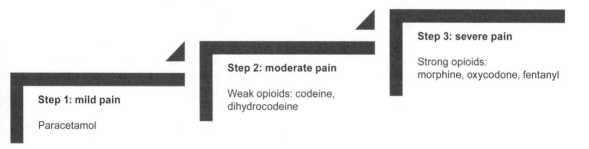

Step 1: mild pain

Paracetamol

Step 2: moderate pain

Weak opioids: codeine, dihydrocodeine

Step 3: severe pain

Strong opioids: morphine, oxycodone, fentanyl

Weak opioids (e.g. codeine or dihydrocodeine) can be useful in moderate pain. These are around 1/10th the potency of morphine and have a ceiling dose of 240 mg. This gives a starting dose for sustained release morphine of 10-15 mg twice daily, which assumes that the ceiling of weak opioid has been reached and pain is not well controlled. There is no benefit in switching between weak opioids if pain is not controlled, although combination products (e.g. co-codamol 30/500) may be useful to help reduce the tablet burden.

Strong opioids (e.g. morphine, oxycodone and fentanyl) are useful in severe pain, especially in malignant disease. The first-line choice is morphine – oxycodone and fentanyl are synthetic opioids which may be useful if morphine is not tolerated, if renal function is compromised, or where the transdermal route is needed to avoid swallowing/absorption problems (fentanyl).[20] Opioids should be titrated carefully and the benefits reviewed regularly. *Box 13.1* details some practice points for managing the use of opioids.

Box 13.1: Practice point: opioids

- Strong opioids should have both a regular (usually an MR preparation) plus a normal release product as a rescue or breakthrough dose.
- Calculate breakthrough (PRN or rescue) as 1/6th of the total daily opioid dose.
- Review breakthrough or rescue doses at any dose change.
- Breakthrough oral morphine or oxycodone can be given up to every hour – in most patients maximum effect is seen after an hour, so further doses can be given. Where more than three repeated doses are needed in 2 hours, reassess the pain – it may not be opioid responsive.
- Warn patients starting opioids of expected adverse effects and how to manage them:
  - Sedation – should wear off after a few days.
  - Nausea – should wear off after a few days. PRN antiemetic can be supplied at the time of prescription.
  - Constipation – a predictable adverse effect which requires regular laxatives.
- All patients on opioids should have a regular laxative and be encouraged to take it.
- Toxicity to opioids is evident when sedation doesn't resolve within about 7 days, or if the patient describes hallucinations.
  - Reassess pain.
  - If pain is well controlled but patient is sleepy (with or without hallucinations) – trial a reduced dose.
  - If opioid responsive but the current opioid is causing toxicity – trial an alternative opioid (check local guidance for equivalent doses).
- If swallowing is a problem, MR morphine can be given as Zomorph capsules which can be opened and mixed with water or soft cold food, or as MST granules which form a long-acting suspension. These are both also licensed for use via PEG tubes.
- Transdermal fentanyl may be a useful alternative. Check local guidance for dose equivalents and appropriate breakthrough doses of morphine or oxycodone.
- Fentanyl transdermal patches will take 36-72 hours to reach their full effect – do not increase dose daily.
- Take care with fentanyl patches – absorption is increased with increasing temperature, so heat pads should be avoided.
- Used patches still contain some drug. Advise that:
  - Patches should be carefully disposed of by folding sticky sides together and discarding in the foil wrapper.
  - Care should also be taken to avoid transfer of patches from the patient to a partner or child with close contact.

For some specific pains, adjuvants such as NSAIDs or neuropathic agents may be more appropriate (see *Table 13.5*). *Box 13.2* details some practice points for managing the use of adjuvant analgesics.

Table 13.5: *Adjuvant analgesics*

Drug class	Example	Indication
NSAID	Naproxen 500 mg twice daily	Bone pain Liver capsule pain
Corticosteroid	Dexamethasone 2-16 mg daily	Headache from brain tumour Liver capsule pain Nerve compression pain
Tricyclic antidepressant	Amitriptyline 10-50 mg daily	Neuropathic pain
Gabapentinoid	Gabapentin 300-1800 mg daily in divided doses	Neuropathic pain

Box 13.2: Practice point: adjuvant analgesics

- Use NSAIDs with caution in people with gastrointestinal disease – gastroprotection may be required with a proton pump inhibitor (PPI).
- Use NSAIDs with caution in people with renal insufficiency.
- The choice of NSAID may vary with local formulary.
- Corticosteroids are used for a wide range of indications in palliative care. The aim is to titrate to the lowest dose needed to control symptoms.
  - They may impair glucose tolerance, requiring adjustment of antidiabetic medication or increased monitoring of blood sugar.
- Tricyclic antidepressants are not licensed for pain, but are useful where night sedation is required.
  - Doses lower than those required for mood are helpful in nerve pain.
- Gabapentinoids (e.g. gabapentin, pregabalin) are usually titrated up to effective dose. Reduced doses are needed in impaired renal function.

Nausea and vomiting

The choice of medicine to manage nausea and vomiting depends on the underlying cause of the symptoms (see *Table 13.6*), and there a number of important considerations to take into account depending on clinical features as well as other medicines the person may be taking (see *Box 13.3*).

Table 13.6: *Choice of antiemetics*

Circumstances	Choice of drug	Dose range
Movement related or brain tumour	Cyclizine	50 mg three times daily orally, or 75-150 mg subcutaneously over 24 hours
Feeling full, bloated or vomiting soon after eating	Metoclopramide	10 mg three times daily orally, or 30-60 mg subcutaneously over 24 hours
	Domperidone	10 mg three times daily orally
Chemical cause (e.g. drug toxicity, uraemia, hypercalcaemia)	Haloperidol	0.5 mg every 8 hours orally, or 1-5 mg over 24 hours by subcutaneous infusion
Multiple causes or cause unclear	Levomepromazine	6.25 mg twice daily orally, or 6.25-25 mg over 24 hours subcutaneous infusion

Box 13.3: Practice point: antiemetics

- Parkinson's disease – avoid dopaminergic drugs if possible. Domperidone, which doesn't cross the blood-brain barrier, may be used if the oral route is available.
  - Cyclizine or ondansetron are suitable alternatives if injectable medication is required.
  - If an antipsychotic is needed for agitation symptoms in the last days of life, levomepromazine is preferred over haloperidol.
- Metoclopramide may be used for more than 5 days and at higher than licensed doses in palliative patients, but they should be monitored closely for signs of parkinsonian side effects.
- Cyclizine may exacerbate heart failure.
- Ondansetron is highly constipating, so is rarely used in palliative care.
- Haloperidol and levomepromazine are unlicensed for nausea – it may be useful to explain the intended indication to patients.
- A regular antiemetic may be required until the underlying cause is treated.
- A change of route may be needed especially if there has been vomiting for a while – consider buccal, subcutaneous or rectal routes.
- Metoclopramide and cyclizine both use the same anticholinergic pathway in the gut, so antagonise each other if used together.
- Corticosteroids may be used – usually dexamethasone 2-4 mg daily for up to 5 days.

Breathlessness

In patients with COPD and heart failure, consider optimising therapy in line with their usual step up, if this is appropriate. Oxygen therapy is only helpful when the patient is hypoxic. Some patients with MND may opt for non-invasive ventilation (NIV), which will be managed by the respiratory specialist team.

Low dose opioids (<30 mg daily) have been shown to reduce the sensation of breathlessness.[21,22] This may be given as 2.5 mg up to hourly as needed as short-acting morphine oral solution, or as a regular sustained release product (MST or Zomorph).

Cough may be helped by nebulised saline (NaCl 0.9%) or low dose oral morphine.

Benzodiazepines are useful in treating the panic which contributes to the cycle of breathlessness. Lorazepam sublingually 0.5-1 mg 8-hourly has benefit in some patients (this is an unlicensed indication/route).

Non-pharmacological interventions are probably the most useful tool. Breathlessness management techniques taught by physiotherapists, occupational therapists and respiratory nurse specialists can give patients control of episodes of breathlessness.

A small handheld electric fan held near the face or sitting near an open window is effective. *Box 13.4* details some practice points for managing breathlessness.

Box 13.4: Practice point: breathlessness

- Carefully explain morphine use for breathlessness, as the manufacturer's patient information leaflets for opioid drugs state that it should be avoided in respiratory disease.
- Genus Pharmaceuticals generic blue lorazepam tablets disperse more effectively sublingually.
- Where frequent lorazepam is needed, diazepam 2 mg twice daily may be helpful.

Constipation

In general, the aim is to promote a good bowel movement at least every second day, but this may be dependent on what is normal for the patient. Laxatives work in a number of different ways and vary in the time taken to produce their effects (see *Table 13.7*). The choice of laxative will depend on a number of factors including:

- Fluid intake – good fluid intake is required for osmotic laxatives to work
- Renal or cardiac function – macrogols have significant electrolyte content which may not be suitable in in impaired renal of cardiac function
- If stool soft but difficult to expel – use stimulant laxatives (e.g. senna)
- If stool hard – use softeners (e.g. docusate) or osmotic laxatives
- Personal choice/experience of patient – taste, ability to swallow large volumes

Significant established constipation may require administration of suppositories or enemas to relieve blockage followed by establishment of a regular oral regimen. *Table 13.7* outlines the mode of action of different classes of laxatives and *Box 13.5* details some practice points for managing the use of laxatives.

Table 13.7: *Laxatives and their effects*

Laxative class	Example	Comments
Stimulant	Senna Bisacodyl	Useful when stool is difficult to pass due to reduced peristalsis
Osmotic	Lactulose	Pull fluid into gut lumen to soften stool and stimulate peristalsis; need to have good fluid intake
Isosmotic	Macrogol preparations	Require ability to take full volume at each dose; may also be used for faecal impaction
Stool softener	Docusate sodium	Detergent action to soften hardened stool

Box 13.5: Practice point: constipation

- Osmotic products will take up to 48 hours to work.
- If the drug regimen is constipating (e.g. opioids and anticholinergic drugs), regular laxative is necessary to avoid constipation.
- Encourage fluid intake and optimise the patient's preferred laxative before adding an additional product.

Anticipatory prescribing for end of life

Pre-emptive prescribing of the injectable drugs required to manage symptoms in the last weeks or days of life is an established practice and includes 'Just in Case' boxes and the MND Association 'Breathing Space Kits'.[23,24]

The oral route is preferable, but when patients are unable to swallow or have poor oral absorption, injectable medicine can be substituted. The aim is to ensure that symptoms can be managed with medicine already stored in the patient's home to avoid potential difficulties obtaining injectable medicines in a community setting at short notice or out of hours. The subcutaneous route is used as this is most easily managed in a non-clinical setting, does not require venous access and is more comfortable for patients.

In the acute setting it can enable nursing staff to quickly control symptoms whilst awaiting medical review. The availability of drugs also facilitates the use of continuous subcutaneous infusions via syringe pump. Careful assessment of the patient's needs is necessary before commencing a continuous infusion.

The choice of drugs may vary locally and may also include some oral or sublingual preparations. The choice may also be guided by individual patient factors such as age, renal function, and pre-existing conditions. *Table 13.8* details some drugs that are commonly available in 'Just in Case' boxes.

Table 13.8: *Injectable drugs for subcutaneous use – ONLY if needed for symptoms*

Drug class	Examples	Usual starting dose	Indication
Opioid	Morphine	This is dependent on the background opioid dose. For opioid naive patients this would usually be 2.5-5 mg morphine up to every hour by subcutaneous injection	Pain or breathlessness
	Oxycodone		
	Diamorphine		
Benzodiazepine	Midazolam	2.5-5 mg up to every 2 hours	Anxiety, distress, breathlessness
Anticholinergic	Hyoscine butylbromide	20 mg up to every 4 hours	Excessive secretions or abdominal colic
	Glycopyrronium	200 micrograms up to every 6 hours	
	Hyoscine hydrobromide	400 micrograms up to every 4 hours	
Antiemetic	Levomepromazine	6.25 mg up to every 12 hours	Nausea or agitation
	Haloperidol	0.5-1 mg up to every 6 hours	

Opioids

It may be necessary to switch from oral medicines to injections, and provide breakthrough pain relief. Ensure you are familiar with the conversions required to calculate equivalent doses and how to titrate doses. Breakthrough doses should be rounded up or down to safely measurable doses.

The breakthrough (PRN or rescue) dose is calculated as 1/6th of the total daily opioid dose. This applies to both oral and subcutaneous routes.

- Oral morphine 60 mg m/r twice daily = 120 mg in 24 hours
- So, the oral breakthrough dose is 120 mg/6, which is 20 mg up to hourly by mouth if needed for breakthrough pain

When converting oral to subcutaneous morphine the ratio is 2:1. You can then calculate the PRN subcutaneous dose.

- Oral morphine 60 mg m/r twice daily = 120 mg in 24 hours
- So, the equivalent subcutaneous does is 120 mg/2, which is 60 mg over 24 hours by subcutaneous infusion
- Plus, a PRN dose of 10 mg (60 mg/6) up to hourly by subcutaneous injection if needed for breakthrough pain

The conversion ratio for oral oxycodone to subcutaneous oxycodone is 1.5-2:1, however this varies locally due to clinical preference. Check your local policy.

- Oral oxycodone m/r 30 mg twice daily = 60 mg oral oxycodone in 24 hours
- So, the equivalent subcutaneous dose is 60 mg/2, which is 30 mg oxycodone over 24 hours by subcutaneous infusion
- Plus, a PRN dose of 5 mg subcutaneous oxycodone if needed for breakthrough pain

The conversion ratio for oral morphine to subcutaneous diamorphine is 3:1.

- Oral morphine m/r 60 mg twice daily = 120 mg oral morphine in 24 hours
- So, the equivalent dose of diamorphine is 120 mg/3 which is 40 mg over 24 hours by subcutaneous infusion
- Plus, a PRN dose of 5 mg subcutaneous diamorphine if needed for breakthrough pain; here the dose is rounded down to 5 mg as a dose of 40/6 = 6.66 mg

When titrating doses, increases should be proportionate and guided by the need for PRN doses. For example, if a patient is receiving morphine 30 mg/24 hours by subcutaneous infusion and has needed 2 × 5 mg subcutaneous injections in the previous 24 hours; an increase of 10 mg in 24 hours to give 24-hour dose of 40 mg would be reasonable.

Generally, increases in the range of 30-50% of the 24-hour dose are acceptable. If PRN use suggests more than this is required, a thorough review of the patient should be undertaken to ensure that the problem is pain and not another cause, such as:

- distress
- full bladder
- constipation
- a need for repositioning in bed etc
- non-opioid responsive pain
- incident pain due to movement or painful dressing changes.

If you are sure that the pain is both escalating and opioid responsive, the dose should be increased with careful monitoring of effect. In this situation it is helpful to discuss with a colleague or with a member of the palliative care team. If rapid escalations of doses are requested from a prescriber, discuss this with them to confirm the doses.[25]

Figure 13.2 illustrates how to manage pain in the last days of life.

Figure 13.2: *Pain management in the last days of life*

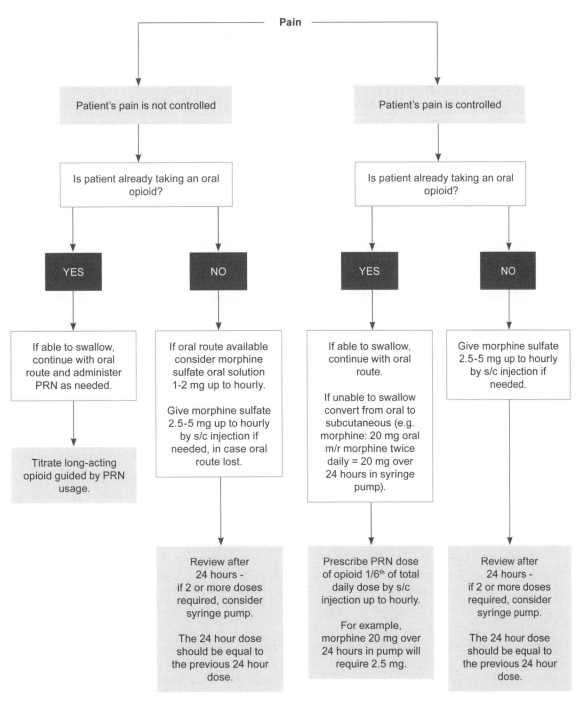

Benzodiazepines

Benzodiazepines are useful to help with symptoms of anxiety, distress and as a replacement for oral anticonvulsants.

Midazolam is suitable for subcutaneous administration (unlicensed route); the 10 mg/2 mL strength is most useful as it allows for a small volume of injection. As with opioids, the dose should be titrated carefully to alleviate symptoms whilst avoiding undue sedation.

For use as anticonvulsant replacement, a dose of 20-30 mg by subcutaneous infusion over 24 hours is recommended as a starting dose. There is no specific conversion from oral anticonvulsants. Doses of 5-10 mg may be required if seizures occur, and these can be used to guide titration of the background dose as required. The aim is for the patient to remain free from seizures.

Buccal midazolam products may also be used to enable families to manage seizures at home. Buccolam is licensed for use in children and the 10 mg dose is recommended (unlicensed) for use in adults. This provides an easier and more acceptable alternative to rectal diazepam.

Low dose lorazepam (0.5-1 mg 8-hourly) may be used sublingually (this is an unlicensed route) for rapid relief of anxiety or breathlessness and is included in some areas for anticipatory prescribing as it is suitable for self-administration.

Anticholinergics

Injectable anticholinergic drugs are used to reduce excessive salivary secretions which may pool in the throat as patients become weaker. These are effective in around 50% of cases, regardless of the choice of drug.

Hyoscine hydrobromide penetrates the blood-brain barrier and can cause hallucinations, so is used less often in end of life.

Doses should be titrated to give acceptable control of secretions whilst avoiding excessively dry mouth – frequent sips of water and use of an artificial saliva product can help with this.

Antiemetics

The choice of antiemetics for anticipatory prescribing is based on a pragmatic choice of the most likely benefit – levomepromazine has a broad spectrum so is often chosen, although haloperidol is less sedating and is a useful alternative. Another reason for choosing antipsychotic medicines is that these can also be used if there is significant agitation or delirium. Higher doses than those used for nausea may be needed for delirium. Dose ranges are detailed in *Table 13.9*.

Table 13.9: *Dose ranges for haloperidol and levomepromazine*

Drug	Antiemetic subcutaneous dose range	Agitation/delirium subcutaneous dose range
Haloperidol	0.5-1 mg up to every 6 hours, maximum 5 mg/24 hours	0.5-2.5 mg every 6 hours, maximum 10 mg/24 hours
Levomepromazine	6.25-12.5 mg up to every 12 hours, usual maximum 50 mg/24 hours	6.25-25 mg every 4 hours, usual maximum 200 mg/24 hours (however doses above 50 mg in 24 hours rarely required)

Syringe pumps for continuous subcutaneous infusions

When the oral route is compromised by poor swallowing or absorption, or when vomiting is prolonged, medicines may be given by subcutaneous infusion to control symptoms. Many patients will not require a subcutaneous pump as they can either manage oral medicines until death, or experience intermittent symptoms which can be controlled by injections when required.

Administration by syringe pump is not only for end of life – some patients will require a short period of subcutaneous administration for control of nausea and then revert to oral medicines.

In the UK the majority of services will use the CME T34 pump. This delivers a small volume infusion over a fixed period of time. For use in palliative care this is usually 10-37 mL over 24 hours. However, check your local guidelines as local services will have their own policy and procedures.

Combinations of symptom control medicine are individualised to help keep patients pain and symptom free, avoid undue sedation, and allow them to eat and drink as they are able. The choice of starting dose and combination are guided by symptoms at the time of assessment. Dose titration is guided by the need for as required medicines, and this should be reassessed daily. *Box 13.6* outlines some useful practice points when managing people at the end of life and *Box 13.7* details some resources that patients, their families and carers may find useful.

Box 13.6: Practice point: pharmacy input

- You will probably be aware of any of your usual patients who are entering the palliative phase of their illness – consider how you could help them and their carers manage their medicines.
- Patients' health often changes rapidly and they may require medicines at short notice – think creatively about how you can quickly fulfil a prescription even if you have to refer to another pharmacy, or contact the prescriber to supply an alternative.
- Good communication is key in supporting patients and families at the end of life. Emotional conversations can be difficult and we all worry that we are going to say the wrong thing – most people will value kindness and honesty.
  - Try to be realistic but kind, focus on what can be done to help symptoms in the absence of cure – 'we can't make the cancer go away, but we can get the pain better controlled'.
  - Ask how carers are coping – you may be the only person they see outside the home that day.
  - Think about resources to help inform patients and carers (see *Box 13.7*).
  - Be aware of local services (e.g. bereavement support or counselling via local hospice).
  - Consider your own further training in difficult conversations (e.g. www.sageandthymetraining.org.uk, or explore locally available options).
- In the community, patients will be under the care of their GP practice and most prescribing will originate there. Specialist teams who know the patient will also be happy to advise, especially if 'hospital only' medication is prescribed.
- Find out if there is a local Community Pharmacist Palliative Care Scheme. These extended roles generally include stocking a locally agreed list of palliative care drugs and a commitment to out of hours.
  - If your pharmacy is not providing the service, it is helpful to be aware of local participants to ensure rapid access to palliative care drugs if you do not have stock. In England, www.lpc-online.org.uk has links to pharmacies holding palliative care drugs.
- Get to know your local palliative care team – they may be based in the hospice or within community services in the Primary Care Trust or CCG. Not all patients will be known to the palliative care team, but most will be happy to give some general advice and support. In many areas there will be a specialist pharmacist attached to the team who will be a good resource for your practice, especially if you are prescribing in this patient group.
- In GP practices, try to go along to the Gold Standards Framework meetings – this is a good opportunity to be aware of patients with palliative care needs and a chance to contribute to the multidisciplinary discussion.
- If you work in a hospital setting, seek out your palliative care team, it is likely they will be seeing patients on your ward and making contact will help you understand the changes they might make to medications.

Box 13.7: Information to support patients and carers

These websites have information sources both for healthcare professionals and for patients and their families. Some will have resources (booklets and leaflets) that you can order for your own use.

- Macmillan Cancer Support
- Cancer Research UK
- Marie Curie
- Dying Matters
- British Heart Foundation
- Motor Neurone Disease Association
- National Multiple Sclerosis Society
- Diabetes UK

Useful resources

- Wilcock A *et al. Palliative Care Formulary (PCF)*, 7th edn. Pharmaceutical Press, 2020
- BNF: Prescribing in palliative care
- Palliative drugs. www.palliativedrugs.com
- Dickman A, Schneider J. *The Syringe Driver*, 4th edn. Oxford University Press, 2016
- The NEWT Guidelines. www.newtguidelines.com
- End of Life Care for All e-learning (e-ELCA). www.e-lfh.org.uk/programmes/end-of-life-care
- Palliative Care Guidelines
    - Scotland: www.palliativecareguidelines.scot.nhs.uk
    - Ireland: www.professionalpalliativehub.com
    - Wales: www.book.pallcare.info
    - England: check local guidance as this may vary

References

1. World Health Organisation (2018). Palliative care: key facts. www.who.int/news-room/fact-sheets/detail/palliative-care
2. Tremel J *et al*. Early palliative care for patients with non-small-cell lung cancer. *N Engl J Med* 2010; 363(8): 733-742.
3. Ali M *et al*. The importance of identifying preferred place of death. *BMJ Supportive & Palliative Care* 2019; 9: 84-91.
4. Office of National Statistics. Rolling annual death registrations by place of occurrence, England (Q3 2018/19). www.ons.gov.uk/file?uri=/peoplepopulationandcommunity/birthsdeathsandmarriages/deaths/adhocs/009673rollingannualdeathregistrationsbyplaceofoccurrenceenglandperiodendingquarter3octtodecoffinancialyear2018to2019/rollingannualq3201819.xls
5. ISD SCOTLAND. www.isdscotland.org
6. Lunney JR *et al*. Patterns of functional decline at the end of life. *JAMA* 2003; 289(18): 2387-2392.
7. Thomas K, Armstrong JA *et al*. The gold standards framework proactive identification guidance (PIG), 6th edn, 2016. www.goldstandardsframework.org.uk/cd-content/uploads/files/PIG/NEW%20PIG%20-%20%20%2020.1.17%20KT%20vs17.pdf
8. NHS Lothian and The University of Edinburgh Primary Palliative Care Research Group (2019). Supportive and palliative care identification tool (SPICT). www.spict.org.uk
9. Smyth JA, ed. The NEWT guidelines for administration of medication to patients with enteral feeding tubes or swallowing difficulties, 3rd edn. North East Wales NHS Trust, 2015.
10. British Association for Parenteral and Enteral Nutrition (2017). www.bapen.org.uk/nutrition-support/enteral-nutrition/medications
11. Guidance on enteral feeding in MND. www.mytube.mymnd.org.uk
12. Macmillan Cancer Support (2019). Primary care 10 top tips. www.macmillan.org.uk/_images/ten-tips-nutrition-at-end-of-life_tcm9-300211.pdf
13. PrescQIPP. Polypharmacy and deprescribing webkit. www.prescqipp.info/our-resources/webkits/polypharmacy-and-deprescribing
14. Care Quality Commission (2018). Polypharmacy and deprescribing. www.cqc.org.uk/guidance-providers/adult-social-care/polypharmacy-deprescribing
15. Todd A *et al*. 'I don't think I'd be frightened if the statins went': a phenomenological qualitative study exploring medicines use in palliative patients, carers and healthcare professionals. *BMC Palliat Care* 2016; 15: 13.
16. Todd A *et al*. Inappropriate prescribing in patients accessing specialist palliative day services. *Int J Clin Pharm* 2014; 36: 535-543.
17. Smith H *et al*. Person centred care including deprescribing for older people. *Pharmacy* 2019; 7(3): 101.1
18. World Health Organization (2010). WHO pain relief ladder. www.who.int/cancer/palliative/painladder/en
19. Scottish Intercollegiate Guidelines (2019). Management of chronic pain. www.sign.ac.uk/media/1108/sign136_2019.pdf
20. National Institute for Health and Care Excellence (2016). Opioids in palliative care: safe and effective prescribing for adults in palliative care [CG140]. www.nice.org.uk/guidance/cg140/evidence/full-guideline-pdf-186485297
21. Ekstrom M *et al*. Effects of opioids on breathlessness and exercise capacity in chronic obstructive pulmonary disease: a systematic review. *Annals of the American Thoracic Society* 2015; 12(7): 1079-1092.
22. Barnes H *et al*. Opioids for the palliation of refractory breathlessness in adults with advanced disease and terminal illness. *Cochrane Database of Systematic Reviews*, 2016. Issue 3.
23. National Institute for Health and Care Excellence (2015). Caring of dying adults in the last days of life [NG31]. www.nice.org.uk/guidance/ng31
24. Amass C *et al*. How a 'just in case' approach can improve out-of-hours palliative care. *The Pharmaceutical Journal* 2005; 275: 22-23.
25. Royal Pharmaceutical Society (2019). Areas for action following the report of the Gosport independent panel. www.rpharms.com/about-us/who-we-are/expert-advisors/hospital-expert-advisory-group/gosport-report

Case studies

Case study 1

Alice, aged 81 years, has type 2 diabetes and COPD. She was diagnosed with lung cancer nine months ago and declined any active treatment. She is in the last few months of life, but is managing at home with the help of her husband. Her daughter and grandchildren live nearby and help out with some of the practicalities of life.

Her medication is as follows:

Regular:

- Metformin – 500 mg twice daily
- Tiotropium (Spiriva) – 2 puffs daily
- Alendronate – 70 mg weekly (Tuesdays)
- Furosemide – 20 mg morning
- Citalopram – 20 mg morning
- Simvastatin – 40 mg night

- Amlodipine – 5 mg morning
- Omeprazole – 20 mg morning
- Paracetamol – 1 g four times daily
- Adcal D3 – 2 tablets daily
- Aspirin – 75 mg morning

PRN medication:

- Morphine sulfate oral solution 10 mg/5 mL – 2 mg up to every hour if needed for pain or breathlessness
- Salbutamol 2 puffs via Volumatic every four hours as needed

She has come to the surgery for review at your regular older people's clinic. She tells you she has been feeling dizzy and a bit sick, which has affected her appetite. She is starting to find the number of tablets she takes a problem and asks if she really needs them all. Otherwise she is feeling well, and does not currently need to use the morphine liquid for her breathlessness or pain.

> **Points to consider**
>
> - How would you answer Alice's query about her medicines?
> - What assessments are appropriate for Alice?

On examination, Alice's blood glucose is 8 mmol/L on finger prick. Alice tells you that she had breakfast of tea and toast about an hour and a half ago. Her blood pressure (BP) is 130/90.

> **Points to consider**
>
> - What, if any, medication changes would you make?
> - What are your reasons?

You decide to stop the following medicines:

- Metformin – this can cause GI upset and nausea. Alice's blood sugar is low, and in the last months of life the desirable range for blood glucose is up to 15 mmol/L. The advantages of tight control of blood glucose are the avoidance of long-term consequences, which are not applicable in Alice's case.
- Simvastatin – this has little benefit for Alice in view of her short prognosis.
- Alendronate – Alice has taken alendronate for the past 4 years to mitigate the risk of her intermittent corticosteroid treatment for exacerbations of COPD. This has a long duration of action once taken up into bone and will persist in its anti-resorption effect for months to years. It is difficult to take and can impact on quality of life.

Points to consider

- How would you involve Alice in this discussion?
- Is it appropriate to continue blood glucose monitoring?
- What follow-up is required?

Alice understands that her blood glucose levels are low, and since she has lost some weight recently and is eating less, the metformin is no longer needed and may be contributing to the nausea. She is happy to trial stopping the metformin. You arrange for her to continue weekly glucose monitoring to make sure this is maintained below 15 mmol/L and that there are no symptoms.

She is happy to stop the alendronate as she finds the need to have this on an empty stomach quite difficult and the tablet itself difficult to swallow. She will continue with her calcium supplements.

You explain to Alice that the simvastatin is probably not needed any more and she is happy to discontinue this.

You make a further appointment with Alice in two weeks to review progress.

Alice tells you that the changes to the medication have made her nausea better, but she still feels a bit dizzy, especially if she stands up too quickly.

You measure her blood pressure and it is 130/90 when she is sitting and 90/75 when standing.

Points to consider

- What are your thoughts on these BP results?
- What management options are appropriate?

You and Alice agree to stop the amlodipine to see if this helps.

After a further review two weeks later, Alice is much happier with her medication, her blood pressure is 132/87 when sitting and 128/86 when standing, and she is feeling less dizzy. Her blood glucose has been maintained between 8–12 mmol/L.

Her current medication is now as follows:

Regular:

- Tiotropium – 2 puffs daily
- Furosemide – 20 mg morning
- Citalopram – 20 mg morning
- Omeprazole – 20 mg morning

- Paracetamol – 1 g four times daily
- Adcal D3 – 2 tablets daily
- Aspirin – 75 mg morning

PRN medication:
- Morphine sulfate oral solution 10 mg/5 mL, 2 mg up to every hour if needed for pain or breathlessness
- Salbutamol 2 puffs via Volumatic every 4 hours as needed

You agree to continue with the current medication and review next month. You advise Alice that there is no need to measure her blood glucose at the moment and she is happy to omit this.

Case study 2

Bob, aged 78 years, has colorectal cancer and brain metastases. He lives with his wife, Susan, and is in the last weeks of his life. He and Susan are keen for him to remain at home. He has a DNACPR (Do Not Attempt Cardiopulmonary Resuscitation) order in place following discussion with the GP. He has regular care visits for personal care and support from the local community palliative care team.

The district nurse asks to discuss the medicines and a plan before she attends a patient. She has been asked to see him as his wife has called the surgery to request a home visit – she reports that he is now struggling to swallow his oral medication, and is taking only small amounts of food and fluids.

You check his medication record:

- Morphine sulfate m/r – 60 mg twice daily
- Lansoprazole – 30 mg morning
- Dexamethasone – 2 mg morning (reducing course due to complete in 4 days)
- Sodium valproate m/r – 300 mg twice daily (commenced following seizures)
- Paracetamol – 1 g four times a day
- Senna – 2 tablets morning
- Isosorbide mononitrate m/r – 60 mg morning
- Morphine sulfate oral solution 10 mg/5 mL – 20 mg (10 ml) up to every hour for pain
- Buccolam 10 mg – to be given for a seizure lasting more than 5 minutes.

> **Points to consider**
>
> - What changes could you make to Bob's medication to help with adherence?

You review the medicines and choose liquid/dispersible preparations to aid adherence.

> **Points to consider**
>
> - Which medicines are available as liquid/dispersible preparations?
> - What dose changes, if any, are required?

Drug	Action
Morphine sulfate m/r 60 mg	Use Zomorph 60 mg – open capsules and mix with water or give on yoghurt/ice cream
Lansoprazole 30 mg	Use orodispersible tablets – review once dexamethasone course complete and stop
Dexamethasone 2 mg	Use dispersible tablets or oral solution
Sodium valproate 300 mg m/r	Switch to oral solution – 200 mg three times daily
Paracetamol 1 g four times daily	Switch to soluble tablets
Senna 2 tablets morning	Switch to senna liquid 10 mL – switch to evening to space out medications
Isosorbide mononitrate m/r 60 mg	Stop – reduced activity so reduced risk of angina Make sure GTN spray or tablets available for PRN use

You arrange for (or prescribe if you are an IP) 'Just in Case' anticipatory medicines – these should include means of managing any seizures. The district nurse should be able to ensure that the sundries required (e.g. sharps bin, needles and syringes) are also all in the home for use. Local paperwork to authorise the use of the medications should also be completed and put in the home.

> **Points to consider**
>
> - What anticipatory medicines would it be appropriate to prescribe?

You prescribe:

- Morphine sulfate injection 10 mg/mL – 10 mg by subcutaneous injection up to every hour if needed for pain. Bob is already taking 60 mg twice daily of oral morphine, with an oral breakthrough dose of 20 mg (120 mg/6), hence the subcutaneous breakthrough dose is 10 mg.
- Midazolam injection 10 mg/2 mL – 2.5-5 mg up to every hour if needed for distress, and 10 mg in the event of a seizure lasting more than 5 minutes.
- Hyoscine butylbromide injection 20 mg/mL – 20 mg up to every four hours if needed for excess secretions.
- Levomepromazine 25 mg/mL – 6.25 mg up to every 12 hours if needed for nausea.
- Water for injections 10 mL – for use as diluent.

Susan comes in to pick up the prescription and you are able to spend time with her to make sure she understands the changes, and that the injections are there in case of any problems, which the district nurses will deal with.

When you ask how she is, she tells you that although she is sad and feeling tired she has help from her family who have arranged a rota to stay over at the house to support her and Bob and she is reassured that things are in place to keep him comfortable. She is grateful that she will be able to keep Bob at home with his family which is what he wants.

Points to consider

- Is there any additional support you can offer Susan?

Two weeks later the district nurse calls to say she is at Bob's home and he is now bed bound, unable to take any oral medication and is only taking sips of fluids. She has given him a 10 mg subcutaneous dose of morphine as he is in pain and didn't manage his morning oral dose of m/r morphine. She now recommends putting his analgesia in a syringe pump and is coming into the surgery to pick one up and to obtain authorisation and a new prescription for further supplies.

Bob's pain has been well controlled on 60 mg morphine m/r twice daily and he will require replacement for his sodium valproate.

A 24-hour continuous subcutaneous infusion via syringe pump will help control Bob's symptoms.

Points to consider

- What dose of morphine should be given by syringe driver?
- What other medication changes are appropriate?

You calculate the morphine dose for the infusion:

- Oral morphine dose 60 mg × 2 daily = 120 mg orally
- 120 mg / 2 = 60 mg subcutaneously over 24 hours

You replace the sodium valproate with midazolam and decide on a pragmatic starting dose of 30 mg/24 hours.

You arrange for a prescription (or prescribe yourself if you are an IP) of the initial infusion on the appropriate local authorisation paperwork:

- Morphine sulfate 60 mg plus midazolam 30 mg in water for injections to a minimum of 10 mL over 24 hours by subcutaneous infusion

This can be made with the medications already in the home (the 'Just in Case' medicines) and a further prescription for more medication can be obtained. The availability of the 'Just in Case' medicines allows prompt control of the symptoms and collection of further supplies within 24-48 hours.

A prescription should be issued for ongoing supplies:

- Morphine sulfate 30 mg/mL injection – use 60 mg to make up subcutaneous infusion over 24 hours × 10 ampoules
- Midazolam 10 mg/2 mL – use 30 mg to make up subcutaneous infusion over 24 hours × 10 ampoules
- Morphine sulfate 10 mg/mL – 10 mg up to hourly if needed for breakthrough pain × 10 ampoules

The district nurse reviews Bob daily and renews the syringe pump each day. Bob remains pain and seizure free and has not required any further medication. The syringe pump prescription remains unchanged and Bob dies three days later.

His daughter comes into the pharmacy a week later with his medication for disposal. She is grateful to the whole team for managing to keep her dad comfortable and in his own home.

CHAPTER 14

Rheumatoid arthritis

Hilary McKee

Overview

Rheumatoid arthritis (RA) is a chronic systemic autoimmune disease in which the immune system, which normally protects the body by attacking foreign substances like bacteria and viruses, mistakenly attacks the body's joints. This creates inflammation that causes the lining of the joints (synovium) to thicken, which results in swelling and pain in and around the joints, especially the fingers, wrists, feet and ankles.

If inflammation is not controlled it can cause damage with eventual loss of cartilage, reduced bone space and joint deformity. Joint damage cannot be reversed and it can occur very early in the disease, so the disease needs to be diagnosed early and treated aggressively to control the symptoms.

The cause of RA is unknown, although several infectious agents have been implicated none have been conclusively linked to RA. In a number of cases, RA begins within a few weeks of an infection and appears to be a consequence of an immune response to the infection.

There is a higher prevalence found in woman worldwide with a ratio of 3:1 women to men – this would suggest a possible hormonal influence. Women who have been pregnant are less likely to develop RA compared to those who have not, and if a woman with RA becomes pregnant, the disease usually improves during the pregnancy (when oestrogen levels increase) but symptoms return postpartum. As oestrogen levels tend to decline after the age of 40, women around this age also have a higher risk of developing RA and indeed those with early menopause are also at increased risk. Although current research does not show a link between female hormones and RA, it appears to be very complex.[1,2]

It has also been shown that there is a genetic influence in the development of RA. Research has shown that people with the HLA Shared Epitope genetic marker have a five times greater chance of developing RA than people without this marker – it is the HLA genetic site that controls immune responses. Other genes connected to RA include STAT4, TRAF1 and C5, which are relevant to chronic inflammation, and also PTPN22, a gene associated with both development and progression of RA. However, not all people with these genes will develop RA and not all people with the condition will have these genes.

Many studies recently have shown that smoking is a risk factor for developing RA. It would appear that cigarette smoking is associated with the production of rheumatoid factor (RF) and positive anti-citrullinated protein antibodies (ACPA) which are both specific and sensitive antibodies associated with developing RA. It is well known that smoking is associated with more severe RA, more active disease and smokers tend not to respond as well to medication.[3] Smoking cessation advice is crucial in patients with RA.

The prevalence of RA appears to vary throughout the world. In European and North American people it has a prevalence of around 0.5-2%, whereas it is rare in less developed and in some rural parts of the world.[1]

Diagnosis

RA can be difficult to diagnose in the early stages, but signs and symptoms include:

- tender, warm, swollen joints
- joint stiffness that is usually worse in the mornings and after inactivity
- fatigue, fever and loss of appetite.

Early RA tends to affect smaller joints first – particularly the joints that attach fingers to hands and toes to feet. As the disease progresses, symptoms often spread to the wrists, knees, ankles, elbows, hips and shoulders. In most cases, symptoms occur in the same joints on both sides of the body.

Diagnosis includes a physical examination to check joints for swelling, pain and heat, and blood tests to check the erythrocyte sedimentation rate (ESR) and the C-reactive protein (CRP) level which provide an indication of inflammation (although they are not specific to RA), as well as tests for ACPA, and RF. X-rays of hands and feet may also be carried out.

A score of 6 or more using the American College of Rheumatology (ACR)/European League Against Rheumatism (EULAR) classification criteria indicates a diagnosis of RA. See *Table 14.1*.

Table 14.1: *ACR/EULAR 2010 classification criteria for diagnosis of RA*[4]

Joint involvement	Score
1 medium-large joint	0
2-10 medium-large joints	1
1-3 small joints	2
4-10 small joints	3
More than 10 small joints	5
Serology	
RF (-) and anti-CPP (-)	0
RF (+) or anti-CCP (+)	2
High RF (+) or anti-CCP (+)	3
Duration of symptoms	
<6 weeks	0
≥6 weeks	1
Acute phase reactants	
CRP and ESR within normal range	0
Elevated CRP or ESR	1
A total score of 6 or more indicates a diagnosis of rheumatoid arthritis.	

Rheumatoid factor (RF)

RF is the autoantibody that was first found in RA. In current practice this test is much less widely relied upon for diagnostic purposes as it is less specific and sensitive for the detection of RA.[5] It is an antibody against the Fc portion of immunoglobulin G (IgG) and is usually composed of immunoglobulin M. However, up to 30% of people with RA will not form RF – they are classified as seronegative.

RF may not be present in early disease but is useful to confirm a clinical picture when it is present. High levels of RF may be present in other diseases, such as Sjorgren's syndrome and other autoimmune or infectious diseases, so is not specific for RA.

Anti-citrullinated protein antibody (ACPA)[6]

Around two-thirds of people with RA have ACPA. It can be detected in blood up to a decade before the appearance of clinical RA and is the antibody of choice to detect early RA in current practice.

Interestingly, around 40% of seronegative RA patients will be ACPA positive. High levels may be predictors of severity of disease.

> ### Box 14.1: Practice point
>
> People with a new diagnosis of rheumatoid arthritis may find this distressing. Referral to one of the arthritis charities, such as Versus Arthritis or National Rheumatoid Arthritis Society (NRAS), for patient peer support and further information can be helpful.

Treatment

There is currently no cure for RA, however, early intervention and modern treatments mean that many people can continue to live healthy, active lives with minimal damage to joints.

The treatment of RA has been revolutionised in the last 20 years with the introduction of biologics. Previously, people were managed with non-steroidal anti-inflammatory drugs (NSAIDs) with disease-modifying anti-rheumatic drugs (DMARDs) added in as the disease progressed.

The goal of treatment is to prevent joint damage, so early DMARD treatment is initiated and dual or triple DMARD therapy is not uncommon.

NSAIDs, both traditional non-selective NSAIDs and COX-2 inhibitors, are widely used for their anti-inflammatory and analgesic effects. They are considered to be a necessary choice in pain management because of the integrated role of the COX pathway in the generation of inflammation and in the biochemical recognition of pain.

Methotrexate has often been considered the 'gold standard' in the treatment of RA and is very often the first choice DMARD. Other DMARDs which are rarely used nowadays include gold, penicillamine, ciclosporin and azathioprine.

Corticosteroids are commonly prescribed in rheumatology and are sometimes administered as 'rescue' during a flare, or are given as cover while waiting for DMARDs to become effective.

If the disease is rapidly progressing and is uncontrolled by DMARDs, the biologics are next in the treatment pathway. There are a number of treatment options available which have different actions, including tumour necrosis factor (TNF) inhibitors, B-cell depletion, interleukin 6 inhibitors, interleukin 17/interleukin 23 inhibitors and Janus kinase (JAK) inhibitors.

If the dominant inflammatory pathway in each person could be determined, a more targeted approach to treatment could be taken, however, this is not yet possible. Currently, all biologics are initiated in secondary care, and in the case of subcutaneous injections, these may be delivered directly to the patient by homecare companies.

Pharmacy input

Pharmacists working in community settings can help to identify people who may have early inflammatory arthritis. For example, people who buy regular topical analgesic preparations may enquire if there is anything stronger for their joint pain – they may complain of stiffness, especially first thing in the morning, and there may be swelling and pain in joints.

Alternatively, sometimes the disease can onset suddenly with only one joint involved.

Questions that pharmacists should ask in these circumstances include:

- Are your joints stiff? If so, are they stiff when you first get up? How long does it take before the stiffness eases?
- Are any joints swollen? Look at the patient's hands for persistent swelling of one or more joints.
- Are your joints painful to squeeze?
- Is there reddening of the skin, or are the joints hot?

People presenting with any of these symptoms should be referred as soon as possible to their GP for assessment and possible onward referral to secondary care. Most rheumatology centres have early arthritis clinics for rapid access for anyone with suspected RA.

Early diagnosis is crucial, it is vitally important to control inflammation as quickly as possible to avoid early joint damage. Once joints have been damaged the clock cannot be turned back and damage cannot be undone with other medications.

Once diagnosed, community pharmacists can encourage lifestyle changes, as smoking cessation and weight management are crucial in managing these patients.[7] In addition, pharmacists can also encourage compliance with treatment, and should know about clinically significant drug interactions.

Pharmacists will have different levels of skill and ability to assess and intervene in the treatment of patients with RA. For this reason, the Professional Expert Practice Guide for Advanced Pharmacy Practice in Rheumatology has been developed.[8]

This document outlines the various competencies required for specialist pharmacists working in rheumatology to allow progression through the skills required in accordance with the Advanced Skills Framework (APF). This expert practice guide provides an overview of the knowledge and skills required to practice at an advanced level in rheumatology pharmacy at three stages:

- Advanced stage I
- Advanced stage II
- Mastery in line with the requirements of the APF

The document is intended to be used by practitioners to support the development of their practice at an advanced level in managing patients with rheumatic disease. It encourages practitioners to think critically and to use knowledge in rheumatic therapeutics, supporting informed decision making using knowledge from this and other related therapeutic areas to promote optimal medicines management for patients. It is intended to be as useful to the wider community working with patients with rheumatic disease from all sectors of care.

See *Table 14.2* for some suggested roles for pharmacists based on their level of knowledge, experience and competence.

Table 14.2: *Pharmacy roles in managing people with rheumatoid arthritis*

Pharmacist	Role in managing rheumatoid arthritis
All pharmacists	<ul><li>Be aware of the signs and symptoms of RA</li><li>Be aware of medicines used to treat RA and their main adverse effects</li><li>Be aware of clinically significant drug interactions (and ones which are not)</li><li>Be aware of the monitoring requirements for RA medicines</li><li>Be aware of early signs of disease flares</li><li>Advise about adverse effects</li><li>Direct patients to sources of information and support (e.g. charities and national support groups)</li><li>Provide lifestyle advice, particularly about smoking cessation and weight management</li><li>Check women of childbearing age are using adequate contraception (if appropriate, depending on the drug)</li><li>Refer to GP if required</li></ul>
Pharmacist with advanced knowledge	<ul><li>Ensure the required monitoring is carried out</li><li>Review monitoring results and understand the significance of slightly abnormal blood results before issuing repeat prescriptions</li><li>Conduct medication reviews<ul><li>– Any suggested changes to medication should be referred to secondary care</li></ul></li><li>Advise about managing adverse effects</li><li>Advise on compliance with medicines</li><li>Advise about contraception if required</li><li>Refer to secondary care when required</li></ul>

Table 14.2: *Pharmacy roles in managing people with rheumatoid arthritis (continued)*

Pharmacist	Role in managing rheumatoid arthritis
Pharmacist with specialist knowledge	• Adjust doses to manage adverse effects • Prescribe alternatives if adverse effects are intolerable or there is no benefit from current medication • Monitor disease progression and adjust treatment regimen • Monitor drug response and initiate change where appropriate • Use clinical examination skills • Manage a patient caseload • Be an integrated part of the multidisciplinary team • Manage patients with complex comorbidities • Refer to rheumatology consultants when required

Box 14.2: Practice point: diagnosis

- Rheumatoid arthritis can develop at any age.
- Be aware of persistently tender, swollen joints and urge referral to secondary care for diagnosis and rapid treatment to minimise damage.
- Encourage positive lifestyle changes, such as smoking cessation and weight management.

Pharmacy review[9,10,11]

In the 1990s, Kurtz and Silverman developed a guide within a practical teaching framework known as the Calgary-Cambridge guide. This guide was developed as a medical model,[12] however it is applicable to pharmacy consultations. It is now used widely to teach consultation skills to healthcare professionals. See *Figure 14.1*.

Figure 14.1: *Step-by-step guide to a consultation[12]*

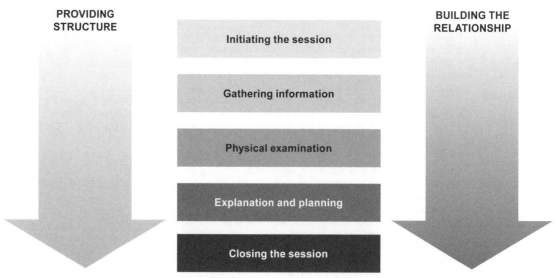

Source: adapted from Kurtz S *et al*, 2003.

Initiating the consultation

Greet the patient, introduce yourself if you are not known to the patient and clarify your role. In community pharmacy this may be as simple as 'I am the pharmacist', in secondary care review clinics it may be necessary to further explain your role in a clinic situation, for example: 'My name is John and I am going to do your rheumatology review today. I am a pharmacist and have had many years of experience working with patients with rheumatoid arthritis'.

You then need to explain the purpose of the consultation, for example: 'I just want to run through your new medicine with you', or 'I just want to make sure your medicines are agreeing with you'.

Be sure the patient can understand you; they have no hearing difficulties, language, or cognition barriers. Do not judge the patient, even if you do not agree with them.

Gathering information

Use appropriate questioning to identify problems and any issues they are having. Ask about:

- General health and joint health
  - If any joints are stiff when they first get up in the morning and how long this lasts for
  - Which joints are painful
- Medication:
  - What medicines they are taking
  - If they are experiencing any side effects they think are related to their medicines
  - If they ever miss medicines
  - If they think the medicines are working
- Monitoring
  - When they last had bloods monitored
- Lifestyle
  - If they smoke and if so, how much
  - If they drink alcohol or take any other substances

  Sometimes it may be necessary to ask: 'If I could only help with one thing, what is it?'

Observe the patient – how they walk, how easily they can get off a chair, watch their body language and listen attentively.

Physical examination

Physical examination by pharmacists will be dependent upon skill levels in individual circumstances. Blood pressure measurements are useful, particularly if a patient is already hypertensive and is starting on a medicine which may cause blood pressure increases, such as leflunomide. Even if a pharmacist does not feel sufficiently confident to undertake a joint count, simple questions as outlined above can be helpful, and joints can be observed for redness and swelling.

Explanation and planning

Always be aware of your limitations in a consultation and know when to refer back to secondary care. Some adverse effects of drugs can be dealt with initially with OTC medicines, for example, loperamide for diarrhoea, antihistamine tablets for itchy skin or injection site reactions.

However, if adverse effects are persistent or severe, a discussion with the prescriber or referral back for specialist opinion may be necessary. Not all drugs are suitable for all patients. Adverse effects can sometimes be managed, but dose alterations or alternative/additional medicines may be required.

Ensure women of childbearing age taking DMARDs have adequate contraception if the drugs are teratogenic, and ensure that they understand and are happy with their treatment plan.

Patient information leaflets are good resources for providing relevant management advice and reiterating when to seek further help.

Closing the session

Make sure the patient understands and is happy with their treatment plan, and ensure the consultation is fully documented and communicated to the relevant personnel. Arrange a follow-up appointment if appropriate.

The principles of medicines optimisation are outlined in *Figure 14.2*. These are easily applied in rheumatoid patients (see *Box 14.3*).

Figure 14.2: *Patient-centred approach*[9]

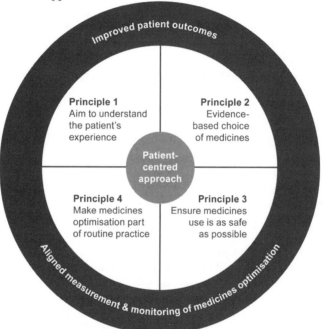

Box 14.3: Practice point: medicines optimisation[9]

Principle 1 – aim to understand the patient experience
- Consider your patients fears of:
  - **Diagnosis** – a lifelong chronic condition; **Disease progression** – disability, loss of function; **Medicines and adverse effects**

Principle 2 – evidence-based choice of medicines
- Consider how your patient feels about being given a particular medicine. Be prepared to answer their questions about treatment choices, for example:
  - **Why am I not allowed glucosamine?; My friend gets a drug every 6 months in the hospital. She says it is great, why can't I have it?; My neighbour told me to take...**

Principle 3 – ensure safe use of medicines
- Be prepared and ready to manage:
  - **Adverse effects; Correct doses; Drug interactions; Temporarily stopping treatment; Pregnancy considerations; Multiple comorbidities**

Principle 4 – make medicines optimisation part of routine practice

Medicines

Medicines for RA are initiated in secondary care but may be managed in primary care under shared care arrangements. In these circumstances, local shared care guidelines should be followed.

Non-steroidal anti-inflammatory drugs (NSAIDs)

NSAIDs are associated with a number of adverse effects; most common are gastrointestinal adverse effects and cardiovascular effects. See *Box 14.4* for information on reducing the risk of adverse effects with NSAIDs.

Non-selective NSAIDs inhibit COX-1 and COX-2 enzymes. COX-1 is present in most tissues and largely governs the homeostatic production of arachidonic acid metabolites including gastro cytoprotection via prostacyclin (PGI2), whereas COX-2 is induced in response to inflammatory stimuli and is responsible for the enhanced production of eicosanoid mediators for inflammation and pain. Inhibition of COX-1 is thought to be responsible for gastrointestinal toxicity. COX-2 specific NSAIDs tend to have less gastrointestinal toxicity.

In general, ibuprofen has the lowest gastrointestinal risk, while diclofenac and naproxen have an intermediate risk, and piroxicam and ketorolac are high risk. However, it should be noted that the advantage of low-risk drugs may be lost when the dose is increased.

At therapeutic doses, COX-2 inhibitors are thought to only inhibit COX-2, which may result in overproduction of harmful by-products that can damage the arterial wall and induce blood clotting. Evidence suggests that this may be a class effect for all NSAIDs, and caution should be exercised in people with cardiovascular disease.[13]

Box 14.4: Practice point: NSAIDs

- Use the lowest effective dose of a traditional NSAID to reduce incidence of complications.
- The analgesic effect has a ceiling, so higher doses do not necessarily result in better analgesia.
- COX-2 inhibitors may be used to reduce the risk of gastrointestinal (GI) adverse events.
- Prophylactic use of proton pump inhibitors (PPIs) is considered appropriate by major treatment guidelines.
- Monitor renal function and blood pressure.
- There is an increased risk of serious GI complications in people:
  - aged over 65 years
  - with a history of peptic ulcer disease
  - taking corticosteroids
  - taking anticoagulants
  - taking aspirin.
- NSAIDs, although useful in controlling pain and inflammation, will not affect disease progression.

Methotrexate

Methotrexate is a disease-modifying anti-rheumatic drug (DMARD), it is not a pain killer. The starting dose varies but is generally between 10 mg and 15 mg. The normal maintenance dose is 5-25 mg once weekly, according to tolerability and effect.

Methotrexate is usually only dispensed in multiples of 2.5 mg tablets in order to reduce the risk of patient error, as the 10 mg and 2.5 mg strength tablets look very similar, and there have been serious incidents where patients have inadvertently overdosed. Methotrexate is also available as a subcutaneous injection, suitable for self-administration, which is useful in people who have a suboptimal response to tablets, or who suffer from nausea as an adverse effect.

Methotrexate is a folic acid antagonist so it is co-prescribed with folic acid 5 mg once weekly (24-48 hours after the dose of methotrexate).

The most common adverse effects are nausea, diarrhoea and mouth ulcers, and this may be dose dependent.

Some patients will suffer from hair loss which is reversible when methotrexate is stopped and methotrexate can also cause abnormal liver function tests; this is usually reversible if methotrexate is withdrawn.

More serious adverse effects include decreased white cell count, platelets and neutropenia, which can affect up to 5% of patients. Around 1% of patients experience lung problems – shortage of breath, cough, so it is essential that a chest X-ray is arranged before starting treatment and some specialists will also check pulmonary function. Patients should be advised that if they have an unexplained cough or shortness of breath which persists, they need to contact their doctor.

Adverse effects should be managed according to the shared care guidelines which may require referral back to the prescriber.

Methotrexate is a potent teratogen and effective contraception must be used in female patients of childbearing age. The general advice is to stop methotrexate for around six months if trying to conceive.

In practice there are very few clinically relevant drug interactions;[14] trimethoprim and sulfamethoxazole should be avoided with methotrexate. There is some concern regarding NSAIDs' link with decreased renal function and increased methotrexate levels. This is very rarely of any clinical significance, even with the use of OTC products, and the combination is often used in the treatment of patients with RA.

Patients should be warned to stop their methotrexate whilst on any antibiotic treatment, and not to restart until signs of infection are resolved.

Box 14.5: Practice point: methotrexate

- Live vaccines should not be administered to people on methotrexate. If these are required, methotrexate should be avoided for at least three months before administration.
  - MMR, varicella (these are attenuated live vaccines), typhoid, Hep A, Hep B and tetanus are safe.
  - Flu vaccine is safe and highly recommended.
  - Varicella zoster immunoglobulin can be given if shingles occurs while on treatment.
- Ensure women of childbearing age are using adequate contraception.
- Nausea associated with methotrexate can sometimes be minimised by taking the methotrexate dose in the evening followed by the folic acid 24 hours later.
  - Antiemetics can sometimes help with nausea.
  - Switching from oral methotrexate to subcutaneous injection can also help with nausea.
- A saltwater rinse or mouthwash may help control mouth ulcers.
- Alcohol intake should be minimised.
- New shortness of breath or persistent cough should prompt referral.
- Advise people to temporarily stop methotrexate if they have an infection or if they are taking antibiotics.
- Methotrexate and NSAIDs are often used in combination and in practice, this rarely causes any problems.

Leflunomide

Leflunomide is a commonly used oral DMARD, and the normal dose is 10 mg or 20 mg once daily. Few centres now use the recommended loading dose of 100 mg daily for three days due to tolerability issues. The drug has a long half-life of around 14 days.

Common adverse effects include diarrhoea and headache – these can be managed with anti-diarrhoeals and analgesics. Blood pressure may also increase, so it is good practice to measure blood pressure before starting treatment and during treatment, particularly if the patient is already taking antihypertensives. Occasionally some patients may experience hair loss, although this doesn't tend to be problematic.

Leflunomide has a long half-life, causing it to persist in the body, but if necessary it can be 'washed out' (e.g. in pregnancy or if there are intolerable adverse effects) with colestyramine 4 g three times daily for 10 days.

Leflunomide is a very potent teratogen and pregnancy should be avoided during treatment and for 24 months after cessation of treatment. Women of childbearing age must have adequate contraception in place, and patients who are on leflunomide and wish to become pregnant should undergo the washout procedure. A blood test is required to check levels once washout has been completed.

Leflunomide can also affect liver enzymes and blood monitoring is required according to shared care guidelines.

Box 14.6: Practice point: leflunomide

- Ensure women of childbearing age are using adequate contraception.
- Monitor blood pressure, particularly if patient is overweight or has hypertension.
  - If the person is responding well to leflunomide, an antihypertensive agent may be added if necessary.
- Nausea and diarrhoea often subside within a few weeks of commencing treatment.
  - Initial diarrhoea may be managed with loperamide, but long-term diarrhoea may necessitate discontinuation of treatment.

Sulfasalazine

Sulfasalazine is available in 500 mg tablets and is normally introduced gradually to reduce the risk of adverse effects. A typical regimen is 500 mg once daily for one week, then 500 mg twice daily for one week, then 500 mg three times daily for one week and then 1 g twice daily. The maximum dose is usually 3 g daily. There is no clinical benefit in increasing dose beyond this, but there is an increased risk of toxicity.

Time to effect is slow – between 4 and 12 weeks. It may be used in pregnancy but should be avoided in people who are sulfa allergic.

Common adverse effects include gastrointestinal problems and rash – depending on the severity, treatment may need to be stopped, but this will be detailed in the shared care guidelines. Discolouration of urine and tears may occur. Other possible adverse effects include agranulocytosis, myelosuppression, hepatitis and azoospermia.

Hydroxychloroquine

Hydroxychloroquine has been used for many years in the treatment of RA. The normal dose is 200-400 mg daily. Time to effect is between 8 and 24 weeks, and it can be used in pregnancy if necessary. Adverse effects include rash, diarrhoea and possible neuromyopathy and retinopathy.

Very detailed guidelines on ocular monitoring have been in place since 2017 and were recently updated in 2020. This involves a baseline examination within 6-12 months of initiation, then annual monitoring for all people who have taken it for more than 5 years. If additional risk factors are present (e.g. impaired renal function), annual monitoring may be required before 5 years.

Corticosteroids

Intra-articular steroid injections may be useful in troublesome inflamed joints, and oral steroids may be used in long-term management, however, long-term use is associated with many adverse effects including osteoporosis, skin fragility, diabetes, Cushing's disease, cataracts and atherosclerosis.

Steroids must not be stopped abruptly; long term use requires careful dose tapering. Patients on long-term steroids must be assessed for osteoporosis risk and treated accordingly.

Box 14.7: Practice point: corticosteroids

Ensure people on long-term steroids are given bone-sparing treatments where appropriate, and that they are adhering to treatment.

Biologics

Anti-tumour necrosis factor (TNF) drugs

Anti-TNFs are normally the first choice of the biologics in the treatment pathway and are normally given with concomitant methotrexate if this is tolerated.[15]

Drugs commonly used include etanercept, adalimumab, infliximab, certolizumab and golimumab – these are all administered by injection, either subcutaneously or by intravenous infusion, as there are no oral formulations.

As they are immunosuppressive, the main adverse effect is increased risk of infection, so patients should be counselled to seek immediate antibiotic treatment if they develop any signs of infection as infections may turn severe very quickly. Patients with known recurrent infections are treated with caution. Other adverse effects include injection site reactions, rare demyelination and there may be a slight increased risk of basal cell carcinoma with some of the anti-TNF drugs.

Patients should be screened carefully before starting treatment. This should include a chest X-ray, pulmonary function tests, screening for tuberculosis (TB), varicella, hepatitis B and hepatitis C. Anti-TNF is known to reactivate latent TB; if any signs of TB are shown on QuantiFERON (a blood test that detects *Mycobacterium tuberculosis*), treatment for TB should be initiated before the anti-TNF is started.

See *Table 14.3* for drugs and dosages for anti-TNF drugs.

Table 14.3: *Dosages of anti-TNF drugs*

Drug	Dose	Type
Etanercept	50 mg subcutaneous (SC) injection every week	Humanised recombinant FC fusion protein
Infliximab	3 mg/kg intravenous infusion every 6 weeks	Chimeric monoclonal antibody
Adalimumab	40 mg SC injection every 2 weeks	Humanised monoclonal antibody
Certolizumab	200 mg SC injection every 2 weeks	Pegol humanised Fab' fragment
Golimumab	50 mg or 100 mg SC injection every month	Humanised monoclonal antibody

Rituximab

Rituximab depletes B cells which results in decreased T cell activation, and downregulation of cytokines IL6, TNF, and IL10. It is normally administered as two IV infusions given two weeks apart and is repeated as required every 6 to 18 months.

Infusion reactions can occasionally be severe, so initial infusions are given slowly with premedication of paracetamol, methylprednisolone and chlorphenamine. If there are any signs of anaphylactic type reaction, the infusion rate is stopped or slowed. Subsequent infusions may be given more quickly if initial infusions are uneventful.

Several cases of progressive multifocal leukoencephalopathy (PML) have been reported in people with lupus from reactivation of JC virus in the central nervous system, so they are counselled about this rare complication. The most prominent symptoms may include paralysis, clumsiness, progressive weakness, vision loss, impaired speech and cognitive deterioration including personality changes. People reporting any of these symptoms should be referred to their doctor at the earliest opportunity.

Interleukin 6 (IL-6) inhibitors

Tocilizumab and sarilumab are both IL-6 receptor inhibitors. In people with RA, IL-6 may be overproduced causing inflammation.

Tocilizumab is administered monthly via a 4-8 mg/kg infusion or by subcutaneous injection every two weeks. The most common adverse effects are injection site reactions, upper respiratory tract infections and hyperlipidaemia. Lipid levels should be checked before starting and periodically during treatment. Neutropenia is also common.

Sarilumab is administered by subcutaneous injection at a dose of 150-200 mg every two weeks and has a similar adverse effect profile to tocilizumab.

Abatacept

Abatacept inhibits the presentation of antigen to T cells. It is particularly useful in patients with high levels of ACPAs. It can be administered by intravenous infusion once a month or as a weekly subcutaneous injection. The most commonly reported adverse effects are headache, nausea and upper respiratory tract infections.

Janus kinase (JAK) inhibitors

These are the most recently developed drugs to help manage RA and they appear to be very effective. They inhibit Janus-associated kinases (JAK1 and JAK3). Current available JAKs are baracitinib and tofacitinib, although there are others in the pipeline. These are small molecules and so are available as tablets, which is preferable to many patients as all other biologics are administered by injection. They also tend to have a very short half-life, which is convenient if infection occurs as the drug is eliminated quickly from the body.

Lipids should be checked before and after initiation as there is a tendency for lipid levels to increase – responsibility for this will be detailed in the shared care guidelines. Other adverse effects include reactivation of herpes, upper respiratory tract infections, headache, diarrhoea, sinusitis and herpes infections. Both should be used with caution in patients with risk factors for deep vein thrombosis/pulmonary embolism.

The dose of tofacitinib is 5 mg twice daily and the recommended dose of baracitinib is 4 mg daily, however, 2 mg daily is appropriate for people aged over 75 years with a history of chronic or recurrent infections and people with reduced kidney function (creatinine clearance between 30 and 60 mL/minute).

Box 14.8: Practice point: DMARDs

- Patients are sometimes co-prescribed non-biologic DMARDs (e.g. methotrexate) with biologics.[10]
- Patients should be advised to temporarily stop treatment if they have an infection.
- Biologics are stopped prior to surgery and after surgery until wound healing is complete. Exact timings depend on the half-life of the drug.

Monitoring

Blood monitoring

All DMARDs require blood monitoring and each drug is monitored according to the British Society of Rheumatology (BSR) recommendations.[16] This may be undertaken in GP practice depending on the treatment and local agreements, but pharmacists may be required to refer to test results if they are involved in prescribing under a shared care guideline.

Blood markers may include full blood count, differential blood count, liver function tests, electrolytes, ESR and CRP, and for some drugs lipids levels may be monitored.

Comprehensive annual review

A comprehensive annual review should be undertaken in secondary care. NICE recommends that people undertaking the review should:[17]

- assess disease activity and damage, and measure functional ability (using, for example, the HAQ)
- check for the development of comorbidities such as hypertension, ischaemic heart disease, osteoporosis and depression
- assess symptoms that suggest complications such as vasculitis and disease of the cervical spine, lungs or eyes
- organise appropriate cross-referral within the multidisciplinary team
- assess the need for referral for surgery
- assess the effect the disease is having on the person's life.

Disease activity

Disease activity is monitored in secondary care at review appointments. A common measurement of disease activity is DAS28 (disease activity score) which looks at 28 joints and is based on the number of tender and swollen joints together with a score of how the patient is feeling. It also takes into account the ESR and CRP. See *Figure 14.3*.

Figure 14.3: *28-joint swollen and tender joint count*

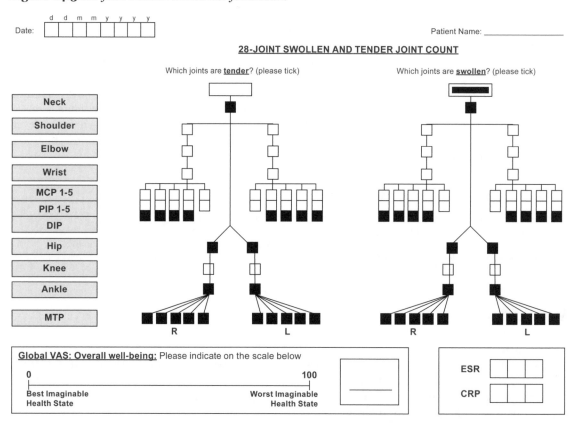

A DAS score of over 5.1 indicates active severe disease and this score is currently used as a marker for starting treatment with biologics. Joints which are examined include the shoulders, elbows, hands (metacarpophalangeal joints (MCPs) and proximal interphalangeal joints (PIPs)) and the knees. This score is combined with the VAS (global wellbeing score) and either ESR or CRP to give the final DAS28 score. The aim of treatment is to see an overall decrease in the score.

Table 14.4: *DAS scoring*[18]

DAS28	Implication
Less than 2.6	Disease remission. Usually no action necessary except remain on current medication.
2.6 to 3.2	Low disease activity. May merit change in therapy for some patients.
3.2 to 5.1	Moderate disease activity. May merit change in therapy for some patients unless mutually agreed to be the best outcome on current treatment.
More than 5.1	Severe disease activity likely to require a change in therapy. This is the current threshold for being considered for biologic treatment as per NICE guidelines.

Referral

Information about when to refer patients back to secondary care will be detailed in the shared care guidelines and may differ depending on the treatment and local arrangements.

Information and advice

In addition to providing information about prescribed medication and lifestyle advice, patients buying herbal products should be counselled about their risks and benefits and drug interactions should be excluded. While it is often assumed that 'herbal' means natural and is therefore always safe, this is not always the case.

Examples of drugs that may be taken to help with RA symptoms include:[19]

- Devils claw – anti-inflammatory properties are not completely understood and are thought to be due to harpagoside; however, devils claw can interact with a number of prescribed medicines including anticoagulants, digoxin and some analgesics
- Echinacea – increased risk of hepatotoxicity
- Ginkgo biloba, garlic – increased risk of bleeding with NSAIDs or steroids
- Cod liver oil – caution is advised when used with antihypertensives and warfarin
- Traditional Chinese medication – these are not recommended
- Turmeric – this has been promoted as an anti-inflammatory agent but has potential for interaction with many medicines including NSAIDs and sulfasalazine

Box 14.9: Practice point: patient advice

- Patients may be keen to purchase OTC herbal medications, assuming that herbal is always safe.
- Be aware of potential interactions with prescribed medications.
- Advise patients that natural products/supplements are not a substitute for prescribed medicines.

Patient information resources

- Versus Arthritis – this is the UK's largest charity dedicated to supporting people with arthritis. It was launched in September 2018, following the legal merger of the two leading arthritis charities in the UK, Arthritis Research UK and Arthritis Care.
- National Rheumatoid Arthritis Society (NRAS) – is a patient-led organisation in the UK specialising in RA and juvenile idiopathic arthritis (JIA). Due to its targeted focus on RA and JIA, NRAS provides truly expert and wide-ranging services to support, educate, provide resources to and campaign for people living with these complex autoimmune conditions. Their websites (www.nras.org.uk/www.jia.org.uk)

provide detailed and credible information about the two conditions. Their frontline services such as a freephone helpline, telephone volunteer support, publications etc. are all free to use.

Resources for pharmacists

- European League against Rheumatism (EULAR). www.eular.org
- American College of Rheumatology (ACR). www.rheumatology.org
- British Society of Rheumatology website for updated guidelines and information. www.rheumatology.org.uk
- Rheumatoid Factor. Medscape. July 2019
- Medicines optimisation: Helping patients to make the most of medicines. 2013. Available at: www.rpharms.com/Portals/0/RPS%20document%20library/Open%20access/Policy/helping-patients-make-the-most-of-their-medicines.pdf

References

1. Smith HR. Rheumatoid Arthritis. Medscape [online] 2020. www.emedicine.medscape.com/article/331715-overview

2. Costenbader KH and Manson JE. Do female hormones affect the onset or severity of rheumatoid arthritis? *Arthritis & Rheumatism* 2008; 59(3): 299-301.

3. Chang K *et al.* Smoking and rheumatoid arthritis. *International Journal of Molecular Science* 2014; 15(12): 22279-22295.

4. Kay J, Upchurch KS. ACR/EULAR 2010 rheumatoid arthritis classification criteria. *Rheumatology* 2012; 51(Suppl 6): vi5-vi9.

5. Street T *et al.* Rheumatoid Factor. Medscape [online] 2019. www.emedicine.medscape.com/article/2087091-overview

6. Cruyssen VC *et al.* Anti-citrullinated protein/peptide antibodies (ACPA) in rheumatoid arthritis: specificity and relation with rheumatoid factor. *Autoimmunity Reviews* 2005; 4(7): 468-474.

7. Bartlett SJ *et al.* Smoking and excess weight attenuate rate of improvement over first 3 years in early RA (abstract). *Arthritis Rheumatology* 2016; 68(suppl 10).

8. Royal Pharmaceutical Society (2016). Expert practice guide for advanced pharmacy practice in rheumatology. London: RPS. www.rpharms.com/development/credentialing/professional-knowledge-guides

9. Royal Pharmaceutical Society (2013). Medicines optimisation: helping patients to make the most of medicines. London: RPS. www.rpharms.com/Portals/0/RPS%20document%20library/Open%20access/Policy/helping-patients-make-the-most-of-their-medicines.pdf

10. Centre for Pharmacy Postgraduate Education (2019). Consultation skills for pharmacy practice: taking a patient-centered approach. CPPE: Manchester. www.consultationskillsforpharmacy.com/docs/docb.pdf

11. Dowdall M *et al.* Making consultations in community pharmacy matter. *The Pharmaceutical Journal* [online] 2019.

12. Kurtz S *et al.* Marrying content and process in clinical method teaching: enhancing the Calgary–Cambridge guides. *Academic Medicine* 2003; 78(8): 802-809.

13. Ong CKS *et al.* An Evidence Based Update on Nonsteroidal Anti-inflammatory Drugs. *Clin Med Res* 2007; 5(1): 19-34.

14. Preston C L. Stockley's Drug Interactions [online]. London: Pharmaceutical Press. www.new.medicinescomplete.com

15. Jani M *et al.* The role of DMARDs in reducing the immunogenicity of TNF inhibitors in chronic inflammatory diseases. *Rheumatology* 2014; 53(2): 213-222.

16. Ledingham J *et al.* BSR and BHPR guideline for the prescription and monitoring of non-biologic disease-modifying anti-rheumatic drugs. *Rheumatology* 2017; 56(6): 865-868.

17. National Institute for Health and Care Excellence (NICE). Rheumatoid arthritis in adults: management. London: NICE; 2018. www.nice.org.uk/guidance/ng100

18. National Rheumatoid Arthritis Society. A patient guide: disease activity score (DAS)28. Maidenhead: NRS. www.nras.org.uk/data/files/Publications/DAS%20patient%20guide.pdf

19. Williamson E. Stockley's Herbal Medicines Interactions [online]. London: Pharmaceutical Press. www.new.medicinescomplete.com

Case studies

Case study 1

Betty, aged 62 years, is a regular in your pharmacy. She has been diagnosed with type 2 diabetes and she also has osteoporosis and hypertension. She weighs 90 kg, smokes around 15 cigarettes per day and is taking the following medicines:

- Ramipril 5 mg daily
- Alendronate 70 mg once weekly
- Calcichew D3 twice daily
- Metformin 500 mg three times daily

Betty asks you to recommend something to help with the pain in her hands. She explains that she has been taking paracetamol and ibuprofen, but they no longer seem effective.

Points to consider

- What questions would you ask Betty?
- What examination, if any, would you undertake?
- What signs would you look for?

You ask Betty if she has pain or stiffness anywhere else and if it is worse at any particular time of the day. Betty tells you that her right knee is also painful, usually first thing in the morning. You examine her hands for swelling, redness and heat.

On examination, there is minimal swelling around her joints, but the second and third metacarpophalangeal joints on both hands are tender. You advise her to consult her doctor to get something stronger for the pain. She returns with a prescription for etoricoxib 90 mg once daily.

Points to consider

- Do you have any concern about the choice of medicine?
- What monitoring is required for this treatment?

You are aware that Betty has hypertension and so need to ensure that her blood pressure is not raised any further by the etoricoxib.

Points to consider

- What lifestyle advice might be appropriate to give Betty?

You advise Betty that it'd be beneficial if she considered losing weight and stopped smoking. Betty returns three months later and tells you she has had a referral to the early arthritis clinic at the local hospital. The presentation at the clinic was as follows:

- Some recent weight loss
- Tried NSAIDs – some relief but had stopped etoricoxib as was 'on too many tablets'
- 6-month history of progressive joint pain:

  - Early morning stiffness
  - Swelling
  - Shoulders, knees, wrists and MCPs
  - Several visits to GP

- On examination:
  - Systems exam: normal
  - BP: 175/95
  - ESR: 52
  - CRP: 43
  - Rheumatoid factor: 1080
  - Anti-CCP >340
  - ANA: negative
  - CXR: normal
  - Hands/feet: no erosions
  - Creatinine: 128
  - eGFR: 44 mL/min
  - LFTs: normal
  - Bone profile: normal

Betty returns to the pharmacy with a prescription for methotrexate tablets 10 mg once weekly, increasing to 15 mg once weekly if tolerated, naproxen 500 mg twice daily and omeprazole 20 mg daily.

Points to consider

- Is this drug regimen appropriate?

You notice that folic acid has been omitted from the prescription and arrange for it to be prescribed and note some concerns about the use of naproxen given her medical history, other medicines and kidney function.

Over the next 6 months, Betty encounters several issues:
- Variable eGFR: 30-50 mL/min
- Significant dyspepsia and diarrhoea
  - Stopped and started MTX
- Trial of sulfasalazine – intolerant
- Naproxen stopped due to variable eGFR and increased blood pressure
- Alendronate stopped due to dyspepsia
- GP referred Betty to gastroenterology for investigations
- Betty was seen by the renal team as she has diabetes, is hypertensive and has CKD
- Gliclazide was initiated after a trial period without metformin (as this was causing GI upset)

Points to consider

- What are appropriate next steps in the management of Betty's rheumatoid arthritis?

Betty has now tried two DMARDS, but the disease is still active, so she needs to progress to effective treatment. At her next six-monthly review Betty had a DAS28 of 6.1.

Points to consider

- What is the relevance of the DAS28 score?
- What does it mean for Betty?

Betty was started on prednisolone 10 mg daily, and the treatment plan was escalated to include biologics.

Points to consider

- Taking into account Betty's medical history and current medication regimen, what concerns do you have?
- Which biologic would you suggest? Remember, she is intolerant of methotrexate, so preference is for a product licensed for use without methotrexate.

Betty has established osteoporosis, but she has stopped bone protection due to intolerability. In addition, she has started prednisolone tablets, so she will need ongoing bone protection (an alternative to the alendronate) and will need to continue with her PPI.

Betty started etanercept 50 mg weekly injections and prednisolone was continued for a further six weeks, then tapered and discontinued.

At her four-month review Betty had two tender joints, one swollen joint, a DAS28 of 3.09 and she felt much better. She had no problems with the injection and generally felt well. Treatment was continued.

CHAPTER 15

Schizophrenia

Nicola Greenhalgh

Overview

Schizophrenia is a serious mental illness involving psychotic symptoms that affect how people think, feel and behave. It is a chronic and debilitating neurodevelopmental disorder that typically develops in adolescence or early adulthood affecting approximately 1% of the population over their lifespan.[1]

Stigma and discrimination are commonly felt by people who are diagnosed with schizophrenia and together with the disease this can affect all aspects of life, including reducing access to appropriate healthcare.[2,3]

The development of schizophrenia is thought to be multifactorial including genetic, biological and environmental factors.[4] Historically, the main theory around the development of schizophrenia involved changes in dopamine pathways, however, now a range of neurochemicals, genes and immune responses have been implicated.[5-8] The genes which have been identified in the development of schizophrenia are likely to play a part along with environmental stressors, particularly those occurring early in life.[5,9,10] People who have risk factors, such as those with a family history, or those exhibiting symptoms of psychosis have a greater risk of developing schizophrenia.[11]

There is a significant association with the use of illicit substances, cigarettes and alcohol in people with schizophrenia.[12,13] Use of illicit substances may be involved in the development of schizophrenia and impacts on patients who have comorbid schizophrenia.[12]

There is a huge health inequality for patients with schizophrenia who are consistently shown to have a significantly shorter life expectancy than is seen in the general population – patients with a serious mental health illness on average live 15-20 years less than the general population.[14,15] Although there are likely to be many factors involved in this, including higher rates of suicide, smoking, alcohol and substance misuse and increased cardiovascular mortality are to play a significant role. Whilst some of this is inherent with the illness itself, medication which increases risk factors, such as weight gain and diabetes, not only increase the development of cardiovascular disease but also cause significant morbidity of their own and affect whether patients will continue taking medicines in the longer term.[16,17]

Box 15.1: Practice point: self-management

- Patients with schizophrenia have consistently been shown to die 15-20 years before the general population.
- Always encourage patients to self-manage their medication and understand their monitoring so that they can take greater control over their health.
- Encourage patients to live healthy lives – provide information on diet, exercise, smoking cessation and alcohol and drug use, and refer to appropriate resources in your area.

Diagnosis

Schizophrenia is diagnosed in secondary care services by a psychiatrist after an assessment that looks at specific positive, negative and cognitive symptoms (see *Table 15.1*) as well as the patient's history.[4] Whilst signs and symptoms are likely to be present in childhood, it is only rarely diagnosed in children, with the majority of patients presenting in adolescence and early adulthood.[18,19]

Table 15.1: *The main symptoms of schizophrenia*[1,20]

Class of symptom	Examples
Positive	• Hallucinations – can be auditory, olfactory, tactile, visual or gustatory. • Delusions – believing things that aren't or can't be true (e.g. that they are someone who they are not or that they have special powers). • Thought disorder – unusual or dysfunctional ways of thinking or disorganised speech. Includes include derailment, poverty of speech, tangentiality, illogicality, perseveration and thought blocking. • Abnormal or repetitive movements.
Negative	• Apathy – lack of interest in everyday activities. • Self-neglect – not eating properly, poor personal hygiene, not attending healthcare appointments. • Withdrawal – not participating with other people and isolating themselves. • Lack of drive – lack of motivation to carry out activities.
Cognitive	• Speed of processing. • Attention/vigilance. • Working memory. • Verbal learning, visual learning. • Reasoning and problem solving. • Social cognition.

Many patients initially present in a prodromal period dominated by negative symptoms which may be confused early on with depression but will develop into more typical psychotic symptoms.[21,22]

Whilst there are some common symptoms, schizophrenia differs from bipolar disorder due to the lack of elevated mood which occurs in bipolar disorder. Schizoaffective disorder occurs where patients experience psychotic symptoms similar to those in schizophrenia along with the changes in effect or mood seen in bipolar disorder. There are many similarities in the way that these disorders are managed pharmacologically and there is much crossover between them.

Treatment

Antipsychotics are used first line in the treatment of schizophrenia and may have already been given to patients to treat psychotic illness or psychosis which has been attributed to other things, such as substance misuse prior to a diagnosis of schizophrenia.[1,23] They are used to treat both the acute positive and negative symptoms and maintain remission. There is no clear first-line antipsychotic and initial treatment is based on patient factors including patient choice, comorbidities, other medication (including potential for use of illicit substances) and the patient's presentation.

It is common for patients to be treated initially with a second- or third-generation antipsychotic rather than the older first-generation antipsychotics[24] (see *Table 15.2* for examples of drugs by classification). It is important to consider the burden of adverse effects when initiating treatment, as for most people treatment with antipsychotics will be lifelong.

Whilst there is a move towards using different classifications based on receptor properties of antipsychotics, which are helpful in understanding the activities of different antipsychotics, they are still often referred to as first- or second-generation and typical or atypical.[25,26] The latter classification is less useful as there is a lot of overlap between typical and atypical antipsychotics in terms of their receptor profiles and therefore adverse effects.[27]

Table 15.2: *Antipsychotics licensed in the UK*

Typical/first generation	Atypical/second/third generation
Chlorpromazine	Amisulpride
Flupentixol	Aripiprazole
Haloperidol	Cariprazine
Levomepromazine	Clozapine
Pericyazine	Lurasidone
Pimozide	Olanzapine
Prochlorperazine	Paliperidone
Sulpiride	Quetiapine
Trifluoperazine	Risperidone
Zuclopenthixol	

Where patients present very agitated and acutely unwell, or for patients who are sleeping poorly, initiation of a sedative in the short time may be considered. This can include the benzodiazepines, z-drugs and promethazine. Use of these should usually be limited and tapered once the patient settles and starts to respond to antipsychotic medication.

Some patients will not respond to treatment or will experience adverse effects which result in them stopping treatment or remaining inadequately treated.[28,29]

Depot or long-acting antipsychotic injections can be helpful to manage patients who stop taking medication because they cannot remember to take them consistently or where they don't believe that they need to take them due either the illness itself or beliefs around the illness. Evidence shows lower relapse rates and longer time in remission for patients who are prescribed long-acting injections over oral antipsychotics.[30,31,32]

Before starting long-acting antipsychotic injections, either a test dose (for the older antipsychotic injections) or a period of oral treatment (with the newer antipsychotic injections) is required to establish tolerance and ideally effectiveness. Information on the use of individual long-acting injections and the differences between them can be found in reference sources such as the Maudsley Prescribing Guidelines and the Psychotropic Drug Directory.[33,34]

Early antipsychotics' main mode of action is antagonism of dopamine D2 receptors, as excess activity in the dopaminergic pathways was thought to be involved in the development of schizophrenia. As well as being involved in mood and psychosis, dopaminergic neurones play a role in many other functions such as movement control and regulation of prolactin; blocking the D2 receptors can, therefore, lead to extrapyramidal side effects (EPSEs) and hyperprolactinaemia.[8]

Many of the second-generation antipsychotics are also serotonin 5HT2A antagonists and affect dopamine receptors to a lesser and varying extent.[35,36] The action at the 5HT2A receptors is thought to be one of the reasons why the atypical antipsychotics are less likely to cause EPSEs, and it may also play a role in the antipsychotic effect.

Whilst the aim of treatment should always be resolution of all symptoms, in some patients complete remission may not be possible.[29,37,38] In these cases it is important to focus on how distressed patients are by their symptoms and how much they impact on their day-to-day functioning. The adverse effects of medication and symptom control also need to be balanced.

Patients may take very different views on how significant adverse effects are compared to their illness and therefore understanding their views is paramount as they may be wary of altering the balance.[39,40]

Psychological treatments should be considered alongside pharmacological management and can be particularly helpful for patients to learn how to cope and manage residual symptoms.[41,42] Patients may also use specific therapies to help them with symptoms such as cognitive impairments.[43,44] All pharmacists should know what is available and encourage patients to access these.

Box 15.2: Practice point: adverse effects

- With the exception of clozapine, there is no evidence to suggest any antipsychotic is more clinically effective than another, therefore you will see a wide range of antipsychotics prescribed in practice.
- Adverse effects are a predominant factor when choosing an antipsychotic.
- Being aware of the main adverse effects and helping patients to understand which ones may be important will help them to make informed decisions about the choice of antipsychotic.

Pharmacy input

Pharmacists can play an important role in optimising treatment, identifying and managing adverse effects, ensuring appropriate monitoring is carried out and also in helping patients access appropriate lifestyle advice and treatment to help them stay healthier for longer.

Whilst many treatments are aimed at positive and negative symptoms, cognitive symptoms can have a huge impact on how patients with schizophrenia function.[45] This can affect their memory, which may impact their ability to take medication, remember information or appointments.[46] Support should be given to help patients manage these difficulties and this is where pharmacists can get involved.

Helping patients to access treatment and support may help reduce the progression of schizophrenia and also help reduce any potential long-term complications. Pharmacy management of people with schizophrenia will depend on your knowledge and skills. Some suggested roles depending on your skill level are outlined in *Table 15.3*. You must always act within your level of competency and know when to refer to a healthcare professional with more experience.

Table 15.3: *Potential roles for pharmacists in managing schizophrenia depending on skills and experience*

	Community pharmacist	Primary care/practice pharmacist	Hospital pharmacist	Specialist mental health pharmacist
Medication review	Undertake medication review of all medication. Help identify ways that patients may self-manage problems, such as adjusting times of day doses are taken. Refer to psychiatry team/GP for further review where required.	Undertake full medication review. Ensure physical and mental health medication is optimised. Support and monitor compliance.	Review whether medication may be contributing to an admission and make immediate changes where necessary. Advise what antipsychotics may be preferable with comorbidities.	Undertake full medication reviews including medication history reviews. Appraise previous treatment and advise on ways to optimise current treatment or on alternatives based on the physical and mental health conditions.
Monitoring	Carry out basic monitoring (e.g. blood glucose, weight, BP) and explain what results mean and whether action is needed. Encourage patients to be involved in their monitoring.	Ensure monitoring has been carried out for patients. Arrange for further monitoring (e.g. blood tests and ECGs as necessary). Identify where results require further investigation or referral.	Ensure all appropriate monitoring is carried out. Advise whether specific further monitoring is required if there are concerns about physical or mental health.	Ensure all monitoring is carried out. Monitor effectiveness, appraise results and advise on changes to treatment, or refer where necessary.

Table 15.3: *Potential roles for pharmacists in managing schizophrenia depending on skills and experience (continued)*

	Community pharmacist	Primary care/practice pharmacist	Hospital pharmacist	Specialist mental health pharmacist
Identifying and managing adverse effects	Talk to patients about adverse effects. Undertake reviews of adverse effects, identify common adverse effects caused by antipsychotics. Identify if over-the-counter or self-management is possible and refer for further review if necessary.	Undertake a more thorough review of adverse effects. Manage adverse effects that can be treated as appropriate. Liaise with psychiatry team.	Advise when immediate discontinuation may be required due to serious adverse effects. Advise on further monitoring or investigations as required. Advise on whether the clinical condition may be impacting on adverse effects.	Proactively review patients for adverse effects, consider the profiles of antipsychotics and review the patient's history to advise on alternative antipsychotics. Advise on management of adverse effects where medication can't be changed.
Managing physical health	Ensure patients are aware of all their medicines and what they are for. Review patients holistically, ensure appropriate monitoring of long-term conditions is undertaken.	Advise on alterations to physical health medication liaising with the psychiatry team where necessary. Be aware of where medication for physical help can impact on mental health and refer for a review. Help patients to manage their medication.	Ensure that physical health conditions are optimised and properly treated. Consider the impact of mental health conditions prior to discharge. Ensure there is good communication between the mental health team and acute hospital about any monitoring. Follow up and what to do should things not go to plan.	Ensure that the psychiatric team are aware of how physical health medication and conditions are affected by mental health medication. Advise on choice of antipsychotics where patients have comorbid physical health conditions. Advise on when referral to a specialist is needed.
Lifestyle intervention	Use opportunities to help patients access support for stopping smoking, drug or alcohol use. Advise on healthy eating and weight loss, and refer to local services depending on availability.			
Interactions	Identify interactions and ensure these have been considered by the prescriber. Advise patients on symptoms they may need to look out for and when to seek further help.	Ensure all patients medication records are up-to-date, particularly medication that isn't obtained from the GP so that any interaction decision software is able to work effectively. Provide more detailed advice to GPs on individual interactions to help manage patients.	Ensure medication provided by secondary care is checked for interactions with mental health medication. Advise on alterations to medication where interactions are identified. Ensure appropriate referral is made to the psychiatry team if medication has to be started which has major interactions with mental health medication.	Advise on managing complex interactions and ensure that the psychiatric team are aware of these. Ensure appropriate monitoring is carried out and patients are counselled appropriately where medication which interacts cannot be avoided. Ensure any other specialists who provide medication are aware of medication for mental health.

Pharmacy review

When undertaking a review of someone with schizophrenia you need to gain an understanding about their knowledge of their diagnosis and medication, how they feel they are getting on with it (benefits and any associated adverse effects) and anything else that can impact on their treatment, such as adherence, drug interactions and monitoring.

Treatment and diagnosis

Asking patients about their understanding of the treatment can be helpful to avoid potential conflict with those who do not understand or who do not agree with their diagnosis.

Some patients may accept the need for the treatment to help with subjective symptoms (for example, they may say that it helps with their sleep or helps them to relax), while others will be able to say whether they have noticed an improvement in direct symptoms such as hallucinations.

So patients may provide a slightly different indication and others may describe their illness by the symptoms (e.g. they may say they take the antipsychotic as they hear voices). In these cases it can be helpful to ask if they have been given a diagnosis by their doctor so that you can gauge their understanding.

It may be useful to prompt patients where they are not sure of their medication or ask if anyone helps them with their medication if they seem unsure.

Where patients don't understand their diagnosis pharmacists can help by offering information, however, where patients seem agitated by this it would be better to refer them to their mental health team for further information.

Questions to ask include:

- What medication do you take?
- How do you take it?
- When do you take it?
- Do you know what you are taking your medication for?
- Would you like some information about your medication?

Benefits and adherence

It is helpful to understand whether the patient is getting benefit from the medication as it is more likely that they will continue to take it if they feel there has been an improvement in their condition.

Not taking medication as prescribed is a common problem in schizophrenia, however, it is essential to ask this in a non-judgemental way and also to try to understand the reasons why patients are not taking their medication.

Lack of understanding or agreement as to why they should take medication, as well as adverse effects, are often major factors in non-adherence. Some patients with schizophrenia also have significant cognitive symptoms which can make remembering medication difficult and finding ways to help support them in this can be very helpful. Questions to ask include:

- Do you think your medication is working for you?
- Do you find that on an average week you miss any of your medication?
- Do you think there is anything that causes you to miss medication?
- Do you feel that you need some help to remember to take your medication?

Other medicines and products

Some patients will get medication from multiple sources, so to ensure a full review of medication is carried out include all other medicines and anything that may have been purchased over the counter.

Other medications that can be used to treat schizophrenia are less evidence-based but may be used either to treat other symptoms or in patients who are treatment-resistant and are being trialled for an individual patient. Benzodiazepines, mood stabilisers and antidepressants are used occasionally.

When carrying out a medication review for a patient with schizophrenia consider the indications and evidence for the indications for which they are being used. Where medication other than antipsychotics are being used, consider the impact of polypharmacy on the patient and whether the medication has been properly reviewed against the treatment goals. Medication that hasn't shown benefit should be challenged.

Complex medication regimes can make it difficult for patients to manage their medicines and there may be additive adverse effects. Ensuring that all prescribers are aware of the medication a patient is taking helps to ensure that appropriate decisions are made. Where a patient consents, providing a copy of any medication review to the mental health team, including a full up-to-date medication list, is helpful. Asking about any medication or herbal medication is important, not only as some medicines may interact, but also because some patients may be using over-the-counter or herbal medicines to self-medicate for either symptoms or adverse effects. Particularly look out for patients who may be trying to self-medicate serious adverse effects such as constipation or unexplained fevers with clozapine.

Questions to ask include:
- Do you take any other medication?
- Have you started any new medication recently?
- Do you buy any medication or herbal medication from pharmacies that you take often?

Box 15.3: Practice point: medication reviews

- It can be difficult for patients with schizophrenia to have a holistic review of their medication as often multiple agencies manage their physical health conditions (e.g. GP, psychiatric team, secondary care teams).
- Wherever possible, prescribers should be encouraged to look at all medicines and not just individual conditions.
- Pharmacists should take opportunities to undertake complete medication reviews, looking at how medications may potentially interact or worsen either mental health or physical health conditions.

Lifestyle

Asking about the patient's lifestyle will help you to understand how it may impact their condition and its treatment. Smoking has a much higher prevalence amongst patients with schizophrenia than the population in general. Opportunities should be taken to encourage patients to stop or reduce their smoking. Stopping smoking can affect some antipsychotics (see the section on interactions), so this should also be considered.

As with smoking, the use of street drugs and alcohol is common amongst patients with schizophrenia. Bear in mind that some people will use alcohol and street drugs to try and self-medicate symptoms that are distressing them, so always ask these questions sensitively. Using drugs or alcohol can worsen both physical and mental health – these patients should be encouraged to seek help. Most drug and alcohol services can be self-referred to by patients.

Many antipsychotics have sedative properties and therefore patients should be made aware that they should not drive if they feel sleepy after taking medication.

Questions to ask about lifestyle include:
- Do you smoke cigarettes?
  - Would you like any help stopping smoking?
- Would it be ok if I asked you questions about your drug or alcohol use?
  - When was the last time you had alcohol, street drugs?
  - Do you feel that this is a problem for you?
  - Would you like some help with this?
- Do you drive?

Adverse effects

A patient's experience of adverse effects can significantly impact on adherence to their treatment regimen, particularly sexual adverse effects and weight gain. Asking patients about adverse effects and using a structured tool can help identify troublesome adverse effects, but may also highlight some issues that the patient may not relate to the medication. It can also help where patients find it difficult to talk about sensitive issues such as sexual adverse effects or constipation. Encouraging patients to talk about their adverse effects and problems they have with medication can reduce the risk of them stopping taking it, which reduces the risk of relapse and improves outcomes. Where the patient consents, pharmacists can directly speak to the team involved in their care to help the patient articulate their concerns.

You can either give the questionnaire to the patient to complete themselves or go through it with them. The Liverpool University Neuroleptic Side Effect Scale (LUNSERS)[47] and the Glasgow Antipsychotic Side effect Scale (GASS)[48] are both available online to download.

Sexual adverse effects are very common with both schizophrenia itself and with antipsychotics, but it can be quite difficult for some patients to talk about it. You can help by opening up the conversation and making patients aware that it is common, but also that there are options available to help manage sexual adverse effects.

As well as affecting dopamine and serotonin receptors, antipsychotics can affect an array of different receptors and this leads to the major differences in their adverse effects.[49] Some adverse effects such as sedation can be beneficial in patients who are unable to sleep or are very agitated, however, the majority of adverse effects can influence whether patients continue with their medicines.[40]

Antipsychotics can affect sleep in different ways; some are very sedating and can make it difficult for patients to wake up in the mornings, while others such as aripiprazole can disturb sleep. You can make patients aware that taking their medication at the right time can help, and if that doesn't work, sometimes the dose can be altered (e.g. to give a greater proportion of a sedative medication at night).

It is important to ask people on clozapine about their bowel habits as clozapine can cause life-threatening constipation. A question about this is specifically asked in the GASS-clozapine[50] adapted scale. If a patient who takes clozapine asks for advice on the use of laxatives, or if they are not passing a stool every 3 days, refer them so that they can be medically assessed.

Stimulant laxatives are used first line, as the main mechanism by which constipation is caused is by reducing bowel activity. It is not sufficient to offer dietary and lifestyle modification alone. If they also have accompanying symptoms such as pain or vomiting then treatment should be sought urgently.

Weight gain can be very problematic with antipsychotics, particularly clozapine and olanzapine but it can occur with any antipsychotic and can be distressing for some patients. It is helpful to be aware of what services are available in your area which may help patients to manage their weight.

Pharmacists can help patients to understand what may be causing adverse effects and whether there are ways to manage them. Knowing which adverse effects can reduce over time helps patients persevere with their medication, and being able to signpost patients who experience more serious adverse effects is equally important. Pharmacist prescribers can help alter the way medicines are prescribed, such as altering the way doses are split or altering the form of the medicine.

The dose-response curve for some antipsychotics is not clear and where doses were escalated quickly on initiation, consideration should be given to reduce the dose to the lowest effective dose once the patient is stable.[51,52] Many adverse effects are dose-related, but there may be some hesitancy to reduce doses, particularly where patients are stable. In most cases, reducing doses of medication will only be done by the mental health team, therefore pharmacists will generally play a role in recognising where doses may be contributing to adverse effects and referring the patient to the mental health team.

The increased risk of cardiovascular death in schizophrenia is thought to be an important reason people with schizophrenia die up to 20 years earlier than average.[14,15] Current antipsychotics can increase the cardiovascular risk in a number of ways, including altering blood pressure, ECG changes, heart rate or rhythm changes, causing weight gain, development of diabetes and lipid changes.[16,17] The last three are often grouped together under the term cardiometabolic changes.

Common adverse effects and how to manage them are detailed in *Table 15.4*.

Table 15.4: *Adverse effects of antipsychotics and how to manage them*[33,34]

Adverse effect	Antipsychotics most likely to cause it	Antipsychotic least likely to cause it	Management
Sedation	Clozapine, chlorpromazine, olanzapine, quetiapine	Aripiprazole, lurasidone, amisulpride	Sedation is often more pronounced early on in treatment or after dose increments – patients can become tolerant to this effect over time. Taking the medicine before bedtime, altering formulations or unevenly splitting doses can help.
Anticholinergic effects (e.g. dry mouth, sedation, constipation)	Clozapine, chlorpromazine	Aripiprazole, lurasidone, amisulpride	Anticholinergic effects are common amongst antipsychotics and are dose related. As many other medicines also cause anticholinergic effects and these are additive, reviewing a patient fully can help identify potential other causes. If problematic, review medication and consider other medicines that may be causing additive effects. Reduce the dose if possible.
Postural hypotension	Clozapine, risperidone, chlorpromazine	Aripiprazole, amisulpride	Hypotension is often more pronounced early on in treatment or after dose increments and can resolve. Review other medication which may cause additive effects. Provide lifestyle advice on how to manage.
Weight gain	Clozapine, olanzapine	Aripiprazole, lurasidone, amisulpride	Weight gain is not clearly linked to dose. Ensure appropriate advice is given on diet and exercise. Ensure weight is being monitored. Once weight has been gained, in most cases switching won't lead to weight loss, but it may reduce or prevent further weight gain. Pharmacological methods of weight loss have limited benefit.
Diabetes	Clozapine, olanzapine	Aripiprazole, lurasidone, amisulpride	Diabetes can occur with all antipsychotics and can occur in the presence or absence of weight gain. Ensure monitoring occurs appropriately. Ensure appropriate advice is given on diet and exercise. Ensure diabetes is treated as per NICE guidelines. Consider alternative medicines with lower risk.
High cholesterol	Clozapine, olanzapine	Aripiprazole, lurasidone, amisulpride	Likely to be linked to weight gain. Ensure advice is given on diet and exercise and that weight gain is managed appropriately. Treat high cholesterol as per NICE guidelines.
EPSEs (extrapyramidal side effects)	First-generation antipsychotics, risperidone, amisulpride	Clozapine, olanzapine, quetiapine, aripiprazole	EPSEs are dose related, therefore, if possible, consider reducing the dose or switching to an alternative with a lower risk of EPSEs. Treat with anticholinergics if necessary.
Hyperprolactinaemia	First-generation antipsychotics, risperidone, amisulpride	Clozapine, olanzapine, quetiapine, aripiprazole	Hyperprolactinaemia is dose related, therefore, if possible, consider reducing the dose or switching to an alternative with a lower risk of hyperprolactinaemia. Consider the longer-term risks of high prolactin. Pharmacological treatment involves dopamine agonists which need to be used very carefully.
Hypertension	Risperidone	Aripiprazole, amisulpride	May resolve with continued treatment but if it does not, consider alternative antipsychotics or treat hypertension as per NICE guidelines.

Questions to ask about adverse effects include:

- Would you be happy to complete a brief questionnaire about side effects that may be related to your medication?
- Lots of people taking these medication notice that they have problems with intimacy or sexual problems, is this something that affects you?
- Have you been sleeping well?
- Do you find it easy to get up in the mornings or do you feel sleepy often?
- How often do you open your bowels (have a poo)?
- Do you think your medication may have caused you to gain weight?
    - Is this something you would like some help with?
    - What do you eat on a typical day?
    - Do you feel that you are eating a healthy diet?
    - Would you like any more information on eating healthily?

Monitoring

Monitoring for antipsychotics generally follows NICE guidelines[1] for schizophrenia: all patients started on treatment, regardless of the type of antipsychotics, should have the same monitoring.

All patients require measurement of creatinine clearance or estimated glomerular filtration rate (eGFR) along with urea and electrolytes (U&Es), liver function tests (LFTs), as well as an assessment of nutritional status, diet and level of physical activity measured at baseline and annually. Other parameters require more frequent monitoring at the start of treatment in addition to measurement at baseline and annually – see *Table 15.5*.

Patients who have other long-term conditions (such as cardiovascular disease, liver disease or renal impairment) or who are on medication that may increase the risk of adverse effects may have monitoring carried out more frequently, but this is considered on an individual basis.

However, most national audits show that across the UK there is still a lot of work to do to ensure that patients are monitored in line with NICE guidelines.[54] Pharmacists can help to reduce this inequality by not only ensuring that monitoring is taking place, but by helping patients understand what it means for them. It is therefore useful to try and engage patients to take an interest in the monitoring that they need.

Engaging patients where possible to monitor their weight and keep records of their physical health monitoring will help them to take ownership of their physical health. Pharmacists in community can talk to patients about their monitoring and encourage them to attend, where they can carry out any additional monitoring. Ensuring that this is communicated with their GP and secondary mental health team is important to ensure that results can be amalgamated and acted upon.

Pharmacists in primary care may carry out monitoring and ensure that tests have been done, but they may also use the results to refer or manage the patient where results are out of range. In acute care, pharmacists may manage more complex comorbidities, however any treatment or concerns with schizophrenia management should be communicated to the mental health team.

Box 15.4: Practice point: monitoring

- Studies frequently show that antipsychotic monitoring is poorly carried out for patients with schizophrenia.
- Poor communication between care providers who carry out monitoring can lead to potential problems if information about a patient's therapy is not shared or acted upon.
- When reviewing patients with schizophrenia, ensure that any monitoring that is undertaken is shared with the patient, their psychiatry team, as well as their GP.

Table 15.5: *Monitoring guidelines for antipsychotics[1,53]*

Parameter	Monitoring frequency after starting treatment
Full blood count	Clozapine requires intensive monitoring on initiation: weekly for 18 weeks, then fortnightly until 52 weeks, and then every 4 weeks thereafter, and for a month after stopping treatment. Monitoring frequency increases based on abnormal results, breaks in treatment and where clinically indicated.
Blood lipids, including cholesterol, triglycerides	At 12 weeks, 6 months and 1 year.
Weight (plotted on a chart), BMI, waist circumference	Weekly for 6 weeks, then at 12 weeks, 6 months and 1 year.
Plasma glucose, glycosylated haemoglobin (HbA1c)	At 12 weeks, 6 months and 1 year.
Prolactin	At 6 months if indicated.
ECG	All inpatients and other patients identified as being at high risk including: ● Presence of specific cardiovascular risk factor, for example, high blood pressure. ● Personal history of CV disease. ● On combination antipsychotics. ● High-dose antipsychotics. ● On other medicines with a risk of CV adverse effects. ● SMPC requirement (e.g. haloperidol, pimozide, sertindole, zotepine). Usually done after medicine is initiated, after medication changes, and then at least yearly (3 monthly for high dose antipsychotics).
Blood pressure/pulse	Frequently during dose titration. Clozapine requires pre- and post-dose monitoring of BP, pulse and temperature during titration.
Smoking status and number/day	Monitor if prescribed specific drugs where cigarette smoking affects metabolism, for example, clozapine, olanzapine and haloperidol.
Creatinine phosphokinase	If neuroleptic malignant syndrome (NMS) suspected.
Adverse effects (e.g. sexual adverse effects, movement disorders)	Movement disorders should be checked before initiation. Monitor for adverse effects frequently during initiation. Consider using a side effect rating scale such as LUNSERS or GASS (GASS-clozapine).

Note: all these parameters should also be measured at baseline and annually in addition to eGFR, U&Es, LFTs, assessment of nutritional status, diet and level of physical activity.

As well as the monitoring required for all people with schizophrenia, additional monitoring is required for people taking clozapine due to its adverse effects (refer to the specific clozapine monographs on www.medicines.org.uk for full information).

In particular, all patients taking clozapine need regular full blood count monitoring due to the risk of agranulocytosis and severe neutropenia. When clozapine is initiated, frequent monitoring of temperature, heart rate and blood pressure is undertaken after every dose due to the risk of serious cardiac toxicity, including myocarditis and cardiomyopathy. Any patient taking clozapine who presents with signs of either cardiac symptoms or neutropenia should be referred for an urgent medical review.[55]

Questions to ask include:

● Are you up-to-date with your monitoring?

● Do you know your results?

Identifying relapse

Pharmacists assessing patients with schizophrenia need to consider both their symptoms and any possible complications of their treatments. Where a patient is well known to a pharmacist, they may be able to pick up on more subtle changes that can occur as they start to relapse.

Patients have different indicators of relapse and understanding these in regular patients is important to help them access prompt care.[29] Patients should have care plans in place which, if they give permission for them to be shared, could be useful for pharmacists to help patients manage their condition. Reducing the amount of time patients remain unwell can help reduce the progression of the illness.

There are a number of structured tools, such as the positive and negative syndrome scale (PANSS)[56] and Brief Psychiatric Rating Scale (BPRS),[57] available to help assess symptom severity for people with schizophrenia, however, the majority of these are mainly used in clinical trials, not clinical practice.

Familiarising yourself with these and the symptoms of schizophrenia can be helpful to understand what to look out for in relapsing patients.

Asking patients how they are feeling and whether they have any symptoms may be useful to keep track of their condition, however, this needs to be carried out sensitively, as some patients may find questioning intrusive or may not have insight into their condition.

Asking open questions, such as 'How are you feeling?' can be a useful start. Some unwell patients may be guarded in their responses to try and mask their symptoms, whereas others may be floridly psychotic and express delusional beliefs or respond to unseen stimuli (visual hallucinations).

It is important to be sensitive to patients expressing psychotic symptoms; for some patients they may manage their symptoms well, however some patients may be quite distressed by their symptoms. The majority of people experiencing psychotic symptoms believe that what they are thinking or perceiving is real. Challenging patients can, therefore, make patients confused, distressed or angry. Supporting them and using phrases such as 'that must be difficult for you' or 'that sounds upsetting' can be helpful without reinforcing that what is happening is real.

Patients who have insight into their condition may recognise their symptoms, be more aware that they are not real and be aware if these are signs of relapse.

Asking if they have seen their GP or mental health team recently can be useful as they are likely to pick up on any signs of relapse. Patients who are inconsistent with requesting or picking up prescriptions may be at a greater risk of relapse. Working with them to find out why they are not taking their medication as prescribed is important as some patients will simply forget, some may experience adverse effects, whereas others may intentionally not take their medication because they don't believe they need it or don't understand their diagnosis.

Drug interactions

There are a number of significant pharmacodynamic and pharmacokinetic drug interactions that can occur between antipsychotics and other medicines. Most antipsychotics are hepatically metabolised, therefore they can be affected by inhibitors and inducers of cytochrome p450 enzymes to varying extents. See *Table 15.6* for details of relevant interactions and how to manage them.

Table 15.6: *Significant drug interactions for antipsychotics*[33,34,58]

Medication or class involved	Antipsychotics	Mechanism	Management
Medicines that cause QTc interval prolongation (e.g. clarithromycin, citalopram, antiarrhythmics)	All antipsychotics can potentially increase QTc interval prolongation, however, they are classified by risk. This can be further impacted where the medicine also inhibits the metabolism of the antipsychotic (e.g. quetiapine and ritonavir).	Potential for additive effect on QTc interval prolongation.	Try to avoid high-risk combinations or in patients already at risk of increased QTc interval prolongation.
Medicines causing blood dyscrasias (e.g. carbimazole, carbamazepine, cytotoxic medication)	Clozapine. Other antipsychotics can also rarely cause blood dyscrasias.	Increased risk of blood dyscrasias. Blood dyscrasias are rarely reported with most other antipsychotics, however, this does not preclude treatment where necessary.	Try to avoid the combination of clozapine with other medicines that can cause blood dyscrasias and particularly agranulocytosis and neutropenia. In many cases, combination is contraindicated. Where combination is essential, specialist advice should be sought. For other antipsychotics monitor full blood count.
Tobacco/cigarette smoke	Clozapine. Haloperidol, olanzapine.	Hydrocarbons in tobacco smoke induce the metabolism of antipsychotics. Levels of antipsychotics increase when smoking decreases and can fall if patients start smoking (e.g. after leaving hospital).	Monitor levels for clozapine and adverse effects/symptoms for all. This is particularly important where offering smoking cessation support or where patients suddenly can no longer smoke as levels can rise significantly.
Anticholinergic medicines (e.g. tricyclic antidepressants, antihistamines, procyclidine, hyoscine)	Potentially all antipsychotics but particularly those which have high anticholinergic activity (e.g. clozapine, olanzapine).	Additive anticholinergic effects such as confusion, constipation, dry mouth.	Where possible try and manage adverse effects without the use of anticholinergic medication. Monitor the patient for symptoms and review as appropriate.
Sedatives (e.g. opioid analgesics, benzodiazepines)	All antipsychotics can cause sedation, but it is more prominent in those that have antihistamine or anticholinergic effects (e.g. olanzapine, clozapine, quetiapine, chlorpromazine, zuclopenthixol).	Additive sedative effects.	Avoid adding sedatives where patients are already sedated. Monitor patients for increased sedation and counsel on the risk, including advise not to drive if sedated.
Antihypertensives or medicines which can lower blood pressure (e.g. diuretics, alpha blockers, ACE inhibitors)	Clozapine, quetiapine, risperidone.	Additive blood pressure lowering effects.	Risk of hypotension with antipsychotics is particularly prominent at the start of treatment and during titration. Monitor BP more closely and titrate slowly.
Dopamine agonists (e.g. medicines used in Parkinson's disease)	All antipsychotics.	Most antipsychotics have a degree of dopamine antagonism, therefore they can exacerbate Parkinsonian symptoms. Dopamine agonists can also cause psychosis.	The use of antipsychotics which have a low affinity for D2 receptors (e.g. clozapine and quetiapine) should be considered in patients with Parkinson's disease. Patients started on dopamine agonists should be closely monitored for relapse of their psychotic symptoms.

Treatment-resistant schizophrenia

Treatment resistance is generally defined as the failure to respond to or tolerate two sequential antipsychotics, where one is a second-generation or atypical antipsychotic, given at an adequate dose for an adequate length of treatment.[1,38,53]

Clozapine is uniquely indicated in treatment-resistant schizophrenia[59,60] as it is the only evidence-based treatment. Patients, and indeed sometimes healthcare professionals, can be resistant to starting clozapine due to the monitoring involved and the complicated titration.[61]

Ensuring clozapine is effectively managed so that patients do not inadvertently miss doses or start medication which may adversely affect their clozapine is paramount. Where patients are admitted to hospital, ensuring supplies of clozapine and that monitoring is maintained can help avoid the need to re-titrate if they miss more than 48 hours of medication.

In most areas, clozapine is only provided by the mental health trust. It is very important to ensure that these details are kept in the patient's medication record or Summary Care Record (SCR) to ensure appropriate prescribing, but also to ensure that wherever the SCR is accessed they are also aware that the patient is on clozapine.

Some patients who are unable to take clozapine, or patients who only have a partial response, may be treated with combinations of antipsychotics or combinations of antipsychotics with other psychiatric medicines (e.g. antidepressants, anticonvulsants, benzodiazepines).[62] The evidence base for these treatments is generally poor. Where combinations of antipsychotics lead to high dose antipsychotic therapy, further monitoring is indicated and it should be reviewed regularly.[63]

Understanding clozapine and being able to talk to patients about its effectiveness to help them make informed decisions is an important role in the pharmacy management of schizophrenia.

Managing special groups

A number of patients, such as those who have significant comorbidities, particularly those with cardiovascular disease or learning difficulties, children and adolescents, the elderly and pregnant or breastfeeding women should be treated cautiously with antipsychotics.

Treatment will often involve starting with lower doses of antipsychotic, titrating more slowly and being cautious when switching medication. Reference sources such as the Maudsley Prescribing Guidelines,[33] Psychotropic Drug Directory[34] and the British Association of Psychopharmacology Guidelines[53] provide information on the use of antipsychotics in specific patient groups.

Switching medication

Antipsychotic switches in schizophrenia are normally driven either by ineffectiveness or adverse effects. It should always be the aim for patients to be symptom-free or, at a minimum, able to function.

Switching should be considered if patients are still symptomatic despite being treated at an effective dose of an antipsychotic for an adequate period, or if they are unable to tolerate adverse effects and dose adjustments are ineffective or lead to re-emergence of symptoms.

The method of switching depends on both the patient and the medication involved.

Medication factors which affect switches include:

- half-life
- route of administration
- receptor and adverse effect profiles
- risk of discontinuation symptoms.

Patient factors which affect switches include:
- how acutely unwell they are
- any adverse effects they are experiencing or have experienced with similar antipsychotics
- other comorbidities
- other medication
- their age and frailty.

Quicker switches may be appropriate in inpatients who can be monitored closely, or where medication is ineffective but the patient has not experienced adverse effects or there is less concern about additive adverse effects.

Slower switches are more appropriate in patients with multiple comorbidities or where patients are struggling with adverse effects. The Psychotropic Drug Directory[34] has information available on specific antipsychotic switches.

Follow-up

Schizophrenia is a lifelong condition and most patients will require lifelong treatment.[18,29] This can be provided by either primary care where patients are stable and responding well to treatment, or secondary care for more complex patients, treatment-resistant patients and those who are acutely unwell or unstable.

The frequency that patients are seen will be mainly determined by whether they are acutely unwell and their risks. Once a patient is stable on medication the frequency of follow-up will reduce but this can vary between individuals.

Monitoring needs to be carried out at least weekly initially and then at 3 months, 6 months, 1 year and annually thereafter for all antipsychotics.

Referral

Many patients with schizophrenia will be managed by a community mental health team and will have contacts available if they need help. Where there are concerns that patients are relapsing or they have problems with their medication, in most cases it would be appropriate to refer them back to their community mental health team. Where possible people should be encouraged and supported to do this themselves, however, in some cases it may be necessary to speak to the patient directly. Where a patient is not involved with a mental health team they should be seen by their GP to assess whether a referral is appropriate.

Whilst most adverse effects can be managed by a GP or mental health team, where patients are showing signs of serious adverse effects, such as severe constipation with clozapine, haematological toxicity or NMS, they should be referred directly to the local accident and emergency department.

Where a patient is very unwell and may be putting themselves or others at risk, for example where they are expressing any thoughts to harm themselves or others, they will need to be referred to either a crisis line at the mental health team or, if that is not available, directly to accident and emergency services.

It is helpful to know what services are available in your area for patients in a mental health crisis so that you can refer them appropriately.

Box 15.5: Practice point: support services
- The services available to patients (e.g. access to help in a crisis, facility to contact mental health services directly) and resources (e.g. a medicines helpline) can differ in each individual mental health trust.
- It is important to be aware of the services available in your locality and how patients can access them.
- Contact your local mental health services to see if they have any leaflets or crisis cards that you can keep for patients in a mental health crisis.

Useful resources

- Rethink Mental Illness is a charity that provides support, advice and information on all aspects of mental health conditions to patients and carers. It has an advice line and can also help people find services that are available to them locally.
- Mind is a charity that provides support, advice and information on all aspects of mental health conditions to patients and carers. It has an online community where patients can access support and an advice line.
- Mental Health Foundation is a charity which has a public health focus on preventing the development of mental health conditions.
- NICE (2014). Psychosis and schizophrenia in adults: prevention and management. www.nice.org.uk/guidance/cg178
- NICE (2016). Psychosis and schizophrenia in children and young people: recognition and management. www.nice.org.uk/guidance/CG155
- Evidence-based guidelines from the British Association of Psychopharmacology on the majority of mental health conditions including schizophrenia, the management of metabolic disorders in patients with psychosis and those taking antipsychotics and use of psychotropic medication in pregnant or breastfeeding patients.
- The Royal College of Psychiatrists provides information for patients and professionals on a range of mental health conditions and their treatment.
- Choice and Medication (access usually available for patients via their mental health service) provides information to patients and healthcare professionals on medication used in mental health, including information on their use, choice in different conditions, use in pregnancy and lactation and adverse effects. Information leaflets are also available in a range of different languages and basic formats.
- YoungMinds provides information on the use of mental health medication and treatment of mental health conditions for children and adolescents.
- MQ is a charity which provides information on mental health conditions, but who aim to drive forward research into mental health conditions. It also provides information on research that it is involved in.

References

1. National Institute for Health and Care Excellence (NICE). Psychosis and schizophrenia in adults: treatment and management. [CG178]. London: NICE; 2014. www.nice.org.uk/guidance/cg178
2. Sibitz I et al. Resistance in patients with schizophrenia. Schizophr Bull 2011; 37: 316.
3. González-Torres MA et al. Stigma and discrimination towards people with schizophrenia and their family members. Soc Psychiatry Psychiatr Epidemio 2007; 42: 14-23.
4. Tsoi D T-Y et al. History, aetiology, and symptomatology of schizophrenia. Psychiatry 2008; 7: 404-409.
5. Hirvonen J, Hietala J. Dysfunctional brain networks and genetic risk for schizophrenia: Specific Neurotransmitter Systems. CNS Neurosci Ther 2011; 17: 89-96.
6. Stone JM. Glutamatergic antipsychotic drugs: a new dawn in the treatment of schizophrenia? Ther Adv Psychopharmacol 2011; 1: 5-18.
7. Parshukova D et al. Autoimmunity and immune system dysregulation in schizophrenia: IgGs from sera of patients hydrolyze myelin basic protein. J Mol Recognit 2019; 32: e2759.
8. Dunlop J, Brandon NJ. Schizophrenia drug discovery and development in an evolving era: Are new drug targets fulfilling expectations? J Psychopharmacol 2015; 29: 230-238.
9. Schizophrenia Working Group of the Psychiatric Genomics Consortium. Biological insights from 108 schizophrenia-associated genetic loci. Nature 2014; 511(7510): 421-427.

10. Comes AL *et al*. Proteomics for blood biomarker exploration of severe mental illness: pitfalls of the past and potential for the future. Transl. *Psychiatry* 2018; 8: 160.

11. Fusar-Poli P *et al*. Development and Validation of a Clinically Based Risk Calculator for the Transdiagnostic Prediction of Psychosis. *JAMA Psychiatry* 2017; 74: 493-500.

12. Volkow ND. Substance use disorders in schizophrenia—clinical implications of comorbidity. *Schizophr Bull* 2009; 35: 469-72.

13. Ziedonis DM *et al*. Improving the care of individuals with schizophrenia and substance use disorders: consensus recommendations. *J Psychiatr Pract* 2005; 11: 315-39.

14. Hjorthøj C *et al*. Years of potential life lost and life expectancy in schizophrenia: a systematic review and meta-analysis. *Lancet Psychiatry* 2017; 4: 295-301.

15. Laursen TM. Life expectancy among persons with schizophrenia or bipolar affective disorder. *Schizophr Res* 2011; 131: 101-104.

16. Ohlsen R, Gaughran F. Schizophrenia: A major risk factor for cardiovascular disease. *Br J Card Nurs* 2011; 6.

17. Cooper S J *et al*. BAP guidelines on the management of weight gain, metabolic disturbances and cardiovascular risk associated with psychosis and antipsychotic drug treatment. *J Psychopharmacol* 2016; 30(8): 717-748.

18. Seppala J *et al*. Definition, epidemiology, clinical course and outcomes in treatment-resistant schizophrenia. *Eur Psychiatry* 2017; 41: S67.

19. Pedersen CB *et al*. A comprehensive nationwide study of the incidence rate and lifetime risk for treated mental disorders. *JAMA Psychiatry* 2014; 71: 573.

20. Green MF. Cognitive impairment and functional outcome in schizophrenia and bipolar disorder. *J Clin Psychiatry* 2006; 67(Suppl 9): 38-42.

21. White T *et al*. Treatment in psychiatry: the schizophrenia prodrome. *Am J Psychiatry* 2006; 163:3: 376-380.

22. Klosterkötter J *et al*. Diagnosing Schizophrenia in the Initial Prodromal Phase. *Arch Gen Psychiatry* 2011; 58: 158.

23. Scottish Intercollegiate Guidelines Network (2013). Management of Schizophrenia: SIGN publication number 131.

24. Keating D *et al*. Pharmacological guidelines for schizophrenia: a systematic review and comparison of recommendations for the first episode. *BMJ Open* 2017; 7: e013881.

25. Zohar J *et al*. A proposal for an updated neuropsychopharmacological nomenclature. *Eur Neuropsychopharmaco* 2014; 24: 1005-1014.

26. Uchida H. Neuroscience-based nomenclature: What is it, why is it needed, and what comes next? *Psychiatry Cli Neurosci* 2018; 72: 50-51.

27. Leucht S *et al*. Comparative efficacy and tolerability of 15 antipsychotic drugs in schizophrenia: a multiple-treatments meta-analysis. *Lancet* 2013; 382: 951-962.

28. Naber D, Lambert M. The CATIE and CUtLASS studies in schizophrenia: results and implications for clinicians. *CNS Drugs* 2009; 23: 649-59.

29. Emsley R *et al*. The nature of relapse in schizophrenia. *BMC Psychiatry* 2013; 13: 50.

30. Olivares JM *et al*. Comparison of long-acting antipsychotic injection and oral antipsychotics in schizophrenia. *Neuropsychiatry* 2011; 1(3): 275-289.

31. Park SC *et al*. Comparative efficacy and safety of long-acting injectable and oral second-generation antipsychotics for the treatment of schizophrenia: a systematic review and meta-analysis. *Clin Psychopharmacol Neurosci* 2018; 16(4): 361-375.

32. Tiihonen J *et al*. Real-world effectiveness of antipsychotic treatments in a nationwide cohort of 29,823 patients with schizophrenia. *JAMA Psychiatry* 2018; 74(7): 686-693.

33. Taylor D *et al*. *The Maudsley Prescribing Guidelines in Psychiatry*, 13th edition. UK: Wiley-Blackwell, 2018.

34. Bazire S. *Psychotropic Drug Directory 2018*. Shaftesbury: Lloyd-Reinhold Publications Ltd.

35. Seeman P. Atypical antipsychotics: mechanism of action. *Can J Psychiatry* 2002; 47: 27-38.

36. Meltzer H. The role of serotonin in antipsychotic drug action. *Neuropsychopharmacology* 1999; 21: 106S-115S.

37. Yeomans D *et al*. Resolution and remission in schizophrenia: getting well and staying well. *Adv Psychiat Treat* 2010; 16: 86-95.

38. Sinclair D, Adams C E. Treatment resistant schizophrenia: a comprehensive survey of randomised controlled trials. *BMC Psychiatry* 2014; 14: 253.

39. Ascher-Svanum H *et al*. Reasons for discontinuation and continuation of antipsychotics in the treatment of schizophrenia from patient and clinician perspectives. *Curr Med Res Opin* 2010; 26: 2403-2410.

40. Dibonaventura D *et al*. A patient perspective of the impact of medication side effects on adherence: results of a cross-sectional nationwide survey of patients with schizophrenia. *BMC Psychiatry* 2012; 12: 20.

41. Jauhar S *et al*. Cognitive-behavioural therapy for the symptoms of schizophrenia: systematic review and meta-analysis with examination of potential bias. *Br J Psychiatry* 2014; 204(1): 20-29.

42. Pilling S *et al.* Psychological treatments in schizophrenia: I. Meta-analysis of family intervention and cognitive behaviour therapy. *Psychol Med* 2002; 32: 763-782.

43. Barlati S *et al.* Cognitive remediation in schizophrenia: current status and future perspectives. *Schizophr Res Treatment* 2013; 2013: 156084.

44. Medalia A, Saperstein AM. Does cognitive remediation for schizophrenia improve functional outcomes? *Curr Opin Psychiatry* 2013; 26: 151-157.

45. Green MF. Impact of cognitive and social cognitive impairment on functional outcomes in patients with schizophrenia. *J Clin Psychiatry* 2016; 77: 8-11.

46. Tripathi A *et al.* Cognitive deficits in schizophrenia: understanding the biological correlates and remediation strategies. *Clin Psychopharmaco Neurosci* 2018; 16: 7-17.

47. Morrison P *et al.* The use of the Liverpool University neuroleptic side-effect rating scale (LUNSERS) in clinical practice. *Aust NZ J Ment Health Nurs* 2000; 9: 166-176.

48. Waddell L, Taylor M. A new self-rating scale for detecting atypical or second-generation antipsychotic side effects. *J Psychopharmacol* 2008; 22: 238-243.

49. Huhn M *et al.* Comparative efficacy and tolerability of 32 oral antipsychotics for the acute treatment of adults with multi-episode schizophrenia: a systematic review and network meta-analysis. *Lancet* 2019; 394: 939-951.

50. Hynes C *et al.* Glasgow antipsychotic side-effects scale for clozapine – development and validation of a clozapine-specific side-effects scale. *Schizophr Res* 2015; 168: 505-513.

51. Davis JM, Chen N. Dose response and dose equivalence of antipsychotics. *J Clin Psychopharmacol* 2004; 24: 192-208.

52. Dold M *et al.* Dose escalation of antipsychotic drugs in schizophrenia: a meta-analysis of randomized controlled trials. *Schizophr Res* 2015; 166: 187-193.

53. Barnes T *et al.* Schizophrenia Consensus Group of the British Association of Psychopharmacology. Evidence-based guidelines for the pharmacological treatment of schizophrenia: recommendations from the British Association for Psychopharmacology (2011).

54. Royal College of Psychiatrists (2014). Report of the second round of the National Audit of Schizophrenia (NAS2). London: RCP.

55. Alawami M *et al.* A systematic review of clozapine induced cardiomyopathy. *Int J Cardiol* 2014; 176: 315-320.

56. Kay SR *et al.* The positive and negative syndrome scale (PANSS) for schizophrenia. *Schizophr Bull* 1987; 13(2): 261-276.

57. Overall, J. E. & Gorham, D. R. The Brief Psychiatric Rating Scale. *Psychol Rep* 1962; 10: 799-812.

58. Pharmaceutical Press. Stockley's Drug Interactions. (2016). Available at: www.medicinescomplete.com/mc/stockley/current/intro.htm

59. Bryan J. After 30 years, clozapine is still best for treatment-resistant patients. *Pharm J* 2014; 292: 58.

60. Mcilwain M E *et al.* Pharmacotherapy for treatment-resistant schizophrenia. *Neuropsychiatr Dis Treat* 2011; 7: 135.

61. Tungaraza TE, Farooq S. Clozapine prescribing in the UK: views and experience of consultant psychiatrists. *Ther Adv Psychopharmacol* 2015; 5: 88-96.

62. Sommer IE *et al.* Pharmacological augmentation strategies for schizophrenia patients with insufficient response to clozapine: a quantitative literature review. *Schizophr Bull* 2012; 38(5): 1003-11.

63. Royal College of Psychiatrists (2014). Consensus statement on high-dose antipsychotic medication College Report CR190. London: RCP.

Case studies

Case study 1

Charles comes to the pharmacy and asks about over-the-counter or herbal weight loss medication as he is worried about the amount of weight he has gained. He has been a regular at the pharmacy for many years and does look considerably heavier than when you last saw him. He used to be on olanzapine but hasn't had that prescription for around four months.

He seems well in himself, although a little drowsy. You speak to him about his lifestyle and diet and carry out basic monitoring of his BP, HR, and BMI. He mentions that he is on medication but can't remember it all, so gives you permission to check his Summary Care Record (SCR) which you do.

He is on some medication for his blood pressure and a statin, but nothing else regularly. You are surprised there is nothing for his schizophrenia and when you ask he mentions that he does take tablets for his mental health, but these come from his psychiatry team directly. He offers to bring them in for you to look at as he would like some help and can't quite remember what they are called. He comes back later with his tablets which include those on the SCR, but also clozapine and hyoscine hydrobromide. You thank him and make a note of the medicine in your PMR, and contact the GP and ask for this medication to be added as a secondary care medication.

> **Points to consider**
>
> - How would you verify what other medicines Charles is taking if it is not on the SCR?
> - Where would you check the monitoring requirements for clozapine?
> - What are the monitoring requirements for clozapine?

He asks you about side effects and you explain that weight gain is very common with antipsychotics (especially clozapine or olanzapine). It can occur early on and lead to significant weight gain if no intervention is made. You explain that weight should be monitored weekly for the first six weeks of treatment.

He mentions his increased drowsiness since starting treatment and you tell him that clozapine sedation can improve over time, but it can also be helpful to take a larger proportion of his daily dose at night.

> **Points to consider**
>
> - What is the normal daily dose of clozapine?
> - What proportion of the daily dose is it safe to take at night?
> - Where would you check for this information?
> - What screening tool could you use to assess adverse effects?

Charles comes back into the pharmacy three weeks later and seems much brighter. His dose has now settled and he has been managing to lose weight. He asks to buy lactulose.

On questioning, he hasn't passed a bowel movement in about a week and it has been getting worse recently. He has been trying to drink more and eat more fruit and vegetables, but it hasn't really helped. He hasn't got any pain or other symptoms. After you refer him back to his GP he is started on senna tablets 15 mg at night and given more advice on his diet which seems to be effective. You continue to question him about his bowel habits at regular intervals so that if he has any concerning symptoms he can be referred appropriately.

Points to consider

- What are the possible consequences of constipation in people taking clozapine?
- What is the mechanism of action of this adverse effect?
- What is the first-line treatment?

Case study 2

Stuart comes in for a review of his blood pressure medication in the pharmacist's clinic. During the review he complains of sexual dysfunction and wonders if it could be due to his medication. On his PMR he is prescribed atorvastatin 40 mg daily, ramipril 10 mg daily and amlodipine 10 mg daily. He then asks about his injection and thinks it started around the time that was increased.

Points to consider

- Are sexual adverse effects associated with the medicines Stuart has mentioned?
- What reference sources would you consult to check this?

There is no mention of an injection on his PMR, but you find a recent letter from his mental health team which notes he's on flupentixol decanoate 100 mg every two weeks, which was increased about three months ago.

Points to consider

- Are sexual adverse effects associated with flupenthixol?
- What monitoring is required for this medicine?
- Given what Stuart has told you, what parameters would you be most interested in?

You look through his results and notice that he has a very high prolactin level, so you write to the mental health team and ask for a review of his medication. You also add the flupentixol decanoate to the secondary care part of his SCR for future reference. The mental health team decide to review his medication due to his high prolactin level that is likely linked to his sexual adverse effects and also poses some long-term risks.

Stuart returns three months later. The mental health team decided to try him on aripiprazole instead of flupenthixol – he has been gradually switched and has been taking 15 mg of aripiprazole once daily for the past week. He has been feeling a bit restless and isn't sleeping well but he has noticed a big improvement in his sexual adverse effects. He was wondering whether to speak to someone to get something for his sleep.

Points to consider

- What is the likely cause of his sleep problems?

On questioning, he explains that he wasn't told when to take aripiprazole as it was just labelled as 'Once a day' and he has always thought you take this sort of medication at night. He also tells you he has got into a routine of playing video games late at night, often in bed which means that frequently he doesn't get to sleep until past midnight.

Points to consider

- What advice would you give Stuart about taking aripiprazole?
- What sleep hygiene advice could you give Stuart to improve his chances of sleeping?

You know that insomnia is quite common with aripiprazole, particularly early on with treatment, so it is helpful to make sure it is taken in the morning. Akathisia or feeling restless is also common in the early stages of treatment, so providing relaxation or distracting techniques can be helpful, although in severe cases short-term management with a benzodiazepine may be needed.

You advise Stuart to try taking aripiprazole in the morning to see if this helps and also go through basic sleep hygiene with him, particularly advising that he tries to switch off the video games before he goes to bed. You also offer some advice around relaxation techniques that can help with both restlessness and insomnia. You advise him that if things don't improve after trying these, get worse, or he is finding it difficult to manage, then he should see his doctor.

When Stuart returns to pick up his next prescription he informs you that these problems have settled down and he is now sleeping much better and thanks you for your advice.

CHAPTER 16

Stroke and transient ischaemic attack

Helen Williams and Rachel Howatson

Overview

A stroke occurs when there is an interruption of blood flow to the brain resulting in death or damage to the brain cells, leading to a neurological deficit lasting longer than 24 hours. Any part of the brain can be affected by stroke and the area of the brain affected determines the symptoms the patient experiences. A stroke is sometimes referred to as a brain attack.

There are two different types of stroke.

- Ischaemic stroke – this accounts for about 85% of all strokes. It occurs if a blood vessel within the brain is blocked and the flow of blood to the brain tissue is interrupted. Ischaemic strokes are most commonly the result of blood clots or atherosclerotic plaques fragmenting and a small piece lodging in the cerebral blood vessels. Other causes of ischaemic stroke include small vessel disease, atrial fibrillation and other heart rhythm disorders and arterial dissection.

- Haemorrhagic stroke – this occurs as a result of bleeding in or around the brain. High blood pressure (BP) leading to rupture of a blood vessel wall is the cause in around half of all haemorrhagic strokes. Other factors implicated in haemorrhagic strokes include cerebral amyloid angiopathy, aneurysms, treatment with anticoagulant therapy and use of illegal drugs, such as cocaine.

Transient ischaemic attack or TIA (also known as a mini-stroke) is the same as a stroke, except that the disruption to the blood flow to the brain is short-lived. The symptoms of TIA are therefore transient, lasting less than 24 hours, with the majority lasting well under an hour. Following a TIA, people often progress to a stroke – 1 in 12 people (8%) will have a stroke within a week of having a TIA, many of these strokes occurring within 24 hours of the TIA.[1]

There are more than 100,000 strokes in the UK each year, equal to around one stroke every five minutes. Stroke is the fourth biggest killer in the UK – in 2016, almost 38,000 people died of stroke in the UK, that's a life lost every 13 minutes, but there are also now over 1.2 million stroke survivors in the UK.[1] Public Health England estimates that improving the management of two of the most common causes of stroke – hypertension and atrial fibrillation (AF) – could prevent 28,000 strokes in England and save approximately £400 million.[2]

Diagnosis

Signs and symptoms of stroke are usually of sudden onset and include numbness or weakness in the face, arm or leg, especially on one side of the body; confusion; trouble speaking or difficulty understanding speech; visual disturbance in one or both eyes; trouble walking, dizziness, loss of balance or lack of coordination; and severe headache with no known cause. The time from symptom onset to treatment is critical, as the outcome is improved if specialist care is accessed as early as possible.

Box 16.1: Practice point: stroke signs and symptoms

The Stroke Association developed the acronym FAST to try to help individuals recognise the signs and symptoms of stroke as early as possible and encourage people to seek urgent medical help. FAST describes:

- Facial weakness – Can they smile? Has their mouth or eye drooped?
- Arm weakness – Can they raise both arms?
- Speech problem – Can they speak clearly, and can they understand what you're saying?
- Time – It's time to call 999 immediately if you see any of these symptoms.

By the time a person with TIA presents for assessment, the symptoms and signs have usually resolved and diagnosis relies on their account of the episode. To identify people presenting with TIA who are most at risk of subsequent stroke, the ABCD² score is sometimes used, although some clinical guidelines now recommend that it should not be used as all people should be seen by a specialist within 24 of onset of symptoms.[3] This score takes into account age, BP, clinical features of the TIA, duration of symptoms and history of diabetes – a high ABCD² score indicates a greater risk of early stroke (within 48 hours) and justifies hospitalisation for monitoring, while lower scores require secondary prevention strategies similar to that of stroke.[4]

It is vital that the person experiencing the stroke or TIA gets timely medical care to improve outcome. Rapid imaging to confirm the diagnosis followed by administration of thrombolysis is essential in patients with acute ischaemic stroke. The aim of thrombolysis is to break up the occluding blood clot and restore blood flow to the ischaemic area of the brain. Alteplase is the only thrombolytic agent licensed for use in acute ischaemic stroke, and the earlier it is administered the better, with the best outcomes if treatment is initiated within the first 1.5 hours after symptom onset, and the poorest outcomes 3-4.5 hour after symptom onset.[3,5,6]

In the acute phase, medical interventions are aimed at keeping the person stable and maintaining oxygenation of the brain to limit further damage (e.g. oxygen therapy, blood sugar management and preventing secondary problems like thrombosis and aspiration pneumonia). People with an acute ischaemic stroke, including those with AF, should be prescribed aspirin 300 mg daily as soon as possible after the onset of symptoms, except in those receiving thrombolysis, when the aspirin should be withheld for 24 hours and reimaging has been performed to rule out haemorrhagic transformation. Haemorrhagic transformation is a frequent complication of acute ischaemic stroke and occurs when there is bleeding into an area of ischaemic brain tissue, often following thrombolytic therapy.

The major risk factors for stroke include:

- hypertension
- diabetes
- CHD, AF, heart valve disease, coronary artery disease
- raised cholesterol
- smoking
- brain aneurisms and other malformations
- increasing age
- combined oral contraceptive pills and hormone replacement therapy, pregnancy and the weeks following birth, pre-eclampsia (this increases the risk of stroke in later life)
- infections and conditions that cause inflammation, such as lupus or rheumatoid arthritis
- ethnicity – stroke risk is higher in people of black African and Caribbean family origin
- family history
- anticoagulant therapy, which increases the risk of haemorrhagic stroke.

One in 8 people (12.5%) who experience stroke will die within the first 30 days, but more than 75% survive for a year and over 50% survive for more than five years.[1] Outcome following ischaemic strokes is better than following a haemorrhagic stroke. It can take weeks, months, or even years to recover from a stroke. Some people recover fully, while others have long-term or lifelong disabilities – around 25% are left living with minor disability and around 40% have more severe disabilities.[1]

Physical disabilities following a stroke include weakness and paralysis, spasticity, difficulty walking and altered sensation. Stroke can also affect cognitive function with impacts on memory, attention and perception. Communication issues include aphasia, dysarthria and dyspraxia. Dysphagia, swallowing problems after stroke, must be taken into account when prescribing.

Box 16.2: Practice point: complications of stroke

- Aphasia affects how a person speaks, as well as their comprehension, reading and writing skills.
- Dysarthria causes weakness in the muscles required to speak, which can change the sound of the voice and cause slurring.
- Dyspraxia describes when the muscles fail to move in the order required to make the sounds needed for speech.

Pharmacy input

All of the consequences of stroke require adjustment for the patient and carer, as well as for the healthcare professionals involved in their care.

The role of the pharmacist in post-stroke care will depend on their knowledge, skills and experience. Patients should be supported by a multidisciplinary team tailored to their needs, which might include physiotherapy, occupational therapy, speech and language therapy and other rehabilitation specialists alongside their GP and wider practice team including the practice pharmacist as well as community pharmacy.

The degree of support required will depend on the severity of the stroke, with some patients returning to normal family life, and others requiring longer-term nursing or residential care to address their needs.

Some aspects of post-stroke care will remain with specialist teams including managing spasticity, controlling seizures and overseeing the rehabilitation programme. Primary care should focus on supporting stroke survivors as they adjust to life after stroke, addressing some long-term consequences, as well as optimising interventions to prevent further vascular events. Key elements of post-stroke care include addressing the emotional impact, cognitive function, mobility and communication issues, swallowing difficulties and nutritional needs of the patient. Consideration should be given to the emotional and psychological effects of the stroke and TIA.

For pharmacists, particular care should be taken to ensure the patient understands, and is able to adhere to, the medication regimen and any concerns or issues that arise are addressed (e.g. the provision of medicines in appropriate formulations which the patients can swallow or receive via other routes if dysphagia is a problem). Practice-based pharmacists and community pharmacists can help identify and address medication-related issues that the patient may be experiencing.

Pharmacy review

The Greater Manchester Stroke Assessment tool, GM-SAT, endorsed by NHS England, gives a framework for a six-month review of a patient post-stroke. See *Box 16.3*.

> ### Box 16.3: Practice point: the Greater Manchester Stroke Assessment tool, GM-SAT
>
> - Medication
> - Assess the degree of disability using the Modified Rankin Scale
> - Review key issues including:
>   - medicines supply and adherence
>   - blood pressure
>   - antithrombotic therapy
>   - lipids
>   - diabetes
>   - alcohol intake, smoking status, diet, physical activity
>   - eyesight, hearing, communication
>   - swallowing, nutritional status, weight management
>   - pain
>   - continence
>   - problems with daily activities of living
>   - mobility issues and falls
> - Assess emotional health and wellbeing including:
>   - mood, anxiety
>   - personality changes
>   - sexual health
>   - fatigue, problems sleeping
>   - memory, concentration, and attention issues
>   - driving, transport and travel
>   - activities and hobbies
>   - working life
>   - money and benefits, housing and carer needs
>
> Source: www.england.nhs.uk/south/wp-content/uploads/sites/6/2017/07/gm-sat-proforma.pdf

Depending on skills and competence, pharmacists can undertake some or all aspects of the review of stroke patients at six months and beyond. Assessment of the post-stroke patient should include:

- measuring weight
- measuring blood pressure
- checking for pulse irregularity (unless AF has been diagnosed)
- taking bloods to assess renal function, lipids and HbA1c
- assessing physical and mental health issues
- reviewing prescribed medication, adherence to therapy and identifying any adverse effects.

Pharmacists should address medication-related issues to support patients to get the most out of their medicines post-stroke or TIA, as well as optimising secondary prevention strategies. See *Table 16.1* which summarises the key issues to consider.

Swallowing difficulties

More than 50% of patients will experience some degree of dysphagia post-stroke.[7] Acute swallowing difficulties will develop into a chronic problem for many patients and may even result in the need for home enteral tube feeding.[8] Speech and language therapists play a key role in assessing swallowing difficulties, but the primary care team may need to adjust medicines to support administration in patients with swallowing difficulties.

Many healthcare professionals assume that patients with dysphagia cannot swallow solid oral formulations and therefore all their medications need to be switched to liquids. However, this is not the case and adjustments to the medication regimen need to be individualised, based on the degree of dysphagia present.

Thin liquid medications can increase the risk of coughing and aspiration, and medication may instead need to be administered with thickened fluids or mixed with textured food. Tablets and capsules should be administered whole with the appropriate food texture and fluid consistency where possible. Where necessary, liquid formulations can be used but must be thickened to the correct consistency, for example, using proprietary thickening agents (e.g. Thick and Easy). Crushing tablets or opening capsules to be administered with modified food or fluid may affect the stability of the medication and renders the formulation unlicensed.[9]

Seek advice from the speech and language team on appropriate liquid consistency or food texture. In people with swallowing difficulties, care should be taken to assess nutritional status and ensure an adequate dietary intake is maintained.

Table 16.1: *Supporting patients to get the best out of their medicines*

Problem	Prompt questions	Relevance
Knowledge	Do you understand what your medicines are for? Do you know why you need to take them long term? Do you have any concerns about your medicines?	Understanding is important to ensure long-term adherence. Addressing this early will ensure optimal stroke prevention.
Adverse effects	Have you experienced any side effects from the medicines (e.g. stomach upset, rashes, headaches, muscle aches, nightmares)?	Ongoing adverse effects will affect the patients' willingness to take their medication long term.
Swallowing	Do you have difficulty swallowing any of your tablets/capsules?	Swallowing difficulties are common in patients following a stroke. Advice such as taking with yoghurts to aid swallowing, or changing to smaller tablets or alternative formulations may be appropriate.
Memory problems	How do you remember to take your medication regularly? How often in a week (or month) do you forget your tablets? Do you find it easy to remember any evening doses?	Infrequent dosing will compromise the effectiveness of drug therapy. The patient may need advice on strategies to aid them in taking their medicines, or require specific medication aids.
Physical disabilities	Do you have any physical disabilities which make it difficult to take your medications: <ul><li>Can you read the label?</li><li>Can you get the tablets out of the blister pack?</li><li>Can you open containers without help?</li><li>Can you manage eye drops? (if appropriate)</li><li>Can you use your inhalers? (if appropriate)</li></ul>	There are a number of devices available to assist patients in taking their medications. Patients can ask for non-child resistant caps to bottles or larger bottles to assist with grip, devices are available to assist using inhalers and eye drops.
Access	Do you have any problems getting your medicines?	Physical disabilities can make it difficult for patient to access medications.

Box 16.4: Practice point: standardised terminology for food textures and thickened fluids

Food textures are:
- B = thin purée dysphagia diet – food needs to be blended to remove all lumps and at the correct consistency will be too runny to eat with a fork and can only be eaten with a spoon
- C = thick purée dysphagia diet – food needs to be blended to remove all lumps
- D = pre-mashed dysphagia diet – food can be eaten with a fork and requires little chewing
- E = fork-mashable dysphagia diet – food requires some chewing, but it is easy for a fork to pass through

Thickened fluids are described as:
- Stage 1: syrup consistency – should pour like single pouring cream
- Stage 2: custard consistency – should drop easily off a teaspoon rather than pour
- Stage 3: pudding consistency – should stay on a spoon like well-whipped double cream

Excessive drooling

Chronic sialorrhoea (excessive salivation and drooling) can occur post-stroke due to residual weakness of the muscles in the mouth and face and is often seen in those with swallowing difficulties.

As well as impacting on oral health, causing bad breath, perioral eczema and eating and speaking difficulties, excessive drooling also has important psychological and social effects including embarrassment, decreased self-esteem and the potential for social isolation.

Refer patients experiencing excessive drooling to speech and language therapy for support. Anticholinergic drugs, such as glycopyrrolate and scopolamine, dry up secretions and may assist with these symptoms. NICE recommends the use of botulinum toxin as an option for treating chronic sialorrhoea caused by neurological conditions in adults.[10]

Dry mouth

Dry mouth (xerostomia) occurs commonly post-stroke, is uncomfortable, leads to increased risk of periodontal disease, and may contribute to dysphagia. Advise that artificial saliva can help to alleviate the symptoms and that maintaining good oral hygiene can minimise the risk of infection.

Depression and anxiety

Approximately one-third of patients will experience depression and/or anxiety post-stroke.[11] The risk factors associated with post-stroke depression include female sex, history of depression or psychiatric illness, functional limitations and cognitive impairment.

Post-stroke depression and anxiety impacts on functional recovery and therefore early detection and management are important. Use a validated screening tool for depression, such as PHQ-2 or PHQ-9, and the Generalised Anxiety Disorder 7-item (GAD-7) to identify those at risk and refer for psychological support and consideration for antidepressant therapy. For more information on assessment and management of anxiety and depression, see **Chapter 1**.

Lifestyle and risk factors

Pharmacists in community and primary care should support stroke patients to address any relevant lifestyle factors to reduce the risk of a recurrent event and aid their recovery. Key lifestyle issues to identify and address include smoking, physical activity (accepting there may be constraints due to any stroke-related disability), dietary intake, weight loss and alcohol intake. Pharmacy teams may be able to offer in-house support, for example, smoking cessation or weight management programmes, or may refer or signpost to other local services.

Physical activity packages will need to be tailored to the individual and may need the support of a physiotherapist.

Medication

Secondary prevention medications are used alongside lifestyle modification post-stroke and TIA to reduce the risk of future vascular events including stroke and myocardial infarction and include antithrombotic therapy, antihypertensives, lipid-lowering therapies and drugs for glycaemic control in diabetic patients.

Antithrombotic therapy

Aspirin therapy is prescribed at a dose of 300 mg daily, usually for the first two weeks post-stroke. At two weeks, the Royal College of Physicians (RCP) recommends that patients should be switched to clopidogrel 75 mg daily which should be continued indefinitely.[3] If clopidogrel cannot be tolerated, aspirin 75 mg daily with modified release dipyridamole 200 mg twice daily should be used. The combination of aspirin and clopidogrel is not recommended unless there is another compelling indication (e.g. acute coronary syndrome or recent coronary stent placement). For more information on anti-platelet therapy see **Chapter 5**.

Post-stroke patients with AF should also be prescribed aspirin 300 mg daily, usually for the first two weeks post-stroke, but at this point, aspirin therapy should be discontinued and anticoagulant therapy initiated with warfarin or a direct oral anticoagulant (DOAC)[3] – for more information on AF and anticoagulation see **Chapter 3**. If anticoagulation is contraindicated, refer the patient to cardiology for consideration of a left atrial appendage occlusion device which reduces the risk of AF-related stroke.[12]

Anticoagulation should not be prescribed for people with stroke or TIA in sinus rhythm unless there is another compelling indication, such as cerebral venous thrombosis or arterial dissection.[3]

Blood pressure and antihypertensive therapy

Hypertension is the most prevalent risk factor for first and recurrent stroke and is present in approximately 64% of patients with stroke.[13,14] Blood pressure reduction is therefore an essential element of secondary prevention post-stroke and TIA. The RCP recommends that BP is lowered to a target of <130/90 mmHg, which has been shown to be safe and to effectively prevent recurrent vascular events, except in people with severe bilateral carotid artery stenosis, for whom a systolic BP target of 140-150 mmHg is appropriate.[3]

The benefits of BP lowering were seen in both hypertensive and non-hypertensive patients and therefore the use of antihypertensives should be considered for all stroke patients aiming for tight BP control of <130/90 mmHg. Due to the concern regarding early BP lowering post-stroke, the RCP recommends that antihypertensive therapies should be initiated prior to the transfer of care out of hospital or at two weeks, whichever is the soonest, or at the first clinic visit for people not admitted.[3] Drug therapy should be initiated in line with the NICE hypertension algorithm, taking into account age and ethnicity to guide drug selection[15] – for more information on the treatment of hypertension see **Chapter 12**.

Treatment should be intensified every two to four weeks until the treatment target is achieved. Adherence should be assessed at each clinic visit. Refer patients for specialist advice if they do not achieve the treatment target.

Lipid-lowering therapy

Lipid-lowering with a statin is indicated in all patients who have an ischaemic stroke, regardless of baseline cholesterol level. In line with NICE guidance, treatment should begin with a high-intensity statin such as atorvastatin 80 mg daily and aim for a greater than 40% reduction in non-HDL cholesterol.[16]

If this is not achieved within three months, discuss adherence and timing of dose, optimise dietary and lifestyle measures and consider increasing to a higher dose if this was not prescribed from the outset. In patients who cannot tolerate a statin or who do not achieve the required reduction in non-HDL cholesterol on statin alone, consider ezetimibe 10 mg daily.[17] Refer patients post-stroke who are not achieving an LDL level <4 mmol/L (<3.5 mmol/L in patients with multiple CV events or vascular disease in more than one bed) despite optimal statin and ezetimibe, for consideration of a PCSK9 inhibitor such as alirocumab or evolocumab.[18,19]

For more information on lipid management for secondary prevention see **Chapter 5**. People with primary intracerebral haemorrhage should avoid statin treatment unless it is required for other indications, due to an increased risk of haemorrhagic stroke seen in clinical studies,

Diabetes

People with type 2 diabetes are two to three times more likely to suffer an ischaemic stroke than those without the condition. Diabetes is a risk factor for carotid atherosclerosis and small vessel cerebrovascular disease and therefore increases the risk of stroke. Patients post-stroke and TIA should be screened for diabetes at least annually and, if identified, therapy initiated to improve glycaemic control. For more information on glycemic control, see **Chapter 9**.

Advice for patients

Advice to patients needs to be tailored to the individual based on the severity of the event experienced and the subsequent consequences on their physical and mental health. Areas to consider include:

- Explore the patient's understanding of stroke/TIA and its consequences
- Identify stroke/TIA risk factors present for the individual and discuss how these can be addressed
- Explore opportunities for lifestyle change to reduce stroke risk and refer or signpost to services for support to address these
- Review physical consequences of stroke and the need for additional support from social care or health care services
- Review prescribed medication, check their understanding of the medicines they are taking, review adherence to prescribed therapy and address any concerns that they may have
- Encourage patients to discuss any impact that stroke/TIA has had on their mental health, particularly any signs of depression

Useful resources

- NICE Clinical Knowledge Summaries (2020). Stroke and TIA scenario: secondary prevention following stroke and TIA .www.cks.nice.org.uk/topics/stroke-tia/management/secondary-prevention-following-stroke-tia/
- NICE (2019). Stroke and transient ischaemic attack in over 16s: diagnosis and initial management [NG128]. www.nice.org.uk/guidance/ng128
- Parmer P. Stroke classification and diagnosis. *Clinical Pharmacist* 2018; 10(1).
- Royal College of Physicians (2016). National Clinical Guideline for Stroke. www.rcplondon.ac.uk/guidelines-policy/stroke-guidelines

References

1. Stroke Association. State of the nation - stroke statistics Jan 2017. London: Stroke Association; 2017. www.stroke.org.uk/sites/default/files/state_of_the_nation_2017_final_1.pdf
2. NHS England. The size of the prize in cardiovascular disease (CVD) prevention. London: NHS England. www.healthcheck.nhs.uk/seecmsfile/?id=983
3. Royal College of Physicians (RCGP). National Clinical Guideline for Stroke. London: RCGP; 2016. www.strokeaudit.org/SupportFiles/Documents/Guidelines/2016-National-Clinical-Guideline-for-Stroke-5t-(1).aspx
4. Johnston SC *et al*. Validation and refinement of scores to predict very early stroke risk after transient ischaemic attack. *Lancet* 2007; 369(9558): 283-292.
5. National Institute for Health and Care Excellence (NICE). Alteplase for treating acute ischaemic stroke [TA264]. London: NICE; 2012. www.nice.org.uk/guidance/ta264
6. Lees KR *et al*. Time to treatment with intravenous alteplase and outcome in stroke: an updated pooled analysis of ECASS, ATLANTIS, NINDS, and EPITHET trials. *Lancet* 2010; 375: 1695-1703.
7. Martino R *et al*. Dysphagia after stroke: incidence, diagnosis, and pulmonary complications. *Stroke* 2005; 36(12): 2756-2763.
8. Broadley S *et al*. Predictors of prolonged dysphagia following acute stroke. *J Clin Neurosci* 2003; 10(3): 300-305.
9. Barnett N and Parmer P. How to tailor medication formulations for patients with dysphagia. *Pharmaceutical Journal* 2016 [online]; 297: No 7892.
10. National Institute for Health and Care Excellence (NICE). Xeomin (botulinum neurotoxin type A) for treating chronic sialorrhoea [TA605]. London: NICE; 2019. www.nice.org.uk/guidance/TA605
11. Towfighi A *et al*. Poststroke depression: a scientific statement for healthcare professionals from the American Heart Association/American Stroke Association. *Stroke* 2017; 48: e30-e44.

12. National Institute for Health and Care Excellence (NICE). Atrial fibrillation: management [CG180]. London: NICE; 2014. www.nice.org.uk/guidance/cg180

13. Feigin VL *et al*. Global burden of stroke. *Circulation Research* 2017; 120: 439-48.

14. O'Donnell MJ *et al*. Risk factors for ischaemic and intracerebral haemorrhagic stroke in 22 countries (the INTERSTROKE study): a case-control study. *Lancet* 2010; 376: 112-23.

15. National Institute for Health and Care Excellence (NICE). Hypertension in adults: diagnosis and management [CG136]. London: NICE; 2019. www.nice.org.uk/guidance/ng136

16. National Institute for Health and Care Excellence (NICE). Cardiovascular disease: risk assessment and reduction, including lipid modification [CG181]. London: NICE; 2014. www.nice.org.uk/guidance/cg181

17. National Institute for Health and Care Excellence (NICE). Ezetimibe for treating primary heterozygous-familial and non-familial hypercholesterolaemia [TA385]. London: NICE; 2016. www.nice.org.uk/guidance/ta385

18. National Institute for Health and Care Excellence (NICE). Alirocumab for treating primary hypercholesterolaemia and mixed dyslipidaemia [TA393] London: NICE; 2016. www.nice.org.uk/guidance/ta393

19. National Institute for Health and Care Excellence (NICE). Evolocumab for treating primary hypercholesterolaemia and mixed dyslipidaemia [TA395]. London: NICE; 2016. www.nice.org.uk/guidance/ta394

Case studies

Case study 1

Penny, aged 72 years, has had an ischaemic stroke, secondary to uncontrolled blood pressure and was recently discharged from the local hospital after an 8-day inpatient stay. Two weeks later she has requested repeat medication from the GP practice.

Her discharge medications were:

- Aspirin 300 mg daily
- Ramipril 5 mg daily
- Indapamide 2.5 mg daily
- Amlodipine 10 mg daily
- Atorvastatin 40 mg daily
- Lansoprazole 30 mg daily

You review her notes and find that pre-stroke she was generally well with a diagnosis of hypertension, previously well controlled, and she has no other long-term conditions. However, Penny has smoked for most of her adult life and her last recorded weight (six months ago) was 82 kg, with a BMI of 27.8.

The discharge summary indicates a rapid recovery with minimal loss of physical function. The local care record shows bloods (renal, liver, FBC) during admission were within the normal ranges. Her total cholesterol on admission was 6.2, with an HDL of 1.1 and non-HDL cholesterol of 5.1.

Points to consider

- What are your priorities in the consultation?

You decide on the following priorities:

- Ensure Penny understands her condition and answer any questions she may have
- Assess how Penny has been managing at home post-stroke
- Review any lifestyle changes that would reduce her risk of recurrent events
- Check her BP and optimise her antihypertensive therapies, if necessary
- Review her antiplatelet therapy
- Assess her lipid-lowering therapy
- Review adherence to drug therapy, identify any adverse effects and address any concerns

Points to consider

- What should you consider when talking with Penny to gauge her understanding of her condition?

Penny has experienced a significant health event and while she appears to have recovered quickly, you know that she is at risk of recurrent events. You are aware that it may take time for her to understand the full implications of experiencing a stroke and so you need to ensure she is supported to come to terms with this.

It is important to take into account the fact that she is likely to have seen patients with significant disability post-stroke during her hospital stay and may be afraid that this will happen to her should she experience a further stroke. You reassure her that there are changes she can make to reduce her risk of another event and that the medicines she has been prescribed will also reduce her risk.

Points to consider

- How would you assess how Penny is managing at home post-stroke?

You ask about:

- Physical limitations – for example, mobility, dexterity, ability to perform activities of daily living.
- Impact on cognitive function – while you may not be able to undertake a full cognitive function assessment in the GP practice, you are aware that stroke can affect concentration, language and memory. These issues may be apparent in the consultation, or the patient, family or carers may become aware of them over time. If there are concerns, the patient should be referred for formal cognitive function assessment.
- Mental health – particularly any signs of depression using PHQ-2/PHQ-9.
- Social circumstances – the support Penny has at home from family and friends.

It is clear in the consultation that Penny has very little physical limitation post-stroke. She is walking well with no obvious impairment, but she does report some weakness in her left hand. She can carry out her usual activities in the home and is going out for a short walk, accompanied by her husband, on most days of the week. She has no signs of cognitive impairment post-stroke and no indication of depression at this time. She is well supported at home by her husband and two adult children, both living nearby. She and her husband are both very pleased with her recovery but do express concerns about the risk of a further stroke in future.

> **Points to consider**
>
> - What lifestyle changes would reduce her risk of recurrent events?

Following her stroke, Penny has stopped smoking and you should congratulate her on that. Bearing in mind that she may need additional support (talking therapies or medication) to maintain this, you advise her to seek help from the practice of the local community pharmacy if needed.

You also highlight that, ideally, she should lose some weight – and she and her husband report that they have been trying to eat more healthily and have started their daily walks to increase their physical activity to address this.

> **Points to consider**
>
> - What medication changes should be considered to optimise therapy?

You check Penny's clinic blood pressure and it is 147/86 mmHg and you decide that it is appropriate to adjust her antihypertensive medication in line with the guidelines. There is scope to increase her ramipril, but you know that her renal function will need to be checked before making any changes.

You review her antiplatelet therapy and she is still taking aspirin – this is usually stopped at discharge from hospital or at two weeks, whichever comes first, and clopidogrel 75 mg started. This should have happened at discharge, but it appears to have been missed, so you change the therapy now.

You assess her lipids and they are within an acceptable range, but you know that the dose of atorvastatin can be increased if there has not been a 40% reduction in her non-HDL cholesterol and that other therapies may be considered if a higher dose statin is not tolerated or does not achieve the required reduction in non-HDL cholesterol.

You review adherence to drug therapy, ask about adverse effects and speak to Penny to see if she has any concerns and ensure that she understands the purpose of the medicines she has been prescribed, particularly those that are intended to reduce her risk of a further stroke.

She reports that she has been reluctant to take her medicines regularly in the past, and she realises not taking her medicine to control her high blood pressure was responsible for her stroke. She tells you that she has been taking her medicines regularly ever since her stroke and her husband helps provide a useful reminder.

You tell her that she can speak to you or her community pharmacist if she has any problems with her medicines, such as adverse effects, so the issue can be addressed.

Points to consider

- What follow-up would you consider for Penny?

You arrange for blood tests and an appointment in two weeks to make any necessary adjustments to her blood pressure and lipid-lowering therapies.

Case study 2

Jay, aged 68 years, has recently been admitted to a local nursing home as a result of a recent move to be closer to his family. He had an atrial fibrillation-related stroke over five years ago and has been left with significant physical impairment which has left him requiring 24-hour care.

He is not mobile, requires a hoist to move from bed to chair, has spasticity to his right arm and leg and is incontinent. Despite this, his cognitive function has not been significantly affected, except for occasional memory lapses. He engages with the nurses and other patients at the nursing home and has good family support from his sons and grandchildren.

The nurses have contacted the practice to ask for help with his medicines as he is having trouble swallowing some of his tablets and they have requested liquid formulation.

His is currently prescribed:

- Apixaban 5 mg twice daily
- Amlodipine 5 mg daily
- Ramipril 2.5 mg twice daily
- Atorvastatin 80 mg daily
- Escitalopram 10 mg daily
- Baclofen 20 mg three times daily
- Sodium docusate 100 mg twice daily
- Lactulose 10 mL twice daily

Points to consider

- What are your initial thoughts about the request to change the formulation?

This may appear to be a simple request to change his medications from tablets/capsules to liquid to make administration easier. However, you know that in people with swallowing difficulties, liquid formulations can cause aspiration.

You are aware that it is important that his swallowing difficulties are fully assessed, particularly if there is evidence of deterioration, so you arrange for a referral to a speech and language specialist. There may implications for his diet as well as his medicines.

Speech and language specialists may advise in the consistency of the diet he should receive, and this will inform how his medicines should be administered.

Points to consider

- What steps can be taken to help Jay take his medicines without changing the formulation?

Depending on the degree of swallowing difficulty, small whole tablets (such as apixaban, amlodipine, ramipril, atorvastatin and escitalopram) may be administered mixed with the appropriate textured food such as a puree or a yoghurt.

Some tablets will disperse quickly in water (amlodipine, atorvastatin) for mixing with diet or thickened fluids.

Other tablets can be crushed and dispersed in water to be given with food – but in some cases, the taste can be very bitter (escitalopram) and care should be taken that this does not affect nutritional intake.

Liquid formulations (baclofen, docusate, lactulose) may be mixed with thickened fluids to achieve the appropriate texture.

You also consider reviewing the dosing to minimise the absolute number of doses prescribed – for example, giving the ramipril as a single daily dose.

Points to consider

- What resources would help when making decisions about administering medicines to people with dysphagia?

Online resources to support the administration of medicines in patients with dysphagia include the Specialist Pharmacy Service website, and advice on opening capsules and crushing tablets can also be sought from the manufacturer.

Points to consider

- How else can you contribute to Jay's care?

As Jay is new to the area and practice, you decide to check that all his other post-stroke needs have been addressed, such as referral to local specialist stroke services support and physiotherapy.

CHAPTER 17

Polypharmacy and multimorbidity

Emyr Jones, Jayne Agnew, Nina Barnett, Paula Crawford, Carmel Darcy, Hilary McKee, Karen Miller, Lelly Oboh and Heather Smith

Overview

The word polypharmacy is derived from the ancient Greek 'polύs' meaning 'many', and 'pharmakeía' meaning 'the use of drugs'. Polypharmacy is now a routine aspect of modern healthcare, driven by an ageing population, combined with innovations in medicine ensuring the prevalence of comorbidities. While there are many definitions of polypharmacy which relate to the quantity of medicines being taken,[1] it has been proposed that polypharmacy is simply more medicines being prescribed or taken than are clinically appropriate in the context of a person's comorbidities.[2]

It is important to bear in mind that the specific number of medicines taken is not an indication of inappropriateness, as all of the medicines may be clinically necessary and appropriate for that person. It has been suggested that the emphasis should be on evidence-based practice[1] rather than a number. Polypharmacy is also categorised in the literature into appropriate and inappropriate and so the context of prescribing in an individual must be taken into account. *Box 17.1* shows the King's Fund definition of appropriate and inappropriate polypharmacy.[3]

Box 17.1: The King's Fund definitions of appropriate and inappropriate polypharmacy[3]

- *Appropriate polypharmacy* is prescribing for an individual for complex conditions or for multiple conditions in circumstances where medicine use has been optimised and the medicines are prescribed according to best evidence. The overall intent for the combination of medicines prescribed should be to maintain good quality of life, improve longevity and minimise harm from medicines.
- *Inappropriate polypharmacy* is where multiple medications are prescribed inappropriately or where the intended benefit of the medicine is not realised.

Appropriate polypharmacy ensures disease states and symptoms are managed effectively. However, as a disease progresses or changes and a person ages, polypharmacy can become inappropriate, leading to potentially problematic polypharmacy which may require medicines discontinuation, dose adjustment or switching of medicines.

Inappropriate polypharmacy occurs when the burden of medicines becomes greater than the burden of the diseases that they are used to treat.[3] Masnoon *et al*[1] concluded that polypharmacy definitions are variable and numerical definitions of polypharmacy do not account for specific comorbidities present and make it difficult to assess safety and appropriateness of therapy in the clinical setting.

Box 17.2: Factors leading to problematic polypharmacy[4,5]

- The medicine combination is hazardous because of interactions.
- The overall demands of the pill burden are unacceptable to the person.
- These demands make it difficult to achieve clinically useful medicines adherence.
- Medicines are being prescribed to treat adverse effects, but alternative solutions are available to reduce the number of medicines prescribed.

Although there is a lack of data on the epidemiology of polypharmacy at the population level, a high prevalence is reported in several countries and it is recognised as an international issue. Morin et al[6] found the incidence in the Swedish population to be 44% (five or more medicines), and the prevalence of excessive polypharmacy was 11.7% (10 or more medicines).

American datasets cite that 30% of older adults take five or more medicines simultaneously and 5% take eight or more medicines,[7] while Guthrie and colleagues[8] cite the numbers of Scottish adults dispensed 5-9, 10-14 or 15 or more medicines in primary care over a 3-month period in 2010 as 16.3%, 4.7% and 1.1% respectively.

The prevalence of polypharmacy is expected to rise as the proportion of older people increases. In one UK study, potentially hazardous prescribing in all people was approximately 5%.[9] Medicines are the most common healthcare intervention and people with multimorbidity are often prescribed medicines by different specialists using disease-specific evidence-based guidelines.[3] This results in polypharmacy which may be appropriate according to the guidelines, but which can cause harm.

Multimorbidity is commonly defined as the presence of two or more long-term health conditions and is common in older people. Conditions can include defined physical and mental health conditions such as diabetes or schizophrenia, ongoing conditions such as learning disability, symptom complexes such as frailty or chronic pain, sensory impairment such as sight or hearing loss and alcohol and substance misuse.[4]

Multimorbidity is associated with decreased quality of life, reduced mobility and functional ability, as well as increases in hospitalisations and use of healthcare resources.[4] The prevalence of multimorbidity increases markedly with age[10], and people are also more likely to demonstrate non-adherence to medicines.[11]

In addition, multimorbidity has also been shown to increase referrals between different sectors of the healthcare system which results in disjointed care, poor communication between healthcare staff, multiple prescribers involved in a person's care, and ultimately the person's safety can be compromised.[10]

Unsurprisingly, the risk of adverse effects and harm increases with increasing numbers of medicines which can lead to drug-drug and drug-disease interactions. Polypharmacy is particularly significant in older people who are at greater risk of adverse events due to decreased renal and hepatic function, lower lean body mass, hearing and visual impairment and impaired cognition and mobility. Polypharmacy is associated with adverse health outcomes[1], impaired medicines adherence and impaired quality of life.[3]

A consequence of polypharmacy is the introduction of unintentional prescribing cascades which occur when a new medicine is prescribed to treat an adverse effect of a medicine that a person is already taking in the mistaken belief that it is a new symptom. There are of course other intentional prescribing cascades which may be introduced to prevent a person from predictable harm that some treatment regimens cause. See Box 17.3 for some examples of intentional and unintentional prescribing cascades and Table 17.1 for the top 10 inappropriate prescribing cascades to be aware of.

Box 17.3: Examples of intentional and unintentional prescribing cascades

Intentional
- A bisphosphonate, calcium and vitamin D for a person on extended prednisolone therapy for vasculitis.
- A laxative for preventing opioid-induced constipation.
- A proton pump inhibitor together with an NSAID as ulcer prophylaxis.

Unintentional
- Antiparkinsonian therapy started in response to someone experiencing extrapyramidal signs and symptoms from antipsychotics. This can then lead to new symptoms, including orthostatic hypotension and delirium.[12]

Table 17.1: *Top 10 examples of inappropriate prescribing cascades*

Initial drug therapy	Adverse drug event	Subsequent drug therapy
Metoclopramide/antipsychotics	Extrapyramidal signs and symptoms	Antiparkinsonian therapy
Amlodipine	Lower limb oedema	Loop diuretic (e.g. furosemide)
Cholinesterase inhibitors (e.g. donepezil, rivastigmine and galantamine)	Urinary incontinence	Antimuscarinic agent (e.g. oxybutynin, tolterodine, solifenacin)
NSAIDs	Increased blood pressure	Antihypertensive therapy
Amitriptyline	Urinary retention	Alpha adrenoceptor blocker (e.g. tamsulosin)
Thiazide diuretics	Hyperuricaemia	Gout treatment (e.g. allopurinol or colchicine)
Digoxin, nitrates, loop diuretics, ACE inhibitors, oral corticosteroids, antibiotics, NSAIDs, opioid analgesics, methylxanthines (e.g. theophylline)[13,14]	Dizziness	Medicine to treat episodes of vertigo (e.g. prochlorperazine, cyclizine)
Vasodilators, diuretics, beta blockers, calcium channel blockers, ACE inhibitors, NSAIDs, opioid analgesics, sedatives, statins[15,16]	Nausea	Antiemetic (e.g. metoclopramide)
ACE inhibitor	Cough	Antibiotic
Paroxetine, haloperidol[13,16]	Tremor	Levodopa-carbidopa

Implementation of single organ clinical guidelines has resulted in the use of polypharmacy and complex treatment regimens that potentially tip the benefit to risk ratio unfavourably in the most vulnerable subpopulations including the 'Very Old, those with COmorbidity, Dementia, Frailty and Limited life Expectancy'.[17] The acronym VOCODFLEX has been proposed to describe circumstances where the benefit/risk ratio of certain treatments may be questionable, and for whom applying, all clinical guidelines may increase adverse drug effects, inappropriate treatment and medicines burden.[18]

Polypharmacy and inappropriate prescribing are well-known risk factors for adverse drug reactions (ADRs).[19]

Pharmacy input

Identifying and addressing problematic and inappropriate polypharmacy is the responsibility of all healthcare professionals and the individuals themselves. Medicines reviews that rely on one profession will fail due to the scale of the problem.[20] Prescribers need to consider the consequences of prescribing more medicines to people already impacted by polypharmacy as this can help prevent inappropriate prescribing cascades.

People at risk of harm need to be identified systematically and opportunistically, and regular patient-facing contact enables pharmacists to identify people who may benefit from an approach to care that takes account of multimorbidity.

Community pharmacists may opportunistically review people when they present with a prescription; ask how they are managing their medicines, and check if any medicines are no longer needed. In addition, they are likely to be aware of people taking a large number of medicines who may benefit from a polypharmacy review, and they can be involved in the important role of discharge reconciliation once people have left secondary care.

Hospital pharmacists may identify people on admission to hospital with problematic polypharmacy, medicine adherence issues or who do not understand how or when to take their medicines. They can also improve the transfer of information about medicines at discharge to people and the healthcare professionals involved in their care.

Pharmacists working in outpatient clinics (e.g. anticoagulant clinics, frailty clinics, falls clinics) can identify people who have difficulty coping with their medicines, while pharmacists working within GP practices can proactively use electronic health records and other systems available to them to identify people taking a large number of medicines or those at greatest risk of harm and conduct more in-depth reviews.

Time is needed to undertake complex medicines reviews, but small steps can be taken by all healthcare professionals that people come into contact with.

Pharmacy technicians can also contribute to reducing the impact of taking multiple medicines and the medicines burden on people, and particularly for vulnerable groups such as older people,[20] and they can be actively involved in undertaking medicines reviews, supporting people to adhere to their medicines, or identifying people who would benefit from a medicines review.[20] Conducting a medicines review is a key role for pharmacists in all settings as part of the multidisciplinary approach to care.

Box 17.4: Knowledge, skills and behaviours that an accomplished pharmacist will possess

- Skilled in reviewing people with complex medicines histories and adopting an individualised, person-centred approach, with a focus on therapeutic areas to target for medicines review.
- Can apply person-centred consultation skills to ensure appropriate, timely medicines review in line with clinical guidelines and evidence-based practice. This ensures a holistic review of medicines taking account of risks versus benefits.
- Can reduce treatment burden by identifying:
  - ways of maximising benefits from existing treatments
  - treatments that could be stopped because of limited benefit.
  - medicines with a higher risk of adverse events (e.g. falls).
- Adept at using screening tools (e.g. STOPP/START[21] tool) in older people to identify medicine-related safety concerns and medicines the person might benefit from, but is not currently taking.
- Can establish and take into account person goals, values and priorities in relation to medicines and their health (e.g. maintaining their independence and reducing harms from medicines).
- Has a key role to play in developing and implementing prevention strategies and standards at person-facing level, as well as corporate and national level, to address the growing burden of polypharmacy and embed principles of medicines optimisation and review within prescribing practices across the health service.

The complexity of review will increase as pharmacists grow in experience and attain the knowledge and skills required (see *Figure 17.1*).

Figure 17.1: *The development of pharmacist practitioners in the management of polypharmacy*

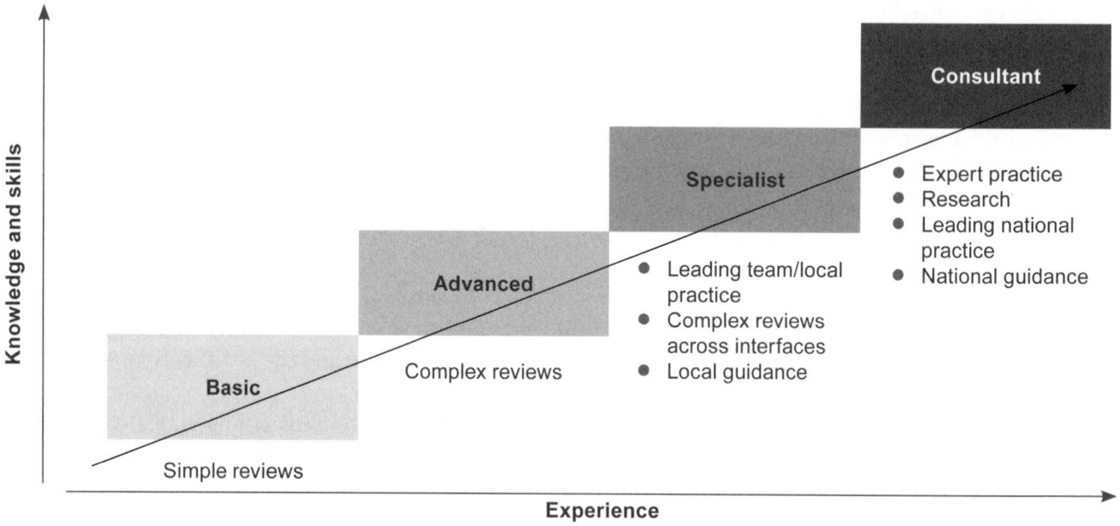

Pharmacy review

Person-centred care

Management of people with multimorbidity is complex and requires a holistic approach, tailored to the person's needs.[22] A 'one-size-fits-all' method does not work and requires care to be personalised based on the individual's preferences, health priorities, lifestyle and goals. People with multimorbidity generally have reduced quality of life and it poses a particular challenge to clinicians as physical and mental conditions can present concurrently.[23]

Good communication is essential; clinicians should avoid overusing medical jargon and should be capable of translating complex medical information into layman's terms. For effective two-way communication, people also need to feel that they've been listened to and understood and have had the opportunity to openly express their views without judgment.

Person-centred care is a philosophy, or way of thinking, that sees clinicians embracing the person as an equal partner and establishing a truly collaborative approach to decision making. This means putting people at the centre of care and taking into account their individual needs and preferences.

Box 17.5: Practice point: good communication

- Listen carefully
- Speak slowly
- Do not use medical jargon
- Explain things clearly
- Repeat points to help improve people's understanding

Investing the time to get to know the person and to understand what is important to them is critical to removing one's preconceived ideas and will lead to more effective conversations.[24] Clinicians' instinctive eagerness to launch into an 'advice giving' role or revert to 'telling' mode is not always helpful. Firstly, the person's current level of understanding needs to be established and also what they want to know or what their beliefs and values are. If this baseline is not achieved initially then there is the risk of a disengaged person with a loss of trust and confidence in the clinician.

Older people are particularly vulnerable to not receiving person-centred care due to clinician assumptions or ageist stereotypes.[25] The role of the clinician is to identify what the older person needs from a consultation and, using an individualised approach, facilitate an interaction that optimises the person's health and wellbeing.[26]

As active partners, the person and clinician should prioritise care based on the preferences and goals of the person. This is the basis of shared decision making.

Shared decision making is a process in which a clinician and the person work together to make the most appropriate decisions about their health and care based on clinical evidence and the person's informed preferences.[26]

Remember, guidelines don't always consider the person's viewpoint. The skill is knowing when to show flexibility within guidelines when a person might benefit from a different approach.

People often have their own agenda which is why it is imperative to understand what's important to them. What are their goals from taking medicines, and do they know why they are taking them? Do they have any concerns or particular worries? By assessing their understanding of the condition and medicines it allows pharmacists to pitch the consultation at the correct level.[27]

To promote the use of shared decision making in routine clinical practice, the process can be broken down into three simple steps based on a 'team talk', an 'option talk', and a 'decision talk'.[28]

Team talk places emphasis on the need to provide support to the person when they are offered different treatment choices, and to use the person's goals to guide decision making. Option talk supports the person to work through and compare the different choices to promote broader understanding and acceptance of risk management decisions. Decision talk refers to the process of reaching a conclusion, which reflects the informed preferences of the person, guided by the experience and expertise of clinicians.

Following an effective shared decision making discussion, as per the international Choosing Wisely initiative,[29] the person should have the following questions answered about their treatment:

1. What are the potential benefits?
2. What are the potential harms?
3. What will happen if nothing is done?
4. Are there any alternative options to consider?

Achieving the person-centred approach isn't always an easy task and can require a fundamental change to a pharmacist's historic practice, but it is something that can be developed and improved with practice, and it is helpful to have a structured approach to a person-centred consultation.

It is important to gain an insight into the person's health literacy skills and their current understanding of their medicine or condition. Using broad probing questions can encourage the person to open up and divulge useful information. Pharmacists may be experts in medicines/health, but the person is an expert in themselves, their social circumstances, psychological state and other factors which may affect their health behaviours.

Developed from the GROW (goal, reality, options, will) model of coaching[30], the 'Four Es'[31] is a useful way for pharmacists to use their expertise to educate the person to alter their health behaviours. This non-judgemental approach avoids using 'Why' questions, such as: 'Why don't you take your medicines regularly?'. 'Why' questions can be perceived as an accusation and can instantly put people on the defensive.

> ## Box 17.6: The four Es — explore, educate, empower, and enable[31]
>
> ### Explore
> - What does the patient know? (about the disease and medicine, about the reason they have been given these medicines)
> - What do they want to know?
> - What worries them about the medicine?
> - What do they want the medicine to do for them?
> - What do they want to achieve by taking the medicine?
> - Find out what the person wants to know and follow their agenda.
>
> ### Educate
> - Talk to them about what they want to know before you talk about what you think they need to know.
>
> ### Empower
> - What do they want to do now?
> - How do they want to manage their disease/medicines taking?
> - Help them to take responsibility for medicines taking.
>
> ### Enable
> - What they have agreed to do.
> - How will they do it?
> - When will they do it?
> - Where will they get help?
> - What will they need to do if this becomes more urgent/who to call?
> - Support behavioural change in order for the person to achieve their aims.
>
> © Nina Barnett

Effective questioning can help people take responsibility for the situation. By exploring and educating them about the pros and cons of the options being offered, they can decide on the best course of action. In partnership, pharmacists can then empower and enable the person to be responsible for taking these actions.

Medicines review

It is important that the person's knowledge, understanding and concerns about medicines are reviewed at regular intervals, as these may change over time. This can be achieved by carrying out a structured medicines review.

Medicines review has been defined as 'a structured critical examination of a person's medicines with the objective of reaching an agreement with the person about treatment, optimising the impact of medicines, minimising the number of medicines-related problems and reducing waste.'[32] To have the optimal health outcomes, medicines reviews should be prioritised to those people who will benefit most, for example:[33,34]

- VOCODFLEX – 'Very Old, those with COmorbidity, Dementia, Frailty and Limited life Expectancy'[35]
- Patients on polypharmacy
- Patients on high-risk medicines
- Care home residents
- Patients with four or more long-term conditions
- Patients with complex neurological conditions (e.g. stroke, Parkinson's disease)
- Housebound patients
- Patients with continuous support needs

Inappropriate polypharmacy can be managed by undertaking regular holistic person-centred, evidence-based medicines reviews.

The person-centred approach to polypharmacy as defined by Barnett et al[36], and shown in *Figure 17.2*, provides practical support for clinicians in embedding medicines optimisation into everyday practice through person-centred, safe, evidence-based medicines reviews.

Using the seven steps ensures that managing polypharmacy and deprescribing is undertaken in a safe, effective, collaborative, coordinated and efficient way. It is more applicable in community settings and can be used in any encounter between a clinician and a person where medicines are being reviewed.

The Scottish Government's national guidance on polypharmacy[33] includes a similar '7-steps' approach to support those carrying out comprehensive face-to-face medicines reviews. This process is also centred on the needs of the person as a whole and is aligned with steps 2 to 5 of Figure 17.2.

Both processes aim to ensure that medicine regimens are optimised for that person to improve clinical outcomes, patient safety, quality of life and reduce adverse drug events and waste from non-adherence to medicines.

Figure 17.2: *A patient-centred approach to managing polypharmacy in practice*[36]

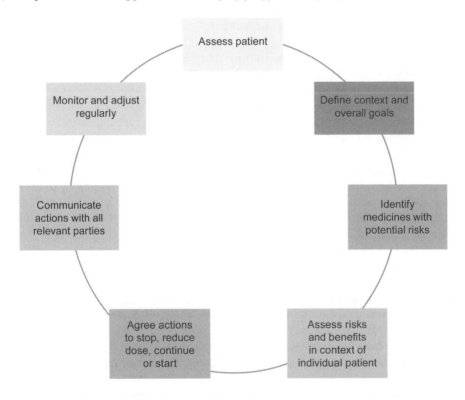

©Nina Barnett, Lelly Oboh & Katie Smith, NHS Specialist Pharmacy Service

The practical steps involved in carrying out a medicines review are:

1. Introduction
   - Ensure you have a private area for the consultation
   - Explain who you are (name, background, and purpose of the consultation)
   - As you are talking to the person, think about sensory, physical and cognitive difficulties (ask if appropriate) and notice clinical signs and symptoms (e.g. obesity, frailty, shortness of breath, cough, mobility, anxiety)

2. Think about what you hear from the person
   - Ask what is important to the person (e.g. a quick fix)
   - Ask what the person wants to achieve from this consultation
   - What do they say about taking their medicines?
     — Do they take medicines regularly?
     — Are there any that they don't like taking, or take only occasionally?
     — Do they feel they are getting benefit?
   - What are the person's perceptions of each medicine?
     — Do they feel it is working? People are more likely to discontinue medicines if they don't see a result (e.g. blood pressure medicines, bisphosphonates)
   - What is their attitude to reducing or adding to their medicines?
3. Are all the medicines necessary and appropriate from a clinical perspective?
   - Identify potentially inappropriate medicines using an evidence-based tool (e.g. STOPP/START[21] or similar)
   - Perform any necessary clinical examinations provided you are competent to do so
   - Do they have other symptoms that may be an adverse effect?
   - What medicines can be reduced, stopped, added or changed?
4. Balance evidence with the person's preferences. Remember guidelines are not intended to be rigid documents
   - Treat what is in front of you. Most will have multiple comorbidities and complex problems
   - Prioritise what is most important for the person, bearing in mind that what may appear to be the best option for you may not necessarily be what the person wants
   - Don't forget that lifestyle interventions (e.g. smoking cessation, weight management) are extremely important and so on can have significant health benefits
5. Agree actions with both the person and the prescriber to stop, start, amend dose or leave unaltered
   - Make sure the person fully understands changes and the rationale
6. Make sure all aspects of the consultation are documented
   - If you have provided written information, document that this has been supplied. Communicate the outcome to all relevant parties (e.g. doctors, pharmacists from other sectors, other prescribers)
7. Review as appropriate and arrange monitoring if necessary (e.g. blood tests)

Table 17.2 outlines further points to consider when undertaking a medicines review and some examples of potential interventions.

The MUST DECIDE to Be SHaRP tool (see *Figure 17.3*) is a combination checklist of medicine prompts and person-centred prompts to help detect inappropriate medicines, whilst ensuring care is focused on the beliefs and preferences of the person.

There is no evidence-based national guidance or literature regarding the most effective method of conducting a polypharmacy review, but there are resources and tools available based on current evidence to support clinicians and patients in the decision making process. Many of the tools help identify potentially inappropriate medicines (e.g. Beers Criteria[37]) and some also identify potential prescribing omissions (e.g. STOPP/START[21]). *Box 17.7* shows some of the tools available.

Table 17.2: *Factors to consider during a medicines review*

Consider	For example
What matters most to the person?	• At the start of the medicines review, identify what the person would like to achieve from the process, what matters most to them and why
Are there any **M**edicines adherence issues? If there are, why? Can they get a regular supply?	• Be aware that the same person can be adherent to one medicine and non-adherent to others • Also, the reasons for non-adherence are multifactorial in older people and can be both intentional and non-intentional
Is there any **U**nmet therapeutic need?	• Bone protection for osteoporosis for people on long courses of corticosteroids • Colecalciferol for people with vitamin D deficiency
Does the person wish to **ST**op any of their medicines?	• Heavy pill burden • Suspected adverse effects • No clinical improvement
Is there any therapeutic **D**uplication?	• Paracetamol and co-dydramol
Are all medicines **E**ffective?	• Docusate for constipation • Antimuscarinic prescribed for urinary frequency without any improvement in the person's symptoms
Is the medicines regimen **C**omplex?	• Consider ease of administration, dosing requirements and frequency to create a simplified medicines regimen
Is there an **I**ndication for all the medicines?	• Diuretics prescribed for oedema in a person without heart failure • PPI for longer than 4 weeks for resolved GORD (in the absence of oesophagitis)
Are there any potential **D**rug interactions?	• Clopidogrel and omeprazole resulting in a potentially reduced antiplatelet efficacy
Do any of the medicines lack clinical **E**vidence?	• Quinine sulfate • Multivitamins
Will the person **B**enefit from a medicine that takes a long time to yield a clinical benefit? Is the duration of treatment beyond the recommended course?	• Bisphosphonate commenced in a severely frail person with a limited life expectancy • Medicines used to treat self-limiting conditions • PPI treatment dose beyond 6 weeks
Are there any **S**ide effects with the current regimen? Have medicines been started as a result leading to a prescribing cascade?	• NSAIDS causing gastrointestinal symptoms • Antihypertensive causing postural hypotension
Are there any **H**igh **R**isk medicines?	• Anticoagulants • Diuretics • NSAIDs • ACE inhibitors • Antidepressants
Is **P**olypharmacy present? Are there potentially inappropriate medicines?	• Inappropriate polypharmacy is associated with increased risk of adverse effects (e.g. people prescribed medicines with high anticholinergic may experience most adverse effects such as falls and cognitive impairment)

Figure 17.3: *MUST DECIDE to Be SHaRP*

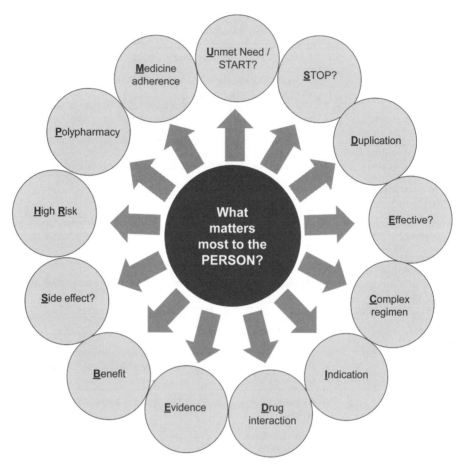

Box 17.7: Resources and tools to support managing polypharmacy and deprescribing

- NHS Scotland Polypharmacy Guidance, Realistic Prescribing 2018[33]
- Royal Pharmaceutical Society: Getting our medicines right[20]
- STOPP/START[21]
- Beers Criteria 2019[37]
- Polypharmacy, oligopharmacy and deprescribing: resources to support local delivery[38]
- NIPOP: Guide to Support Medication Review in Older People[39]
- All Wales Medicines Strategy Group: Polypharmacy: Guidance for Prescribing[40]
- Medstopper (Canada)[41]
- RxISK Polypharmacy Index[42]
- PrescQIPP Polypharmacy and Deprescribing webkit[43]
- Deprescribing.org (Canada)[44]
- Priscus List (Germany)[45]
- FORTA (Fit fOR The Aged) classification (Germany)[46]
- STOPPFRAIL[47]
- CRIME (CRIteria to assess appropriate Medication use among Elderly complex patients) (Italy)[48]

Tools to aid the medicines review process can be explicit criterion-based or implicit judgement-based. Explicit tools such as STOPP/START contain a list of specific recommendations validated by consensus panels to help clinicians detect inappropriate use of medicines. Implicit tools, on the other hand, rely on the clinician's expert professional judgement to guide decision making. This includes the Medication Appropriateness Index (MAI)[49], which is a validated tool that requires the user to answer 10 questions regarding a medicine to determine its appropriateness for a patient. It helps to detect potentially inappropriate prescribing and is a useful tool to quantify the impact of medication changes. The Good Palliative-Geriatric Algorithm[50] and the NOTEARS[51] tool are other tools designed to aid the medication review process and help the clinician gauge the appropriateness of the prescribed medicines.

Drug interactions

An unsurprising consequence of polypharmacy is an increased risk of drug-drug and drug-disease interactions (see *Table 17.3*) which can put the person at risk of serious adverse events. The risk of these adverse drug events (ADE) increases as the number of co-existing conditions and prescribed medicines increases.[52-55]

A person taking two medicines has a risk of 13% of having an ADE, but this rises to 58% when taking five medicines and taking seven or more medicines increases the risk to 82%.[56] It is also important to consider if the person is using over-the-counter, herbal and complementary treatments in addition to their prescribed medicines as this may further compound the risks.

Table 17.3: *Drug-disease interactions*

Disease	Medicines	Potential consequence
Chronic kidney disease	• NSAIDs • Furosemide	• Worsening of renal function • Acute kidney injury
Dementia	• Anticholinergics • Antipsychotics • Benzodiazepines • H_2 receptor antagonists	• Increased risk of CV event and mortality • Increase CNS adverse effects • Worsening cognition
Gastrointestinal ulcers	• Antiplatelets • Anticoagulants • NSAIDs • SSRIs • Corticosteroids	• Gastrointestinal inflammation, exacerbation of ulcers, bleeding
Asthma	• NSAIDs	• Asthma attack

An interaction is said to occur when the effects of one medicine are changed by the presence of another medicine, herbal medicine, food, drink or by some environmental chemical agent.[57]

There are different mechanisms by which drug interactions can occur and these are classified as either pharmacodynamic or pharmacokinetic. Pharmacodynamic interactions are where the effects of one medicine are altered by the presence of another medicine with either additive or opposing effects, for example, an increase in bleeding risk when anticoagulants and NSAIDs are taken together. The other mechanism is pharmacokinetic interactions where absorption, distribution, metabolism or excretion are affected, such as when warfarin metabolism is altered by other interacting medicines resulting in unstable INRs.[57]

The most clinically significant drug interactions are those that result in either enhanced medicine activity leading to adverse effects and/or toxicity, or reduced efficacy due to a reduction in medicine activity. Medicines with narrow therapeutic windows such as lithium, digoxin, warfarin or gentamicin are often associated with these types of reactions.

In terms of adverse clinical effect, the most problematic pharmacokinetic interactions are caused by those medicines which induce or inhibit the cytochrome P450 system, thereby affecting the metabolism of another medicine (see *Table 17.4* for examples and *Box 17.8* for details on how to manage drug interactions).

Table 17.4: *Inducers and inhibitors of cytochrome P450*

Inducers	Inhibitors
Barbiturates	Amiodarone
Carbamazepine	Cimetidine
Omeprazole	Disulfiram
Phenobarbitone	Fluoxetine
Phenytoin	Grapefruit juice
Rifampicin	Itraconazole
Smoking	Ketoconazole
St John's wort	Macrolides

Box 17.8: Practice point: how to manage drug interactions

- Take a good history
- Involve the person in shared decision making about medicine choice
- Check medicines information sources for interactions (e.g. SPCs, Stockley's Drug interactions, BNF)
- Avoid drug interaction combinations if possible and prescribe an alternative
- Continue the interacting medicines were the interaction is not clinically significant
- Take care when starting and stopping medicines – adjusting doses may compensate when initiating or stopping interacting medicines
- Allow 2-3 hours between interacting medicines may reduce the effects (e.g. a 2-hour dosing interval between levothyroxine and iron supplements can reduce the effects on the absorption of levothyroxine)
- Educate the person to be vigilant about potential adverse effects and adverse drug interactions (e.g. bleeding or bruising when on warfarin)
- Advise people to seek guidance if they plan to stop smoking or start a herbal remedy
- Monitor the person (e.g. desired clinical effect achieved, laboratory tests such as INR, U&Es, LFTs, serum levels of medicines)
- Report suspected drug interactions for new medicines using the Yellow Card Scheme

Pharmacists have a major role to play in relation to prevention, detection and reporting of ADEs which can have a big impact on patient safety. Through advanced knowledge of medicines' adverse effect profiles, pharmacists can identify potential prescribing cascades by linking unexpected symptoms experienced by patients to possible adverse effects.

High-risk medicines

It is helpful for pharmacists to be aware of high-risk medicines or combinations of medicines that should be targeted during medicines reviews. People on these medicines are more likely to suffer adverse outcomes.

Researchers[58] have identified examples of six high-risk medicines or combinations of high-risk medicines that should be targeted in medicines reviews. These are detailed in *Table 17.5* along with suggested management options.

Table 17.5: *Six key high-risk medicines to target in regular medicines reviews*[58]

High-risk medicine	Additional factors	Potential harm	Suggested action
'Triple whammy' combination: NSAID plus diuretic plus ACE inhibitor	People of all ages, although the elderly are at higher risk	All these medicines have the potential to decrease renal function; when these medicines are prescribed together the risk of acute kidney injury is increased	Stop NSAID
NSAID	Reduced renal function	NSAID may precipitate acute renal failure and the risk is increased in the elderly	Stop NSAID
NSAID	Aged over 75 years with no PPI	NSAID use has been associated with potentially serious gastrointestinal (GI) complications, such as upper GI bleeding	Stop NSAID or add PPI
Hypnotic/benzodiazepine	Aged over 60 years	Risks include falls, cognitive impairment and withdrawal symptoms	Reduce or stop hypnotic/benzodiazepine
Tricyclic antidepressant	Aged over 60 years	Risks include postural hypotension which can lead to falls, cardiac conduction abnormalities, and antimuscarinic side effects	Reduce or stop tricyclic antidepressant
Antipsychotic	Aged over 60 years	Risks include decrease in cognitive function, postural hypotension, parkinsonian events and cardiovascular effects	Reduce or stop antipsychotic

Monitoring

Monitoring a person after the medicines review and once a plan has been put in place is an essential step in confirming a comprehensive person-centred approach to tackling polypharmacy. A clear monitoring plan ensures that optimisation of medicines is carried out in a safe, effective, coordinated and efficient way.[36]

Monitoring can occur face-to-face in the clinic, in the person's own home, via telephone or electronic platforms and should be documented, communicated and shared with the person, family or carer (with the person's consent) and relevant health and social care professionals.

Box 17.9: Advantages of regular monitoring

- Ensures continuity of care
- Maintains patient contact and confidence
- Allows an opportunity to make appropriate adjustments to medicines
- Reduces risk of medicines-related harm
- Allows assessment of patient and therapeutic goals
- Maintains professional responsibility

The frequency of monitoring is determined by either the person's conditions or the medicine, and in many cases by a combination of both. In some instances, the person's condition may be unstable (changes in blood pressure or pain) and regular contact with shorter time intervals between follow-up needs to be established. The frequency can also be determined by the person's preference or expectations (some need shorter time intervals than others), potential emergence of withdrawal symptoms, or need for therapeutic drug monitoring (TDM) requiring drug levels/biochemical markers to be sampled.

The NHS Specialist Pharmacy Service produces comprehensive guidance on TDM in adults in primary care which can be used to guide how to monitor commonly prescribed high-risk medicines as shown in *Table 17.6*.[59]

Table 17.6: *Example of drug monitoring: apixaban*[59]

Tests prior to starting treatment	• Renal function • Body weight • Baseline clotting screen • Full blood count • Liver function tests (LFTs) • BP (needed in conjunction with renal and liver function if want to calculate HAS-BLED score)

Monitoring until patient is stabilised	• No routine anticoagulation monitoring is needed
	• First follow-up appointment should be after one month, then ideally assess patient every three months to:
	  – assess compliance and reinforce advice regarding regular dosing schedule
	  – enquire about adverse effects such as bleeding
	  – assess for the presence of thromboembolic events
	  – enquire about other medicines, including OTC medicines

Ongoing monitoring	• No routine anticoagulation monitoring is needed
	• Patient compliance should be assessed every three months ideally
	• Enquire about presence of any adverse effects, in particular signs and symptoms of bleeding and anaemia, every three months ideally
	• Renal function may decline whilst on treatment so it should be monitored:
	  – annually if CrCl >60 mL/min
	  – every 6 months if CrCl 30-60 mL/min
	  – every 3 months if CrCl 15-30 mL/min
	• The European Heart Rhythm Association (EHRA) guidance suggests retesting every x-months (where x = CrCl/10) (e.g. if CrCl 30 mL/min every 3 months, if CrCl 20 mL/min every 2 months)
	• LFTs annually
	• CrCl and LFTs should be performed more often if there is an intercurrent illness that may impact renal or hepatic function
	• Full blood count annually
	  – A low haemoglobin may suggest that occult bleeding is occurring and may require further investigations

Action required if abnormal results	• If CrCl <15 mL/min – stop apixaban, assess for bleeding and seek advice regarding alternative anticoagulation therapy
	• If CrCl is 15-29 mL/min, the following recommendations apply:
	  – For prophylaxis of recurrent DVT or PE, and treatment of DVT or PE, use apixaban with caution
	  – For prophylaxis of stroke and systemic embolism in a person with AF, reduce the dose to 2.5 mg twice daily if CrCl is 15-29 mL/minute, or if serum creatinine is 133 micromol/litre or greater and the person is 80 years of age or older or weighs 60 kg or less
	• If liver enzymes are elevated (ALT/AST >2 × ULN or total bilirubin ≥1.5 × ULN), apixaban should be used with caution
	• If the patient's HASBLED score is more than 3, then the patient is at a high risk of bleeding and apixaban should be used cautiously, with regular reviews

TDM may also be useful to guide dosage adjustment of certain medicines. Medicines with a narrow therapeutic index (where therapeutic drug levels do not differ greatly from levels associated with serious toxicity) should be monitored; examples include lithium, phenytoin and digoxin. Patient compliance is essential if drug monitoring data are to be correctly interpreted.[59]

In addition to TDM, the effectiveness of prescribed medicines can be measured objectively using a variety of tools. *Table 17.7* outlines some of the tools used to review commonly prescribed medicines.

Table 17.7: *Tools used in review of commonly prescribed medicines*

Medicine class	Examples of commonly used tools
Antipsychotics used to treat behaviours that challenge in dementia	ABC behaviours chart
Analgesics	Pain charts (e.g. Bolton/Abbey pain chart) for people living with dementia unable to verbalise pain
Antidepressants	Depression scales (e.g. geriatric depression scale)
Sedatives	Sleep charts
Antihypertensives	Blood pressure monitoring charts
Antimuscarinics used to treat lower urinary tract symptoms (LUTS)	Bladder fluid charts Urinary incontinence questionnaires International Prostate Symptom Score (I-PSS)
Laxatives	Bristol Stool Chart
Acetylcholinesterase inhibitors	MMSE, the Mini-Addenbrooke's Cognitive Examination (M-ACE score)
Inhaled therapies	COPD Assessment Test (CAT)

Person-centred approach to adherence

Pharmacists are key players in helping people to make person-centred decisions about the treatment options available to them and consequently in enhancing medicines adherence.

Adherence is defined as 'the extent to which the person's behaviour matches agreed recommendations from the prescriber'.[60] The World Health Organization (WHO) reported that global medicines adherence among people with chronic diseases averages 50%, and that adherence rates decrease as the number of comorbid diseases increases.[61]

Non-adherence is problematic for healthcare delivery because it is one of the major reasons for poor treatment outcomes resulting in an avoidable health burden to society and reduced quality of life for the person.[61]

There are many causes of non-adherence but they fall into two overlapping categories: intentional and non-intentional.[62]

- Intentional non-adherence is when people choose not to take their prescribed medicines for a variety of reasons, and this also includes when people self-adjust their regimens because of side effects, toxicity or personal beliefs, resulting in a reduced motivation to adhere.
- Non-intentional non-adherence occurs when the person wants to follow the general treatment plan but can't because of barriers beyond their control, for example, they experience difficulty accessing the medicines from blister packs or operating inhaler devices or they find it hard to order and collect their prescriptions. These people have a reduced capability or opportunity to adhere.

It has been suggested that increasing the effectiveness of adherence interventions may have a far greater impact on the health of the population than any improvement in specific medical treatments.[62]

Deciding on the best treatment can be very difficult, especially when there is more than one option on the table and when neither is clearly better, or there is a lack of clinical trial evidence for that particular population (e.g. frail older people). The key skill is to achieve a balance between clinical decision making and person expectation.

Patient decision aids can be used in consultations to support people to make informed choices by describing the treatment options available, and the outcomes of these options, so that complex health information can be displayed in a simpler patient-friendly format.

The number needed to treat (NNT) is used to report the outcomes of clinical trials in terms of patient numbers. Pharmacists can coach the person through the process by explaining the chance of benefit and the risk of harm from medicines. This allows the person to decide for themselves if the benefits outweigh the potential harm, allowing a fully informed decision to be made.

The effectiveness of patient decision aids has been extensively researched and a Cochrane systematic review[63] concluded that their use improved people's knowledge and perceptions of risk, with more people achieving decisions that were informed and consistent with their values.

Adherence can be promoted by using effective communication skills as part of a person-centred approach, however, it needs to be recognised that most people are non-adherent at times.

Medicines' taking is a complex human behaviour[62], with a plethora of influencing factors, however, the magnitude of the problem reflects a fundamental communication problem between clinicians and people.[64]

Non-adherence is multifaceted with many factors influencing a person's decision or ability to take their prescribed medicines. Factors include the person's beliefs and views, previous experiences, emotional and mental health, disability and understanding of the intended purpose of the prescribed treatment, and unsurprisingly as the number of prescribed medicines increases adherence decreases.[65]

In reality, not taking prescribed medicines may be a combination of both intentional and non-intentional non-adherence on the part of a person. The COM-B model[66] (see *Table 17.8*) can be employed as an approach to exploring the determinants of behaviour to identify the root causes of non-adherence. The COM-B model understands that a person should have adequate Capability, Opportunity and Motivation for a Behaviour to change. Where a person has a deficit in one or more of these factors then the desired change in behaviour is unlikely to occur.[67]

Chronic disease management is a particular challenge due to the lack of 'apparent' benefits of medicines and the need to continue with therapy long term. Tackling the motivation to take a medicine is one of the most difficult aspects as it often relies on eliciting behaviour change as opposed to a practical intervention.

Non-adherence should be assessed in a non-judgemental way during every interaction with a person. Using the mantra 'making every contact count' and by using simple behavioural nudge theories, pharmacists have an opportunity to make a huge contribution to support people to make positive changes to get the most out of their medicines.

It is of utmost importance that the pharmacist assesses the person's adherence through cautious questioning without being seen to apportion blame. This can be done by asking the person if they have missed any doses of medicines whilst explaining the rationale of the question i.e. not to 'police', but rather to find out whether they need more information and support. Mentioning a specific time period such as 'in the past week' is helpful. Looking for clues such as prescribing/dispensing dates and patterns can be a useful way to identify non-adherence.

Box 17.10: Practice point: simple questions that can be asked routinely about adherence

- How many doses of your medicines have you missed in the past week?
- How are you taking your medicines?
- Have you ever forgotten to take your medicines?
- Are you experiencing any side effects?
- How are you feeling since you started taking the medicine?
- Have you stopped or reduced any of your medicines?

Table 17.8: *The COM-B model for medicines adherence*[66]

COM-B	Points to consider	Examples of interventions to increase adherence
Capability	<ul><li>Can the person get to the pharmacy or to the doctors? Can the person carry a large supply home?</li><li>Does the person have the manual dexterity to open the medicines package or use a device inhaler?</li><li>Does the person have the skills to calculate the appropriate combinations of tablets for the required dose?</li><li>Can the person remember to take their medicines?</li><li>Does the person have the health literacy to understand the instructions on the medicines?</li><li>Does the person understand why they are taking the medicines and what they do?</li></ul>	<ul><li>Deliver and collect prescription.</li><li>Supply medicines in more accessible containers.</li><li>Supply screw caps instead of child-resistant caps.</li><li>Supply a device to aid medicines administration (aid for instilling eye drops).</li><li>Label medicines in a more legible way (e.g. large fonts).</li><li>Suggest the person records their medicine-taking or identify ways to prompt, such as a reminder chart or mobile phone alarm.</li></ul>
Opportunity	<ul><li>Does the person have the opportunity to discuss any medicines related problems or have access to a medicines review?</li><li>Is the high pill burden a contributing factor?</li><li>Does the person have sufficient social resources to support them to take medicines?</li><li>Does the person have faith in healthcare professionals?</li></ul>	<ul><li>Ensure there is a robust recall system for medicines reviews.</li><li>Suggest ways to simply the regime (e.g. switching to once-a-day preparation or combination therapy).</li><li>Identify if any medicines can be safely discontinued.</li><li>Consider interventions aimed to promote social support.</li><li>Promote a person-centred approach and establish a truly collaborative approach.</li></ul>
Motivation	<ul><li>Does the person have sufficient knowledge of the disease and the perceived need for treatment? (N.B this is often low when a person is currently well)</li><li>Does the person suffer from or have concerns about adverse effects?</li><li>Is there an underlying mental health disorder to consider? (e.g. depression)</li></ul>	<ul><li>Address any beliefs and concerns that the person may have that result in reduced adherence.</li><li>Suggest ways to manage or reduce adverse effects – change the dose or timing.</li><li>Discuss the benefits, adverse effects and long-term effects with the person to allow them to make an informed choice.</li></ul>

Non-adherence is very common, so adopt a no blame, frank and open approach. *Box 17.11* suggests some ways to support people with medicines adherence.

> ## Box 17.11: Practice point: how to support people with medicines adherence[68]
>
> *Involve the person in decision making by:*
> - using communication appropriate to the person's need
> - encouraging people to ask questions about their medicines and acknowledging the person's views[1]
> - asking if they have any concerns and what matters to them most by exploring their perspective and reasons for non-adherence
> - providing evidence-based information on the medicines in an appropriate format so that the person can make informed person-centred decisions based on likely benefits and risks
> - offering advice, options, possible solutions, negotiate trade-offs
> - respecting the person's decisions
> - encouraging people to seek assistance if anything changes in the future (e.g. adverse effects emerge, circumstances or medicines change)
>
> *Offer practical solutions such as:*
> - encouraging people and/or carers to maintain up-to-date lists of their medicines, (including OTC medicines) allergies or adverse reactions
> - undertaking evidenced-based medicines reviews to address inappropriate polypharmacy
> - simplifying dosing regimens where possible
> - providing reminder cards or devices
> - offering alternative packaging/formulation or a compliance aid if the person has a problem accessing the medicines (e.g. tablet popper for medicines packaged in blister strips)
> - checking if the person needs help to order or collect prescriptions or deliver their medicines
> - signposting the person to support groups/other healthcare professionals if appropriate[1]
>
> *Follow up and review any solutions suggested by:*
> - arranging an adherence review at an agreed interval
> - recording details of the medicines adherence review
> - ensuring communication of any agreed changes with relevant healthcare professions
>
> Adapted from RPS Medicines Adherence – a quick reference guide. Jan 2013.

Person-centred approach to deprescribing

If inappropriate polypharmacy is identified, deprescribing of the inappropriate medicines should be considered. Deprescribing is the process of withdrawing inappropriate medicines, supervised by a healthcare professional, with the goal of managing polypharmacy and improving outcomes.[69]

To ensure that deprescribing is successful, it is key that the person (and sometimes the carer) is actively involved in the process and that the person's preferences and choices are taken into account.[70]

During the medicines review, pharmacists may identify more than one medicine that may be considered for deprescribing. In these circumstances, it is best to prioritise the order in which medicines should be stopped. Withdrawing one medicine at a time allows the effects to be monitored and any problems identified. When deciding the order, the following criteria may be useful:[71]

- Medicines that the person is most willing to discontinue
- Medicines with the most harm and least benefit
- Medicines that are the easiest to withdraw (e.g. less likely to cause withdrawal effects)

Almost all medicines acting on the brain or heart can increase the risk of falls and should be reviewed to ensure they are appropriate and not causing unwanted adverse effects. People taking four or more medicines[72] are at increased risk of falls, especially if they include centrally sedating and antihypertensives medicines. Proactive review of people at risk of falling should aim to reduce the quantity and dosage of medicines known to contribute to falls. Some medicines carry a higher risk than others when used individually or in combination.[73] *Table 17.9* is not a comprehensive list of all medicines, but is intended to raise awareness of high-risk medicines that can cause falls.

Table 17.9: *High-risk medicines that can cause falls*

High-risk medicines	Mechanism	Examples
Antidepressants	Can cause drowsiness, impaired co-ordination, poor balance and confusion	Amitriptyline, dosulepin, trazodone, venlafaxine, duloxetine, sertraline, citalopram
	Monoamine oxidase inhibitors (MAOIs) cause severe orthostatic hypotension	Moclobemide, phenelzine, isocarboxazid
Antimuscarinics	May cause acute confusional states in the elderly, especially those with pre-existing cognitive impairment	Oxybutynin
Antipsychotics (including atypical)	Can cause sedation, slow reflexes and loss of balance. All have some alpha receptor blocking activity and can cause orthostatic hypotension which is dose related	Chlorpromazine, haloperidol, risperidone, quetiapine, prochlorperazine
Benzodiazepines and hypnotics	Can cause drowsiness, slow reactions and impaired balance	Temazepam, diazepam, chlordiazepoxide, zopiclone
Dopaminergics used in Parkinson's disease	Falls are common as reduced mobility, stability and orthostatic hypotension (OH) are part of the disease. Sudden excessive daytime sleepiness can occur with levodopa and other dopamine receptor agonists	Levodopa, ropinirole, pramipexole, selegiline

Frailty is a state of increased vulnerability that, although not necessarily part of the ageing process, will become more prevalent as the population ages.[74,75] Pharmacists have a significant role to play in assisting with the recognition and management of the five frailty syndromes (see *Table 17.10*) by conducting person-centred medicines reviews that incorporate evidence-based tools such as STOPP/START criteria[21] and Beers Criteria[37] to optimise medicines.

Older people can be considered as a special population because of the physiological changes that occur during ageing. These natural age-related changes result in older people living with more multimorbidities, greater polypharmacy, frailty and enhanced susceptibility to ADRs due to altered pharmacokinetics and pharmacodynamics responses.[76]

The effect of ageing changes how medicines are handled in older adults, resulting in alterations to the process of distribution, metabolism and elimination. Medicines may have longer half-lives and cause more toxicity due to altered serum levels and interactions with other medicines. Medicine clearance is often reduced in older people, as during healthy ageing liver size decreases by 25-35%[77] and hepatic blood flow by 40%.[76]

Similarly, renal function declines steadily through life which can have a significant effect on renally excreted medicines such as digoxin, lithium and methotrexate. This is further complicated by changes that occur to body mass with ageing resulting in decreased skeletal muscle, and consequently less creatinine is produced as a by-product of muscle metabolism. It is often the case that the serum creatinine levels in older people are misinterpreted as representing a satisfactory renal function when in fact the renal function is significantly impaired, resulting in decreased drug excretion leading to the potential for toxicity and ADEs.

Identifying ADRs in older people is challenging because often the symptoms reflect common problems that they present with, such as dizziness, confusion and falls. Moreover, polypharmacy increases the risk of drug interactions, poor outcomes and an unnecessary treatment burden. These risks are all amplified in the presence of frailty and warrant an effective deprescribing plan.[70]

Table 17.10: *Medicines associated with the frailty syndromes*

Frailty syndrome	Medicines that trigger frailty syndrome
Falls	<ul><li>Antipsychotics</li><li>Antidepressants</li><li>Anticholinergics</li><li>Opioids</li><li>Antihypertensives</li></ul>
Delirium	<ul><li>Sedative hypnotics</li><li>Antipsychotics</li><li>Benzodiazepines</li><li>Antiepileptics</li></ul>
Incontinence	<ul><li>Diuretics</li><li>Muscle relaxants and sedatives</li><li>Antihistamines</li><li>Alpha adrenergic antagonists</li><li>Anticholinergics</li></ul>
Immobility (or reduced mobility)	<ul><li>Medicines that contributes to falls and subsequent fracture leading to immobility and increased dependence (e.g. inability to collect prescriptions or medicines or inability to access toilets leading to incontinence).</li><li>Antihypertensives</li><li>Antipyschotics</li><li>Benzodiazepines</li><li>Diuretics</li></ul>
Susceptibility to the adverse effects of medicines	<ul><li>General consequence of age-related physiological changes</li></ul>

Anticholinergic medicines in the elderly

Anticholinergic medicines are known to be associated with impaired cognition and physical decline, and targeted deprescribing of these medicines may need to be considered. Older adults are more susceptible to these adverse effects because they are more likely to be prescribed these medicines due to their multimorbidity, an age-associated decline in hepatic and renal drug metabolism, an increase in blood-brain barrier permeability and a reduction in central cholinergic activities.[78]

There are a number of tools available to measure potential anticholinergic effects. The anticholinergic burden (ACB)[79] and the anticholinergic effect on cognition (AEC)[80] are available as online calculators. Medicines are assigned a score: the higher the score the greater the anticholinergic burden or effect. The score can be used to identify high-risk medicines and to discuss the benefits and harms with the person and then make an informed decision as to whether to completely stop the medicines or to change to a different medicine with less anticholinergic effects.

Deprescribing in end of life

For many older adults and people at end of life, symptom control, quality of life and decreased burden of care are valued more than the aim to prevent disease progression or prolong life. Studies have consistently reported the unnecessary treatment burden, still present at the end of life, which should be scrutinised through structured deprescribing.[81,82,83]

Todd *et al*[84] presented five recommendations to support deprescribing in people with limited life expectancy:

1. Shared decision making when initiating medicines to discuss benefits and harms
2. Not prescribing a medicine should be presented as a reasonable alternative for patients late in life, when appropriate
3. Deprescribing is part of prescribing – prescribing a medicine should always include a consideration of how long it will be continued for and how it will be discontinued
4. Prescribers have to embrace uncertainty
5. Difficult discussions now simplify difficult decisions in the future – when a medicine is started, a discussion about when, why, and how to stop should be initiated with the person

Evidence-based tools such as the STOPPFrail tool,[47] presents an explicit list of potentially inappropriate prescribing indicators which can be used to support decisions to deprescribe at the palliative stage or end of life. Patient criteria are described in *Box 17.12*.

Box 17.12: STOPPFrail patient criteria[47]

Older patients (≥65 years) who meet ALL of the criteria listed below:
1. End-stage irreversible pathology
2. Poor one-year survival prognosis
3. Severe functional impairment or severe cognitive impairment or both
4. Symptom control is the priority rather than prevention of disease progression

The decision to prescribe/not prescribe medicines to the person should also be influenced by the following issues:
1. Risk of the medicines outweighing the benefit
2. Administration of the medicines is challenging
3. Monitoring of the medicines effect is challenging
4. Medicine adherence/compliance is difficult

Referrals

Onward referrals are usually made to another health or social care professional directly related to the condition and/or medicines being reviewed, or by the identification of an immediate need for investigation, treatment and management by a specialist team, or to the community and voluntary sector to support people with complex needs. Examples of support from the voluntary or community sector include social prescribing which can divert the need for further pharmacological prescribing to manage specific conditions (e.g. a befriending service to tackle loneliness in place of a prescription for an antidepressant or the use of technology to prompt medicine administration or reminders in place of a monitored dosage system).

The Academy of Medical Royal Colleges in the UK published guidance[85] on the best practice for onward referrals (see *Box 17.13*).

Box 17.13: Practice point: good principles for onward referral[85]

- Just like the review process, people remain at the centre of the referral process: personal choice and understanding of the reason for referral must be recognised.
- The person's experience and safety must be considered at all times.
- Depending on management pathways, processes and clinical judgement, onward referral may be appropriate without going via the person's GP.
- At all times, the referrer should ensure the person's GP, who has detailed knowledge of the person, retains appropriate clinical involvement and responsibility.
  - Good communication is considered to be at the heart of good referral practice – copy the GP in to any onward referral.

References

1. Masnoon N *et al*. What is polypharmacy? A systematic review of definitions. *BMC Geriatrics* 2017; 17: 230.

2. Zarowitz BJ *et al*. Reduction of high-risk polypharmacy drug combinations in patients in a managed care setting. *Pharmacotherapy: The Journal of Human Pharmacology & Drug Therapy* 2005; 25(11): 1636-1645.

3. Duerden M *et al* (2013). Polypharmacy and Medicines Optimisation Making It Safe and Sound. London: The Kings Fund.

4. National Institute for Health and Care Excellence (NICE). Multimorbidity: clinical assessment and management [NG56]. London: NICE; 2016. www.nice.org.uk/guidance/ng56

5. National Institute for Health and Care Excellence (NICE). Multimorbidity and polypharmacy. Key therapeutic topic [KTT18]. London: NICE; 2017. www.nice.org.uk/advice/ktt18/chapter/Evidence-context

6. Morin L *et al*. The epidemiology of polypharmacy in older adults: register-based prospective cohort study. *Clinical Epidemiology* 2018; 10: 289-298.

7. Quinn KJ, Shah NH. A dataset quantifying polypharmacy in the United States. *Scientific Data* 2017; 4: 169.

8. Guthrie B *et al*. The rising tide of polypharmacy and drug-drug interactions: population database analysis 1995-2010. *BioMed Central Medicine* 2015; 13: 74.

9. Stocks SJ *et al*. Examining variations in prescribing safety in UK general practice: cross sectional study using the Clinical Practice Research Datalink. *BMJ* 2015; 351: h5501.

10. World Health Organization (2016). Multimorbidity: Technical Series on Safer Primary Care. Geneva: World Health Organization.

11. Mantelli S *et al*. How general practitioners would deprescribe in frail oldest-old with Polypharmacy – the LESS study. *BMC Family Practice* 2018; 19(1): 169.

12. Rochon PA (2019). Drug prescribing for older adults. www.uptodate.com/contents/drug-prescribing-for-older-adults#H15

13. Kalisch LM *et al*. The prescribing cascade. *Aust Prescr* 2011; 34: 162-6.

14. Bytzer P, Hallas J. Drug-induced symptoms of functional dyspepsia and nausea. A symmetry analysis of one million prescriptions. *Aliment Pharmacol Ther* 2000; 14(11): 1479-84.

15. Caughey GE *et al*. Increased risk of hip fracture in the elderly associated with prochlorperazine: is a prescribing cascade contributing? *Pharmacoepidemiol Drug Saf* 2010; 19: 977-82.

16. Mallet L *et al*. The challenge of managing drug interactions in elderly people. *Lancet* 2007; 370: 185-91.

17. Garfinkel D *et al*. Routine deprescribing of chronic medications to combat polypharmacy. *Therapeutic advances in drug safety* 2015; 6(6): 212-233.

18. Garfinkel D *et al*. Inappropriate medication use and polypharmacy in end- stage cancer patients: Isn't it the family doctor's role to de-prescribe much earlier? *Int J Clin Pract* 2018; 72: e13061.

19. Scott I, Jaythissa S. Quality of drug prescribing in older patients: is there a problem and can we improve it? *Internal Medicine Journal* 2010; 40: 7-18.

20. Royal Pharmaceutical Society (2019). Polypharmacy. Getting our medicines right.

21. O'Mahony D *et al*. STOPP/START criteria for potentially inappropriate prescribing in older people. *Age Ageing* 2015; 44(2): 213-218.

22. Moffat K, Mercer S. Challenges of managing people with multimorbidity in today's healthcare systems. *BMC Fam Pract* 2015; 16: 129.

23. Navickas R *et al*. Multimorbidity: What do we know? What should we do? *J Comorb* 2016; 6(1): 4-11.

24. Hafskjold L *et al*. A cross-sectional study on person-centred communication in the care of older people: the COMHOME study protocol. *BMJ Open* 2015; 5: e007864.

25. Barnett N. Improving pharmacy consultations for older people with disabilities. *Journal of Medicines Optimisation* 2016; 2(4): 72-76.

26. Coulter A, Collins A (2011). Making shared decision making a reality. No decision about me, without me. London: The Kings Fund.

27. Smith H *et al*. Person-Centred Care Including Deprescribing for Older People. *Pharmacy* 2019; 7: 101.

28. Elwyn G *et al*. A three-talk model for shared decision making: multistage consultation process. *BMJ* 2017; 359 : j4891.

29. Choosing Wisely UK (2019). About choosing Wisely UK. www.choosingwisely.co.uk/about-choosing-wisely-uk

30. Whitmore J. *Coaching for Performance*. London: Nicholas Brealey, 1992.

31. Barnett N. The new medicine service and beyond - Taking concordance to the next level. *Pharm J* 2011; 287: 653.

32. Task Force on Medicines Partnership, The National Collaborative Medicines Management Service Programme (2002). Room for Review. A guide to medication review: the agenda for patients, practitioners and managers. Medicines Partnership: London.

33. Scottish Government (2018). Polypharmacy guidance, realistic prescribing. 3rd edn. Edinburgh: Scottish Government. www.therapeutics.scot.nhs.uk/wp-content/uploads/2018/09/Polypharmacy-Guidance-2018.pdf

34. NHS England (2017). Toolkit for general practice in supporting older people living with frailty. www.england.nhs.uk/wp-content/uploads/2017/03/toolkit-general-practice-frailty-1.pdf

35. Garfinkel D *et al*. Routine deprescribing of chronic medications to combat polypharmacy. *Therapeutic advances in drug safety* 2015; 6(6): 212-233.

36. Barnett N *et al*. Patient-centred management of polypharmacy: A process for practice. *Eur J Hosp Pharm* 2016; 23: 113-117.

37. American Geriatrics Society 2019 Updated AGS Beers Criteria® for Potentially Inappropriate Medication Use in Older Adults. *J Am Geriatr Soc* 2019; 67(4): 674-694.

38. Specialist Pharmacy Service (2017). Polypharmacy, oligopharmacy and deprescribing: resources to support local delivery. www.sps.nhs.uk/articles/polypharmacy-oligopharmacy-deprescribing-resources-to-support-local-delivery

39. Northern Ireland Pharmacists working with Older People (2017). A guide to support medication review in older people 2017. www.pfni.org.uk/wp-content/uploads/2017/05/Pharmacy-Forum-Support-NEW-OCT-2017.pdf

40. All Wales Medicines Strategy Group (2014). Polypharmacy: Guidance for Prescribing. www.awmsg.nhs.wales/medicines-appraisals-and-guidance/medicines-optimisation/prescribing-guidance/polypharmacy-guidance-for-prescribing

41. McCormack J *et al*. Medstopper. University of British Columbia. www.medstopper.com

42. Healy J *et al*. RxISK Polypharmacy Index. Data Based Medicine Americas Ltd. www.rxisk.org/tools/polypharmacy-index

43. PrescQIPP. Polypharmacy and deprescribing webkit. Improving Medicines and Polypharmacy Appropriateness Clinical Tool (IMPACT). www.prescqipp.info/our-resources/webkits/polypharmacy-and-deprescribing

44. Farrell B, Tannenbaum C. Deprescribing.org. Bruyère Research Institute (Ottawa) and Université de Montréal. www.deprescribing.org

45. Holt S *et al*. Potentially Inappropriate Medications in the Elderly: the PRISCUS list. *Dtsch Arztebl Int* 2010; 107(31-32): 543-551.

46. Pazan F *et al*. FORTA (Fit fOR The Aged) list 2018: third version of a validated clinical tool for improved drug treatment in older people. *Drugs Aging* 2019; 36(5): 481-484.

47. Lavan AH *et al*. STOPPFrail (Screening Tool of Older Persons Prescriptions in Frail adults with limited life expectancy): consensus validation. *Age and Ageing* 2017; 46(4): 600-607.

48. Fusco D *et al*. Development of criteria to assess appropriate medication use among elderly complex patients (CRIME) project: rationale and methodology. *Drugs Aging* 2009; 26(Suppl1): 3-13.

49. Hanlon JT *et al*. A method for assessing drug therapy appropriateness. *J Clin Epidemiol* 1992; 45(10): 1045-51.

50. Garfinkel D, Mangin D. Feasibility study of a systematic approach for discontinuation of multiple medications in older adults. Addressing polypharmacy. *Arch Intern Med* 2010; 170(18): 1648-1654.

51. Lewis T. Using the NO TEARS tool for medication review. *BMJ* 2004; 329: 434.

52. Vazquez SR. Drug-drug interactions in an era of multiple anticoagulants: a focus on clinically relevant drug interactions. *Blood* 2018; 132: 2230-2239.

53. Najjar MF *et al*. Predictors of polypharmacy and adverse drug reactions among geriatric in patients at Malaysian hospital. *HealthMed* 2010; 4(2).

54. Nguyen JK *et al*. Polypharmacy as a risk factor for adverse drug reactions in geriatric nursing home residents. *Am J Geriatri Pharmacother* 2006; 4: 36-41.

55. Johnell K, Klarin I. The relationship between number of drugs and potential drug-drug interactions in the elderly: a study of over 600,000 elderly patients from the Swedish Prescribed Drug Register. *Drug Saf* 2007; 30(10): 911-918.

56. Davies EA *et al*. Adverse drug interactions in special populations - the elderly. *Br J Clin Pharmacol* 2015; 80(4): 796-807.

57. Preston C L. Stockley's Drug Interactions [online]. London: Pharmaceutical Press. www.new.medicinescomplete.com

58. Morrison C, MacRae Y. Promoting safer use of high-risk pharmacotherapy: impact of pharmacist-led targeted medication reviews. *Drugs Real World Outcomes* 2015; 2(3): 261-271.

59. NHS Specialist Pharmacist Services (2018). Suggestions for Therapeutic Drug Monitoring in Adults in Primary Care. www.sps.nhs.uk/wp-content/uploads/2017/12/Drug-monitoring-2017.pdf

60. Bell JS *et al*. Concordance is not synonymous with compliance or adherence. *Br J Clin Pharmacol* 2007; 64: 710-711.

61. Sabaté E (2003). Adherence to Long-Term Therapies: Evidence for Action. Geneva: World Health Organization.

62. National Institute for Health and Care Excellence (NICE). Medicines adherence: involving patients in decisions about prescribed medicines and supporting adherence [CG76]. London: NICE; 2019. www.nice.org.uk/guidance/cg76

63. Stacey D *et al*. Decision aids for people facing health treatment or screening decisions. *Cochrane Database Systematic Reviews* 2017, Issue 4.

64. Martin LR *et al*. The challenge of patient adherence. *Ther Clin Risk Manag* 2005; 1(3): 189-199.

65. Hincapic A *et al*. Understanding reasons for non-adherence to medicines in Medicare part A Beneficiary sample. *J Manag Care Spec Pharm* 2015; 21(5): 391-399.

66. Jackson C *et al*. Applying COM-B to medication adherence. *The European Health Psychologist* 2014; 16 (1): 7-17.

67. Easthall C *et al*. Using Theory to Explore the Determinants of Medication Adherence. *Pharmacy (Basel)* 2017; 5(3): 50.

68. Royal Pharmaceutical Society (2013). Medicines Adherence - a quick reference guide.

69. Reeve E *et al*. A systematic review of the emerging definition of deprescribing with network analysis: implications for future research and clinical practice. *Br J Clin Pharmacol* 2015; 80: 1254-1268.

70. Frailty, polypharmacy and deprescribing. *Drug Ther Bull* 2016; 54(6): 69-72.

71. Scott IA *et al*. Reducing Inappropriate polypharmacy. The process of Deprescribing. *JAMA Int Med* 2015; 175(5): 827-834.

72. Department of Health (2001). National Service Framework for Older People, London.

73. Royal College of Physicians. FallSafe. www.rcplondon.ac.uk/projects/fallsafe

74. Kojima G *et al*. Frailty syndrome: implications and challenges for health care policy. *Risk Manag Healthc Policy* 2019; 12: 23-30.

75. The British Geriatrics Society, the Royal College of General Practitioners, and Age UK (2014). Fit for Frailty: recognition and management of frailty in individuals in community and outpatient settings.

76. Davis EA, O'Mahony MS. Adverse drug reactions in special populations - the elderly. *Br J Clin Pharmacol* 2015; 80(4): 796-807.

77. Schmucker DL. Liver function and phase 1 metabolism in the elderly. *Drugs Aging* 2001; 18: 837-851.

78. Boustani M *et al*. Impact of anticholinergics on the aging brain: A review and practical application. *Aging Health* 2008; 4: 311-320.

79. Anticholinergic Burden Scale. www.acbcalc.com

80. Anticholinergic effect on Cognition. www.medichec.com/assessment

81. Cardona *et al*. Non-beneficial treatments in hospital at the end of life: a systematic review on extent of the problem. *International Journal for Quality in Health Care* 2016; 28(4): 456-469.

82. Morin L *et al*. Polypharmacy increases significantly during end of life. *Am J Med* 2017; 130(8): 927-936.

83. McNeil M *et al*. The burden of Polypharmacy in Patient Near the End of Life. *J Pain Symptom Manage* 2016; 51(2): 178-183.

84. Todd A, Holmes HM. Recommendations to support deprescribing medications late in Life. *Int J Clin Pharm* 2015; 37(5): 678-681.

85. Academy of Medical Royal Colleges (2018). Clinical Guidance: onward referral. www.aomrc.org.uk/reports-guidance/clinical-guidance-onward-referral

Case studies

Case study 1

Nan, aged 87 years, lives in a residential care home for people with dementia. Her key worker referred her to the care home pharmacist for a medicines review as she was very drowsy and was sleeping all the time. Nan has mixed dementia (vascular dementia and Alzheimer's disease), hypertension, type 2 diabetes mellitus, chronic kidney disease stage 3 and has had a previous transient ischaemic attack (TIA).

Nan's regular medicines are:

- Gliclazide 80 mg in the morning
- Aspirin 75 mg in the morning
- Omeprazole 20 mg twice a day
- Memantine 20 mg in the morning
- Mirtazapine 45 mg at night
- Paracetamol 1 g every 4-6 hours when required

- Risperidone 250 micrograms in the morning and 500 micrograms at night
- Cetirizine 10 mg in the morning
- Lactulose 10 mL twice a day
- Amlodipine 5 mg in the morning
- Cyclizine 50 mg three times a day

Points to consider

- How would you start to assess Nan and her medicines?
- Would this require a face-to-face consultation?

Her latest blood pressure (BP) reading was 151/76 mmHg and her heart rate was 73 bpm. She weighed 64.9 kg. Her eGFR was 45 mL/min/1.73 m^2 from her last U&Es result and her calculated creatinine clearance was 33 mL/min. Nan's last glycated haemoglobin (HbA1c) result was 49 mmol/mol.

Points to consider

- Is there anything of significance in the results of Nan's most recent tests that you need to consider?

The care home pharmacist arranged to visit Nan and undertake the review. The primary aim was to determine if any of Nan's medicines were contributing to her drowsiness and what changes could be made to try to resolve this. Nan was unable to be involved in the review as she lacked capacity due to her cognitive impairment.

Points to consider

- What does capacity mean?
- What are your options if the person lacks capacity?

Her son and daughter-in-law agreed to take part in the review as they had power of attorney for health. All issues identified were first discussed with the care home and Nan's family, and their consent obtained. The proposed changes to Nan's medicines were then discussed with Nan's GP and the practice-based pharmacist, who then actioned the changes that were agreed.

Points to consider

- Are there any medicines that you think could be contributing to the symptoms Nan is experiencing?
- What reference sources and guidelines would you consult?
- What relevant issues did you identify?
- What suggested changes to Nan's medicines would you recommend?

Gliclazide – Nan's last HbA1c result was 49 mmol/mol. NICE recommends a target HbA1c level of 53 mmol/mol for individuals on a medicine associated with hypoglycaemia. It also suggests relaxing the target in frail older people who are unlikely to achieve longer-term risk-reduction benefits. The International Diabetes Federation recommends that a HbA1c target up to 70 mmol/mol may be appropriate in dementia.

The care home staff and family were willing to try to reduce the dose of gliclazide to prevent hypoglycaemia. Nan's GP agreed to reduce the gliclazide dose to 40 mg in the morning and to recheck the HbA1c level in three months. The repeat HbA1c level was 58 mmol/mol and the gliclazide was discontinued.

Memantine – Nan has impaired renal function. The SPC (Summary of Product Characteristics) for memantine recommends that in people with moderate renal impairment (CrCl 30-49 mL/min), the daily dose should be 10 mg per day. If tolerated well after at least seven days of treatment, the dose can be increased to 20 mg/day according to the standard titration scheme. A common adverse effect of memantine is somnolence. As Nan's behaviour was currently manageable, it was agreed with the family, care home and GP to reduce the dose to 10 mg daily based on Nan's decreasing renal function and sleepiness.

Risperidone – Nan had been prescribed this for 18 months for behavioural and psychological symptoms of dementia (BPSD). Risperidone should not be used for more than six weeks in people with BPSD, and during treatment, people must be evaluated frequently and regularly, and the need for continuing treatment reassessed. Risperidone can cause drowsiness. The family and care home were willing to trial a reduction in the risperidone dose. If Nan became agitated, the dose could be increased again – the GP agreed the trial. The risperidone was initially reduced to 250 micrograms twice a day. Nan was reviewed over the next couple of weeks and she was slightly less drowsy. The risperidone was then reduced to 250 micrograms at night for a couple of weeks. Nan was not agitated and was not sleeping as much during the day. The risperidone was then stopped.

Amlodipine – Nan's last BP reading was 151/76 mmHg. NICE guideline recommends a target BP of <150/90 mmHg if aged over 80 years. The European Society of Cardiology and the European Society of Hypertension recommend a threshold of ≥160/90 in people aged over 80 years for hypertensive treatment. It is good practice to check sitting and standing blood pressure to exclude postural hypotension, which could lead to falls.

It was decided to leave the dose the same and to continue to monitor Nan's blood pressure.

Aspirin – this was prescribed for Nan's vascular dementia, prevention of TIAs and secondary prevention of cardiovascular disease. The Royal College of Physicians recommends clopidogrel monotherapy for the prevention of further vascular events. The aspirin had been commenced prior to this change in the guidelines.

Nan had not had any further vascular events and the GP preferred to continue the aspirin 75 mg in the morning.

Mirtazapine – an adverse effect of mirtazapine is drowsiness. The clearance of mirtazapine may be decreased in people with moderate to severe renal impairment (CrCl <40 mL/min). Nan has a long history of depression and anxiety. Her family felt that the mirtazapine had made a significant difference to Nan's symptoms and wanted this to continue. However, after seeing how some of Nan's other medicines had been stopped or the dose reduced, they were willing to trial a dose reduction.

The GP agreed to reduce the dose to 30 mg daily. There was no deterioration in Nan's mood with the dose reduction.

Cetirizine – can cause fatigue and drowsiness. Nan's family and the care home did not know why this had been started and were willing to stop it. There was no documented indication in the GP medical record.

The GP agreed to stop the cetirizine.

Cyclizine – an adverse effect of cyclizine is drowsiness. Nan was not displaying any symptoms of nausea and had a good appetite. Nan's family and the care home staff did not know why cyclizine was being used on an ongoing basis and agreed that it could be stopped.

Nan's GP agreed to trial stopping the cyclizine for two weeks and then review if Nan was suffering from any nausea. The cyclizine was stopped after two weeks as Nan was not suffering from nausea.

Omeprazole – Nan had been prescribed the full therapeutic dose of omeprazole for five years. This was prescribed for gastro-oesophageal reflux disease. Nan's family thought that the dose had been increased when Nan was very anxious and were willing to reduce the dose.

The care home and the GP agreed with this and the omeprazole dose was decreased to 20 mg daily with the understanding that if Nan showed any signs and symptoms of reflux or dyspepsia, that the dose would be increased again. One month after reducing the dose Nan had not shown any change in her condition and the lower dose was continued (as gastroprotection for aspirin). The choice of proton pump inhibitor was compliant with the local formulary recommendations.

Paracetamol – Nan could not communicate that she was in pain due to her cognitive impairment, but did not display any signs of being in pain (e.g. grimacing, fidgeting, guarding part of her body or agitation).

Following a risk benefit assessment, the paracetamol was continued.

Lactulose – Nan was prone to constipation and the twice a day dose was currently working. The lactulose was continued.

Following the pharmacist's medicines review with the care home, Nan's family and her GP, risperidone, cetirizine and cyclizine were stopped and the dose of gliclazide, memantine, mirtazapine and omeprazole were reduced. Nan's drowsiness did slightly improve and there was no deterioration in her condition.

Case study 2

Tony, aged 84 years, is a frail gentleman with multiple comorbidities. He lives alone in a bungalow and has two carers four times a day. He manages his own medicines which are packaged in a multi-compartment compliance aid (MCA). The acute care at home team referred Tony for a pharmacist medicines review for polypharmacy.

Tony suffers from recurrent urinary tract infections (UTIs), gout, hypopituitarism and acromegaly (post removal of a pituitary tumour), tubulovillous ademona, osteoarthritis in both shoulders, type 2 diabetes mellitus, atrial fibrillation, heart failure, hypertension, lymphoedema, hiatus hernia, gallstones, previous cerebrovascular accident (CVA), irritable bowel disease, nocturia, history of cellulitis in both legs, widespread pain in both shoulders and hips, knees and lower legs and obesity.

Tony is only able to mobilise short distances within his home with the use of a walking frame.

The specialist heart failure nurse was managing Tony's heart failure. His latest blood pressure (BP) reading was 130/80 mmHg and his heart rate was 80 bpm. He weighed 124 kg. His eGFR was 49 mL/min/1.73 m^2 from his last U&Es result and his calculated creatinine clearance for adjusted body weight was 52 mL/min. His BMI was 42 kg/m^2.

> **Points to consider**
>
> - Is there anything of significance in the results of Tony's most recent tests that you need to consider?
> - Are there any additional test(s) results you would need to enable you to conduct a medicines review?

Tony's regular medicines are:

- Linagliptin 5 mg in the morning
- Mirabegron MR 25 mg at night
- Atorvastatin 20 mg at night
- Adcal-D3 (Calcium carbonate 1.5g and cholecalciferol 400 units), one twice a day
- Metformin MR 500 mg twice a day
- Sertraline 150 mg at night
- Furosemide 80 mg in the morning and 40 mg at lunchtime

- Paracetamol 1 g four times a day
- Mebeverine 135 mg twice a day
- Ranitidine 150 mg at night
- Carbocisteine 750 mg twice a day
- Oxycodone MR 20 mg twice a day
- Ispaghula husk, one sachet once a day
- Omeprazole 20 mg in the morning
- Temazepam 10 mg at night

- Macrogols, one sachet twice a day when required
- Apixaban 2.5 mg twice a day
- Ferrous sulfate 200 mg in the morning
- Oxybutynin MR 5 mg in the morning
- Allopurinol 100 mg in the morning
- Hydrocortisone 20 mg in the morning and 10 mg at night

Tony participated in the medicines review. All possible changes were discussed with Tony and the changes he agreed to were then discussed with the GP and practice-based pharmacist who actioned the changes.

The most important thing to Tony was the management of his pain. He was also keen to reduce the number of tablets he had to take every day.

Linagliptin and metformin – Tony's latest HbA1c was 51 mmol/mol. The NICE type 2 diabetes guideline recommends aiming for an HbA1c level of 53 mmol/mol, and to consider relaxing the target HbA1c level on a case-by-case basis, with particular consideration for people who are older or frail. The International Diabetes Federation recommends that an HbA1c target up to 70 mmol/mol may be appropriate in frail elderly people.

Tony's GP did not agree to reduce the diabetes medicines at this time. The HbA1c was to be rechecked in three months; if it decreased to 50 mmol/mol or less, then the linagliptin was to be stopped and the metformin reviewed.

Mebeverine and ispaghula husk – Tony was prescribed mebeverine and ispaghula husk for irritable bowel syndrome. Tony liked taking the ispaghula husk and was able to drink sufficient water to take the medicines as recommended by the manufacturer. He was willing to try stopping the mebeverine under the proviso that if he suffered from abdominal cramps it could be restarted or he could be switched to a mebeverine/ ispaghula husk combination product.

The mebeverine was stopped without any change to Tony's symptoms.

Macrogols – this was prescribed to treat opioid-induced constipation. An osmotic laxative is recommended for the management of opioid-induced constipation. Tony only took this occasionally and was not troubled with constipation.

The macrogols was continued when required.

Oxybutynin and mirabegron – Tony had initially been prescribed oxybutynin for nocturia and urgency of micturition. The mirabegron was added by a consultant urologist until he underwent a flexible cystoscopy and urodynamic studies. When the pharmacist first met Tony, a temporary catheter had been inserted two days previously for urinary retention. Tony was suffering from a dry mouth but was fluid restricted due to his heart failure.

The pharmacist contacted the consultant urologist to check if the oxybutynin could be stopped. The consultant agreed and advised that if Tony's symptoms worsened, the mirabegron dose could be increased to 50 mg at night. Tony was monitored over the next month. His dry mouth improved. After two months it was decided that Tony required a permanent catheter. The mirabegron was then stopped.

Sertraline – Tony had been started on sertraline several years ago. The dose had been increased after the death of his wife two years previously. Tony was willing to trial a reduction of the sertraline. It was agreed to reduce the dose to 100 mg daily.

After two months on the reduced dose, Tony requested to reduce the dose further. It was successfully reduced to 50 mg daily.

Ranitidine and omeprazole – these medicines had been recommended by a gastroenterologist for longstanding reflux and dyspepsia. His symptoms were controlled on both agents but previous attempts to reduce doses had resulted in symptoms recurring.

Tony wished to continue both medicines.

Apixaban – this was prescribed for prevention of stroke in atrial fibrillation. Tony is over 80 years of age and his serum creatinine is greater than 133 micromol/L.

The dose of 2.5 mg twice a day was appropriate and was continued.

Allopurinol – this was prescribed for gout prophylaxis. The dose had been commenced at 100 mg daily to reduce the risk of adverse effects. The serum urate had decreased to a normal level of 341 micromol/L.

The allopurinol was continued as Tony was concerned about the gout returning.

Atorvastatin – was initially started for primary prevention due to his type 2 diabetes. Tony then had a CVA. NICE recommends a dose of 80 mg atorvastatin for secondary prevention in people with cardiovascular disease. Tony's lipid profile has never been elevated. His latest cholesterol result was 3 mmol/L, HDL 1.3 mmol/L, LDL 1.2 mmol/L, cholesterol/HDL ratio 2.31 and non-HDL cholesterol 1.7 mmol/L.

The atorvastatin was continued at the same dose.

Furosemide – this was prescribed for Tony's heart failure. The dose had recently been increased. The heart failure specialist nurse was currently monitoring Tony and adjusting his diuretic dose.

Carbocisteine – Tony could not recall when or why the carbocisteine had been commenced. He is an ex-smoker but does not have COPD.

Tony agreed to try stopping the carbocisteine. The carbocisteine was successfully stopped with no increase in sputum amount or viscosity.

Temazepam – Tony has taken this for the last six years. He currently sleeps in a recliner and would often wake several times during the night. Initially, Tony wanted to continue his sleeping tablet but after stopping some of his other medicines without any untoward effect, he asked to trial stopping the sleeping tablet.

The temazepam was removed from the MCA. It was supplied in a separate container and the frequency was changed to when required so that Tony could choose not to take it. Tony tried a night without taking a sleeping tablet to see if this had any effect on his sleeping pattern. Tony felt that the temazepam did not improve his sleep pattern. He repeated this for several more nights and decided himself to stop the sleeping tablet.

Ferrous sulfate – Tony has been taking this for five years. His most recent haemoglobin level was 113 g/L and his ferritin was 222.6 micrograms/L.

After discussion with Tony and his GP, it was agreed to try stopping the ferrous sulfate and recheck his full blood picture and iron profile in three months.

Hydrocortisone – this was prescribed for corticosteroid replacement due to hypopituitarism. It was continued at the same dose.

Adcal-D3 – a DEXA scan taken 12 months previously showed that Tony had osteoporosis (T score right hip -3.4). This is most probably corticosteroid induced. Tony had never been prescribed a bisphosphonate. This was discussed with Tony's GP.

Due to his immobility it was decided not to prescribe a bisphosphonate and to continue the Adcal-D3.

Paracetamol and oxycodone – these were prescribed for Tony's widespread pain. His leg pain troubled him the most. Tony's pain relief was very important to him.

Both medicines were continued at the same dose.

Hypertension is listed in Tony's medical history, however he is not on any antihypertensive medicines and his BP was 130/80 mmHg. Treatment is not currently indicated.

Following the pharmacist's medicines review with Tony, and with the agreement of his GP, mebeverine, oxybutynin, mirabegron, carbocisteine and ferrous sulfate were stopped and the dose of sertraline was reduced. Tony stopped the temazepam himself without the need to gradually wean him off the benzodiazepine. Tony will be followed up to ascertain if the ferrous sulfate needs to be recommenced.

In both case studies the issues were not addressed in one visit. It was a gradual process involving the person and their family, taking small steps and gaining the person and their family's confidence and the confidence of other healthcare professionals involved in their care.

Key priorities for pharmacist medicines review

- Listen to the person (what is important to them about their medicines).
- Involve the person and/or their family/carer and the relevant healthcare professionals.
- Focus on a small number of key concerns (go slow, don't try to fix everything at once).
- Trial and review – if symptoms return or worsen, the drug or an appropriate alternative can be restarted, or the dose can be increased again.

Index